Encyclopedic Dictionary of
Sports Medicine

Encyclopedic Dictionary of Sports Medicine

DAVID F. TVER
HOWARD F. HUNT, PhD

CHAPMAN AND HALL

NEW YORK   LONDON

First published 1986
by Chapman and Hall
29 West 35th St. New York, NY 10001

Published in Great Britain by
Chapman and Hall Ltd
11 New Fetter Lane, London EC4P 4EE

© 1986 Chapman and Hall

Printed in the United States of America

Library of Congress Cataloging-in-Publication Data

Tver, David F.
    Encyclopedic dictionary of sports medicine.

    Bibliography: p.
    1. Sports medicine—Dictionaries. I. Hunt, Howard F.
II. Title. [DNLM: 1. Sports Medicine—dictionaries.
QT 13 T968e]
RC1206.T88   1986   617'.1027   86-11725
ISBN 0-412-01361-4

Acknowledgements

Grateful thanks are due to Mr. Basil Helal MCh(Orth), FRCS, Chairman of the British Association of Sports Medicine and Orthopaedic Advisor to the British Olympic Association, for contributing some of the entries relevant to non-American sports. Thanks also to Kenneth A. Anderson for invaluable editorial assistance.

Foreword

Since President John F. Kennedy sparked a national interest in health and fitness in 1960, the number of people participating in different types of physical exercises and sports-related activities has grown from thousands into millions. As a result of that increased interest, there has been a steady rise in physical and sports-related injuries. This volume provides a quick, up-to-date, reliable, and accurate reference to assist those interested in the latest technologies about sports medicine. Readers will be able to find state-of-the-art information when it comes to the identification, diagnosis, and understanding of physical and sports conditions and injuries.

This is not just a technical encyclopedia for the sports physician or allied health professionals. The volume is a must for anyone interested in understanding, preventing, or treating physical activity or sports-related injuries. It is a ready reference for the lay person participating in physical and sports-related activities. It should be read by everyone involved in a vigorous exercise or physical fitness program. Most physical or sports-related injuries can be prevented if proper attention is first given to the basics of optimal health and fitness levels followed by adequate reasonable activity limits, stress management and good common sense. Violation of those basics is the most probable cause of physical and sports-related pains or injuries.

As the number of people interested in health and fitness has continued to rise, the number of sports physicians and health professionals, leaders, teachers, trainers, and supportive personnel has also increased. Many corporations now have health promotion programs that include physical activities and exercise classes. Some companies have their own health professionals, such as health and fitness directors, worksite wellness coordinators, health promotion leaders, health engineers, among others. The number of organizations providing health and fitness information, programs, equipment, and services has also dramatically grown until it has become one of the fastest-growing industries of modern time. This growing cadre of interested exercise and health professionals is in need of such a book as the *Encyclopedic Dictionary of Sports Medicine*.

The authors, Dr. Howard Hunt, chairman of the Physical Education Department at the University of California, San Diego, and David Tver, author of several widely published books, are to be congratulated for having come up with a most valuable resource and contribution to this field. As more and more people worldwide join the health and fitness revolution, this book should become their Bible.

E. Lee Rice, D.O., F.A.A.F.P.
Director of the San Diego Sports Medicine Center
Team Physician, San Diego Chargers

Preface

In the last decade, the number of people interested and participating in sports both recreationally and competitively has risen dramatically. Physical activity of some kind is now the rule for more than 100 million Americans. The President's Council on Physical Fitness and the Department of Commerce estimates that there are 25 million Americans who are jogging or running. Similar figures are thought to apply to other sports.

With the increase in participation there has also been a rise in the number of sports-related injuries and deaths. In the United States alone, in one year approximately 700 deaths occurred in bicycling, compared with 4,500 deaths from tuberculosis.

"Physical fitness" has been defined by the Committee on Exercise and Physical Fitness of the American Medical Association as "the general capacity to adapt and respond favorably to physical effort. The degree of physical fitness depends on the individual's state of health, constitution, and present and previous physical activity."

Physical activity and its applied combinations (sports, athletics, recreation, etc.) assume an important role in the cultures of the modern world. Hardly a person is not influenced by physical activity either directly or indirectly. Research programs in the science and medical management of sports and physical activity have increased materially in the last decade. Their importance in television, radio, newspapers, and space gives evidence of that increasing influence.

Sports, athletics, and physical activity have become important factors in the United States culture not only for reasons of fitness and health but also for economic reasons. Commercial sports are a big business. Professional football, basketball, baseball, and soccer are all well established economically. Physical activities and physical education represent one of the largest and most expensive parts of school budgets. Athletics have become large factors in the politics of a culture and a nation.

Organized athletics now involve a major segment of the young. In many areas such activity starts during grade school years with the Little Leagues such as soccer, football, and baseball. Health clubs, hiking clubs, bicycle clubs, walking tours, tennis clubs, golf clubs, etc., are continually growing. Competitive athletics have a great appeal to the mass of the people. Unfortunately the inclination by the masses is to look at the score, to observe the outstanding players, and to foster competition rather than to direct attention toward those facets in sports that will do the most good to the greatest number.

The tangible health benefits to be derived from athletic competition greatly outweigh the elements of risk. The athlete develops a stronger body and mind. The trained athlete is superior to his or her more sedentary counterpart in both drive and stamina and is thus better fitted for work or play. The ex-athlete who "turns to fat" has at least postponed his impending adiposity throughout his years of activity and training. Competitive athletics also have a positive salutary effect upon the character of the participant.

The medical management of athletes requires a greater understanding of general medical principles as applied to athletics. Norms accepted for the general population do not always apply to trained athletes. New standards of physical measurements are constantly being established, and what might have been considered abnormal in an athlete several years ago is not understood to be physiologic.

Attention to the importance of nutritional values is part of the total athletic concept. Basic cardiology for competence in cardiac rehabilitation programs and even ingenuity to unravel dermatologic problems in athletes are all necessary. Fitness and optimal health are best achieved by understanding how the body and mind respond to proper nutrition and adequate exercise programs.

The extent and significance of injury have great variability from individual to individual. In certain individuals an injury is a single chance even with no untoward sequela and no psychologic or financial complications. However, in the serious amateur and professional athlete, every injury is viewed as a "career-threatening event."

Sports medicine deals with the science and medical treatment of the human organism in sports and physical activities. The objectives are prevention, protection, and correction of injuries and preparation for physical activity in its full range of intensity. The profession of sports medicine utilizes the basic principles of the sciences, particularly physiology and psychology, and the various aspects of medicine correlated with the requirements of physical activity. Until recently comparatively little attention outside of the sport itself has been paid to conditioning or to prevention of injury. The greater emphasis has been placed on the "injury" itself.

The literature pertaining to sports medicine and injuries has not kept pace with the growth of knowledge concerning athletic training and performance. Publications on the effects of sports on the fitness and health of large participating groups, heretofore not athletically inclined, have been scarce or confined to technical or scientific periodicals.

With the resurgence of active participation in many different sports by huge numbers determined to improve their appearance and well-being, sports medicine has become an important subject for study and knowledge.

As participation in many leisure time activities increases, many physical problems have arisen. One of the present-day issues that will demand attention is the rise of physical injury associated with all sorts of recreation. There is no sport that is entirely without risk.

This book is an examination of the injuries and illnesses that may occur in physical activities and sports of all kinds. It also describes certain parts of the body that receive a greater proportion of injuries. No study in 1 volume can contain everything that can be said on this subject. There are also various opinions on the importance of different subjects and what should be stressed from a physiological to a psychological viewpoint. Therefore, there are bound to be certain omissions in this volume owing to lack of space.

The definitions are in alphabetical or dictionary form and have been made as short as possible with sufficient detailed explanation for complete understanding. Each definition basically gives the explanation of the injury and its related symptoms. No attempt is made to suggest or prescribe any type of treatment. It is felt that with the constant changing concepts of treatment in sports medicine, the main purpose of this encyclopedia is to make the reader aware of the injury and its nature and symptoms. Once it is recognized, a determination can be made to find suitable medical treatment.

This book should be of interest to anyone in any way involved in sports—from the professional and the weekend athlete, from coaches, instructors, medical professionals, schools, colleges, and universities to athletic clubs and fitness and sport medicine centers.

David F. Tver
Howard F. Hunt, Ph.D.
San Diego, Calif., March, 1986

NOTE: The glossary in the rear section is more than a glossary. In addition to explaining terms that appear in the main section, it also has many short terms and definitions related to athletic health and activity. Since those terms and definitions were too short to include in the main section, they are nevertheless important in understanding athletic health and well-being.

Contents

xvi • **Contents**

A

abdominal injuries. The position of the abdomen (in the middle of the body) with its contained viscera makes it vulnerable to direct blows during most sporting activities. Many injuries of the abdominal wall are superficial and may lead to conditions such as contusion. Relatively fixed organs are the most frequently damaged. Liver injury may follow a blow to the right lower ribs; a spleen may be injured with a blow on the left lower ribs. Kidneys, intestines, testicles, and urethra may also be damaged in a similar manner. If the contusion is large, it may be associated with muscular damage, rupture of the rectus abdominis being the most common type. That results in severe pain and disability, and associated with the condition there may be a tear of the inferior epigastric artery. Profuse bleeding may occur in the lower abdominal wall, resulting in shock. A large tender mass can be palpated. Some muscular injuries may result from direct trauma, such as avulsion of the anterior superior iliac spine (occasionally experienced in adolescents). Traction injuries of the rectus abdominis can cause a painful lesion localized at the pubic bone, where persistent pain and tenderness result in considerable functional disability. More serious abdominal injuries result from trauma to underlying viscera. Even the most minor injury may at times cause enough damage to lead to a serious abdominal emergency and perhaps death. The most common injury from an abdominal blow is acute winding. That results in neurogenic shock because of stimulation of the solar plexus. When that occurs, the athlete doubles up with severe pain, finding difficulty in breathing. The abdominal wall can then become rigid, and the diaphragm may spasm. The individual feels faint and is pale and clammy. Immediate treatment is to loosen any restrictive clothing and encourage circulation. In the situation where symptoms or signs persist, there may be serious injury and the athlete should be kept under the observation of a physician. Of more significance, the athlete may appear to recover but later has increasing abdominal pain or may even collapse. That could be due to a delayed hemorrhage or even intestinal damage.

abrasion. A scraping injury to the skin. It may be of any grade of severity, from a simple excoriation of the skin by the opponent's headgear to very extensive damage. The major abrasions will occur over those parts of the body where there is a firm underlying tissue, particularly bone. Areas commonly injured are the shin, knee, iliac crest, elbow, and back of the hand. Abrasions in themselves are not particularly serious, but their complications may become a problem. Once injury to the deeper structure has been ruled out, the most immediate consideration is the prevention of infection.

abscesses. Abscesses, boils, carbuncles, and pimples are essentially identical localized infections that differ only in size. They are almost all caused by staphylococci, which are frequently resistant to antibiotics. Those organisms release enzymes that cause clotting and obstruction of the blood vessels and lymphatics surrounding the site of the infection. The vascular obstruction inhibits the spread of the bacteria so that the infection remains localized. But the obstruction also prevents antibiotics, antibodies, and other protective substances in the blood from reaching the infecting organisms. Other enzymes released by the bacteria destroy the tissues in the area of infection, producing a cavity that is filled with a mixture of bacteria, white blood cells, and liquified, dead tissues commonly known as "pus." The treatment for such disorder consists primarily of drainage and is similar to the treatment for infected wounds.

abscess, palmar space. Infection, usually staphylococcal; portal of entry, blister, callus, punctured wound, as in rowing and gymnastics. There is local pain, weakness of grip, perhaps malaise. Physical signs include tenderness, rapid swelling of palmar space, abscess pointing dorsally between metacarpals; indurated palm with loss of concavity; hand swollen dorsally; limited motion; pain elicited by extension of fingers, and fever. Complications can involve extension to adjoining tissue space, joints, tendon sheaths, lymphatic system (vessels), osteomyelitis, or contracture.

accessory tarsal navicular fracture. Forcible eversion with tight posterior tibial tendon. Symptoms are pain over medial aspect of navicular. Signs are tenderness sharply localized to medial aspect of navicular, pain elicited under forced passive eversion, undue prominence of medial aspect of navicular. Complications may result in a persistent disability.

acetabulum fracture (direct blow). Symptoms include pain localized in the hip, accentuated by motion, inability to bear weight, or disability. Signs are tenderness, muscle spasm about hip, laxity of tensor facia lata, or in leg position of external rotation.

Achilles tendon rupture. Injury occurs in the very heavy and older athletes primarily. When the athlete is supported on the toes of one foot, the force exerted on the tendon is a multiple of the ratio of the distance from the points of support on the ball of the foot to the midpoint of the ankle and from the midpoint to the attachment of the tendon to the calcaneus. The heavy, tall athlete with long feet, such as a defensive tackle in football, is at the greatest risk. The tendon of the older athlete often ruptures as the result of chronic strain and the gradual weakening of the tendon that usually accompanies the aging process.

Achilles tendon strain. Pulled heel cord. Forced dorsiflexion of ankle when calf muscles contracted. It may result from vigorous exercise with muscular incoordination. Symptoms include severe pain (especially on motion) and disability. Signs are graded by degree of severity, such as tender thickening over tendon about an inch above insertion, if complete rupture, *palpable* defect at musculotendinous junction, inability to walk on tiptoe, minimal or no plantarflexion caused by squeezing calf; pain elicited on active plantarflexion or passive dorsiflexion. Complications may lead to persistent disability. An X ray may show soft tissue defect in region of Achilles tendon.

Achilles tendinitis. Pain at the Achilles tendon attachment to the os calcis is a common problem in runners. The athlete complains that aching starts in the area of the Achilles tendon after running a short distance. The same complaint is heard from tennis players and basketball players. Repetitive overextension or overuse of the Achilles tendon may cause the overlying sheath to become inflamed and thickened, resulting in chronic pain and tightness over the Achilles tendon. The condition may be chronic and incapacitating, usually coming on insidiously from a change in training, such as hill running or increasing speed too rapidly. The predisposing problem in almost all cases is excessively tight gastrocnemius-soleus muscles, but tibia varus, cavus foot, heel, and forefoot varus deformities may also be predisposing factors. Symptoms include pain both during and after running and with any stretching of the tendon. Examination reveals either diffuse or localized swelling and tenderness to palpation of the tendon. Continuing to participate in athletics with the tendon inflamed may result in a complete rupture of the tendon. Acute rupture of the tendon usually occurs 1 or 2 inches above the insertion of the tendon on the calcaneus, with the athlete feeling a sudden tearing sensation and severe pain, with sudden loss of function and inability to stand on the toes. Active plantar flexion is weakened but may still be present because of action in the posterior tibial and flexor hallucis longus muscles. An Achilles tendon rupture is disabling.

Achilles tendon tenosynovitis. Caused by excessive repetitive running or jumping, unaccustomed activity, or wearing of tight shoes during an activity. Symptoms include local pain and discomfort especially on motion. Signs are tenderness and swelling over Achilles tendon, crepitus, pain elicited on active plantar-flexion and passive dorsiflexion. Complications may be persistent disability.

achillobursitis. Comes from too much repetitive walking or running, especially in cleated athletic shoes; congenitally enlarged poster-superior angle of calcaneus may be predisposing. Symptoms include pain (localized usually proximal to insertion and anterior to tendon) or disability. Signs may be confused with Achilles tendon strain or tenosynovitis. Active contraction of calf does not increase symptoms, while local pressure does. Pain is usually elicited by pressure in the space anterior to Achilles tendon

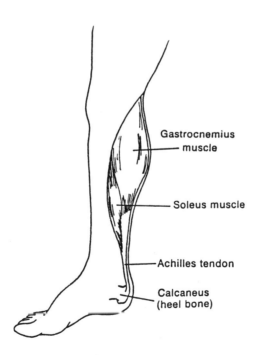

Gastrocnemius muscle

Soleus muscle

Achilles tendon

Calcaneus (heel bone)

Achilles tendinitis.

or between skin and calcaneal tuberosity. Retrocalcaneal bursitis rarely permits palpation of fluid, but superficial calcaneal bursitis may show cystic mass. Complications are chronicity; calcific deposits in retrocalcaneal area. X ray will show enlarged postersuperior angle of the calcaneus or calcific deposits if present.

acne. A disorder or disease of the oil glands of the skin. Common acne, or acne vulgaris, is found most often in individuals between the ages of 14 and 25. The infection of the oil glands takes the form of pimples, which may surround blackheads. Acne is usually severe at adolescence because certain glands in the body that control the secretions of the sebaceous glands are particularly active at that timie. For an athlete, acne can be a serious problem since he may actually become disabled from secondary infection. The vigorous physical activity of sports seems to increase sebum secretion, probably through some endocrine mechanism. The heat and perspiration of exercise aggravate existing acne unmercifully.

acromioclavicular dislocation. This injury is usually produced by a fall on the tip of the shoulder but may occur when the shoulders are pinned to the floor in wrestling. Reduction is difficult to maintain because of the obliquity of the articular facets. In subluxation the superior and inferior capsule is torn, but the main stabilizing ligament (the coracoclavicular ligament) remains intact. In a dislocation, the coracoclavicular ligament is ruptured, thus permitting wide separation of the 2 fragments. Clinical appearance shows an elevation of the outer aspect of the clavicle, but that may be masked by edema.

acromioclavicular sprain, 1st degree. Caused by a fall on a point of the shoulder, such as a leveraged force, as in a fall on an adducted (folded) arm. Symptoms include local pain (especially on motion) and some loss of shoulder function. Signs are tenderness localized over and behind joint, no deformity, and slight swelling.

acromioclavicular sprain, 2nd degree. Produced by a fall on a point of the shoulder, such as a leveraged force, as in a fall on an adducted arm. Symptoms include local pain and moderate disability. Signs are prominence of joint, local tenderness, ligamentous and capsular laxity with increased mobility about the joint. Complications may be permanent deformity, disability, or traumatic arthritis. X ray will show outer end of clavicle displaced slightly upward or backward.

acromioclavicular sprain, 3rd degree. Comes from a major fall on a point of the shoulder, such as a leveraged force, as in a fall on an adducted arm. Symptoms include severe pain and marked disability. Signs are obvious deformity, local tenderness, ligamentous and capsular laxity with increased mobility about the joint. Complications are permanent deformity, disability, or traumatic arthritis. X ray may show increased distance between clavicle and coracoid process or outer end of clavicle displaced upward or backward.

adductor longus strain (forced abduction of thigh). Symptoms include localized pain in ischiopubic region or upper medial aspect of thigh and disability. Signs are graded by degree of severity: ecchymosis, swelling, tenderness in ischiopubic region, pain elicited by passive abduction of thigh, tender firm mass more noticeable on active abduction against resistance, palpable defect between puboischium and muscle belly, bunching of muscle a short distance away from pelvis.

adductor magnus strain. A forced straddling injury, caused by a sudden violent muscular contraction, as in running out of crouched position. Symptoms include acute pain in ischiopubic region, possibly radiating along medial aspect of thigh down to medial femoral condyle. Signs are graded by degree of severity: swelling, ecchymosis, tenderness localized along medial aspect of the thigh with possible palpable defect in the muscle belly, pain elicited by passive abduction and active adduction of thigh X ray may show avulsion of bone fragment downwardly displaced from ischiopubic rami.

adenosine triphosphate. The immediate source of energy for any muscle activity is adenosine triphosphate (ATP). It is stored in limited amounts in striated muscles and replenished as needed from substances stored in the body for future energy use. ATP can be provided to muscle cells in 3 ways; 2 of them are anaerobic (oxygen is not absolutely necessary in the production of ATP), and the 3rd is aerobic (requiring oxygen to manufacture ATP). For brief bursts of energy (e.g., up to 10 seconds), ATP is immediately available from phosphocreatine (PC), a substance normally stored in skeletal muscles. Training can be expected to increase the amounts of ATP and PC available for brief, high output needs for energy in sprints, throwing and jumping events, and explosive movements in football, basketball, and similar sports. The disadvantage is that the total amount of stored ATP and PC is always extremely small.

aerobic. Basically means living or working with oxygen. Aerobic exercise is performed at an intensity moderate enough to keep the energy requirements of the exercising muscles from exceeding the ability of the lungs, heart, and blood vessels to bring enough oxygen to them. If enough oxygen is present, the energy sources in the muscles (carbohydrates and fats) are burned completely to carbon dioxide and water, which are easily excreted by the body. During more intense exercise, energy requirements may be so high that not enough oxygen is available. Incomplete burning of carbohydrates then occurs. The products of incomplete burning are toxic and interfere with normal function. Aerobic exercise is not concerned mainly with developing muscle strength, nor is it related to learning a skilled act, such as hitting a tennis ball or swinging a golf club. It is the running in tennis and walking on the golf course that make aerobic activities useful in developing cardiovascular fitness. Exercises of higher intensity that require more energy for muscle work than can be derived from aerobic metabolism are called anaerobic exercise. Fat cannot be utilized as an energy source for anaerobic muscle work; only carbohydrates of sugar can be used. Anaerobic metabolism can produce energy for muscular work fairly quickly, but it is very inefficient, and the lactic acid or lactate that is the end product builds up and causes muscle pains and cramps and interference with muscle formation. Because of its high intensity and high energy requirements, anaerobic exercise can be performed for only short periods, far too short to produce cardiovascular fitness.

age effects. Age effects are due to the ravages of time and poor diet and to the buffetings to which everyone, to some extent, is exposed, but the loss of condition caused by decreased physical activity also contributes. Generally, maximal exercise ability decreases progressively with age, partly because of a general reduction in the number of active body cells in the muscles and elsewhere. There is, for example, a reduction in the basal metabolism and in the volume of the intracellular water in the body. In the lungs there is less elastic supporting tissues available to hold open the small air passages. As a result of the diminution in elastic recoil, the caliber of the airways at a given lung volume decreases and the airway resistance rises so that the maximum breathing capacity is reduced. On expiration, the airways close completely at a progressively increasing lung capacity and the volume of the residual gas in the lung rises. At the same time, the fine balance between pulmonary ventilation and perfusion is disturbed, so that more air is needed for a given uptake of oxygen (i.e., the ventilation equivalent increases) and the pulmonary diffusion capacity diminishes because of loss of alveolar capillaries. Those changes affect all aspects of lung function and explain the reduction of exercise capacity with age. But they do not occur in isolation. Similar changes affect every tissue of the body. The heart's output decreases, both at rest by a reduction of stroke volume and on exercise by reduction of the maximal obtainable pulse frequency. The smaller cardiac output lessens heat tolerance, and lactic acid appears in the blood at a lower level of exercise. The ability to accumulate oxygen reserves also decreases with age, so that the highest attainable blood lactic acid concentration falls. In the central nervous system, the time taken to react to a stimulus increases, and there is a reduction in the rate of transmission of impulses up to the individual nerve fibers. Coordination is impaired, and that in turn may affect exercise performance.

agility. Difficult to define but basically refers to the maneuverability and flexibility of the individual, i.e., the ability to shift the direction of movement rapidly, without loss of balance or sense of position. Agility is a combination of speed, strength, quick reactions, balance, and coordination. It can refer to the total body or to a specific part, such as the hands or feet. Agility reflects the ability of athletes to perform with a smoothly balanced and fluid motion. It is exemplified by the gymnast who performs a complex routine on the balance beam. Agility is partly an inherited trait, but it can be substantially improved by repeated practice of a specific skill or move.

air pollution. Air pollution is a mixture of atmospheric contaminants that can be categorized into 2 major types. The sulfur oxide and hydrocarbons (particulate complex) produced by the combustion of fossil fuels affect the industrialized urban areas of many parts of the country. Photochemical pollution, or smog, results principally from motor vehicle emissions. Effects of pollutants are usually observed only at levels several-fold higher than those normally encountered in ambient air. Certain people, such as those suffering asthma, may be more sensitive to pollution. Carbon monoxide is of particular importance for the endurance athlete because of its effects on oxygen transport and the exposure of urban athletes to motor vehicle exhaust. Carbon monoxide limits oxygen transport by combining with hemoglobin to form nonfunctional carboxyhemoglobin and by limiting tissue oxygen availability by increasing hemoglobin affinity for oxygen. Exercise increases the rate at which hemoglobin achieves equilibrium with inhaled carbon monoxide. Carbon monoxide pollution that limits the maximal performance of normal individuals rarely occurs.

air temperature and humidity. Outdoors, moderate temperatures between 65° and 75°F are most suitable for peak human performance. As air temperature rises, it becomes more difficult for the body to cool itself during exercise, with the result that extra energy is expended to facilitate the cooling process. As air temperature rises above mean body temperature, the body begins to store heat, cutting down on the efficiency of its working processes and posing the danger of heat exhaustion or stroke. A high relative humidity, which may lead to heat stroke through hydromeiosis, is more critical than the air temperature.

airway maintenance. The mouth and nose, throat, larynx (voice box), trachea, and bronchi form the passages through which air moves into the lungs and are known collectively as the airway. The mouth, throat, and tongue are so constructed that the base of the tongue can move backward and obstruct the opening to the trachea. In swallowing, the tongue and epiglottis block the airway to prevent food or fluids from entering the lungs. Partial obstruction of those passages during sleep results in snoring. However, the obstruction that produces snoring is only partial because the muscles that hold the tongue and structures of the throat are not totally relaxed during sleep. In contrast, disorders resulting in unconsciousness can produce complete relaxation of those muscles, permitting the tongue to totally obstruct the passage of air into the lungs. The adequacy of the airway is very easily checked. If the individual is breathing quietly, the airway is open. Snoring or noisy breathing, labored respirations, or the absence of respiratory movements indicate partial or complete airway obstruction. A tracheostomy is an opening in the trachea, usually in the lower portion of the neck, which allows the individual to breathe without having the air pass through the upper air passages, the mouth or nose, throat, and larynx. An individual whose airway is blocked by the tongue may be "saved" by properly repositioning the lower jaw forward, a technique easily learned in basic first aid.

alcohol. Has been used for years by competitors in 3 ways in sports competition: as a tranquilizer in shooters, as a source of energy in cyclists, and as a stimulant by athletes in several categories. Alcohol is a depressant and may decrease performance by prolonging reaction time and slowing neuromuscular response. However, scientists believe that alcohol (such as beer) is not harmful and appears to protect the heart. One study, which covered a 6-year period, reports that moderate beer drinkers had half as many heart attacks compared with those who totally abstained. It is still unclear whether alcohol itself has some protective value or whether the teetotaler represents a rigid personality type that may predispose to heart attack. Beer has long been a favorite thirst quencher for many distance runners, and it is popular as a replacement solution during long-distance runs, including marathons. Beer has been credited with keeping the kidneys functioning during endurance exercises by blocking antidiuretic hormone (ADH) secretion and thus preventing kidney stones and hematuria from bruising the bladder. Beer has a high potassium and sodium ratio, making it a safe sweat replacement preventing hypokalemia. It also replaces silicon and raises the level of high-density lipoproteins. Alcohol is high in caloric content, 7 calories per gram. Only fat with 9 calories per gram has more by comparison (protein and carbohydrates each contain only 4 calories per gram). While moderate alcohol consumption (3 to 4 beers per week), especially beer, is certainly not harmful and may even protect the heart, heavy drinking is very hazardous, being toxic to the brain, heart, and liver.

alkalinizers. Their use involves the ingestion of an alkaline salt following meals for a few days before and after athletic performance. It has been suggested that alkalinizing drugs, by producing an elevated pH at the beginning of exercise, allow an athlete to tolerate higher levels of lactic acid before exhaustion and thus achieve greater work output. The Medical Commission of the International Olympic Committee has reported that the use of alkalinizers can, by raising the urine pH, reduce the urinary excretion of the by-products of certain stimulants used by athletes. Alkalinizing agents have been used to mask the appearance of stimulant by-products in the urine.

allergic dermatitis. Lesions are fairly common in the popliteal and antecubital fossae. The skin is dry, flaky, and easily irritated. The hands and feet are common areas of involvement. Allergic dermatitis causes severe itching. Heat, sweat, cold, and excitement can aggravate the dermatitis, leading to increased scratching and secondary infections. Coaches should be aware of the seriousness of the condition and the discomfort and embarrassment it can cause, and they should arrange or suggest medical care.

allergy. The tendency of some individuals to react unfavorably to the presence of certain substances that are normally harmless to most people. The substances are called allergens and, like any antigen, are often of a protein nature. Examples of typical allergens are pollens, house dust, dog hair, and horse dander. When the tissues of a susceptible person are repeatedly exposed to an allergen, for example, the nasal mucosa to pollens, those tissues become sensitized; that is, antibodies are produced in them. When the next invasion of the allergen occurs, there is an antigen-antibody reaction. Normally that type of reaction takes place in the blood without harm, as it does in immunity. In allergy, however, the antigen-antibody reaction takes place within the cells of the sensitized tissues with often exaggerated reactions and results that are disagreeable and sometimes dangerous. In the case of the nasal mucosa that has become sensitized to pollen, the allergic manifestation is hay fever, with symptoms much like those of the common cold. Many drugs temporarily relieve the allergic state, but that form of protection does not last long. Some allergic disorders are strongly associated with emotional disturbances. Asthma and migraine, or sick headache, are good examples of that type. In such disorders, the interaction of body and mind still is not fully understood.

altitude medical problems. Medical problems caused by high altitude basically result from a decrease in oxygen concentration in the blood caused by the low atmospheric pressure at high altitudes. Altitude effects result from the lower oxygen content of the air, not the lower barometric pressure. At 18,000 feet, the atmospheric pressure is half that at sea level, and any given volume of air contains half the amount (by weight) of oxygen it does at sea level. However, the proportion of oxygen in the atmosphere does remain constant at approximately 20 percent. The body (resting or active) requires as much oxygen at high altitude as at sea level but cannot store oxygen as it stores water or nutrients. High altitude alone is not dangerous for the heart. Heavy exercise puts a greater strain on the cardiovascular system at higher altitudes. Maximal exercise at sea level is limited by the heart's ability to pump blood. At high altitude exercise is limited by the ability of the chest muscles and diaphragm to move air in and out of the lung. At sea level the lung's capacity to deliver oxygen to the blood maintains a normal blood oxygen concentration even during exhausting exercise. During heavy exercise at high altitude that capacity of the lungs can be exceeded, and the oxygen concentration of the blood can fall. The magnitude of the fall in oxygen concentration is related to the severity of the exercise and the altitude level and is an important factor in limiting exercise performance at very high altitudes. Breathing requires work both by the muscles connecting the ribs and by the diaphragm. The oxygen required for such work is small, accounting for only about 3 percent of the total body oxygen consumption. At high altitudes the work of breathing, especially during exercise, is greatly augmented. The increase in the rate and depth of breathing requires the use of muscles of the neck, shoulders, and abdomen. With heavy effort at very high altitudes, the oxygen required for breathing may be so great that it significantly reduces the amount left for climbing. Supplemental oxygen at very high altitude helps prevent a fall in oxygen concentration during exercise and also decreases the amount of oxygen required for the work of breathing, making more available for climbing.

altitude sickness (mountain sickness). An acute respiratory failure, often but not always caused by pulmonary edema occurring at high altitudes. Without proper acclimation at altitudes as low as 8,000 feet, symptoms may occur rapidly in hours or over several days and often without warning. The condition occurs in the healthy but may be predisposed by chronic lung or heart disease. The common complaints are headache, malaise, nausea, and vomiting. Early symptoms include dyspnea on exertion and fatigue with ordinary effort. Signs include rapid respiration, rales, tachycardia, coughing, cyanosis, apprehension, distended neck veins, arrhythmia, hypotension, and disturbed consciousness leading to coma. In severe cases a bloody sputum will be exhibited.

anal fissure. A cracklike sore in the anus or rectal opening that can be caused by constipation, as in dehydration from wrestling; infection; trauma; or diarrhea. Symptoms include burning pain initiated by defecation. Signs are fissure usually in midline posteriorly, spasm of anal sphincter, or bleeding. Complications may be infection, disability, chronicity.

aneurysms of the hand. In sports where the hand is used as a bat, such as in handball and karate, or struck or crushed, aneurysms and thrombosis of the palm may occur. The 2 common sites are at the hook of the hamate and at the base of the thenar eminence where branches of the radial and ulnar arteries are relatively unprotected from injury.

angina pectoris. A particular form of chest discomfort caused by narrowing of the coronary arteries that supply the heart muscle itself with blood. The narrowing is the result of arteriosclerosis, which consists of deposits of lipids (cholesterol and other fats) in the inner lining of the arteries. Rupture of the fat deposits on clotting in the narrowed artery may cause the onset of angina, an increase in the severity of preexisting angina, or an acute myocardial infarction (heart attack or coronary thrombosis). The discomfort of angina pectoris consists of a pressurelike sensation or a deep-seated pain beneath the breastbone (sternum) appearing on effort and usually disappearing after a few minutes of rest. The discomfort may be described as a sensation of squeezing, a weight on the chest, a band around the heart, or a deep burning sensation. The discomfort may be felt in the neck, jaws, or arms. If effort is continued, the discomfort increases. Angina pectoris with effort may frequently be accompanied by shortness of breath, which subsides as the chest discomfort eases. Individuals with a history of angina attacks should participate in sports and/or physical conditioning programs only under the direction of a physician.

angling injuries.   This is a popular and very widely practiced sport. There are basically 3 sites for angling, sea, river, and lake. The former may subject the sportsman to all the sea-going hazards, navigational and environmental, when exposure, hypothermia, and drowning are possible. Freshwater fishing can be of 2 types—dry fly casting and using bait. The bait can give rise to sensitivities and allergies in the fishermen. The hooks can cause severe eye injury and can become embedded in the skin and should be pushed through the nearest surface. No attempt should be made to pull them out against the barbs. The line can become enwrapped around a finger and pulled extremely tight by a fighting fish with varying degrees of damage. Shoulder and elbow strains may follow prolonged and frequent casting. Bites can occur in handling fish caught, such as congers and shark, which can inflict severe damage to the fingers and hand in particular.

ankle.   The ankle is made up of 3 bones, the tibia and fibula (both leg bones) and the talus. The tibia and fibula converge together from the leg to cup the talus bone, which is the bone of the foot. The ankle is a saddle-type joint, the talus resembling a saddle with the body pivoting over it. The ankle joint is supported by gravity and joint congruity, strong ligaments, and muscle tendons. Body weight or gravity helps maintain joint alignment as long as there are no postural or structural defects that may favor joint misalignment. Ligaments are the ankle's mainstay of stability. Both the inside and outside of the joint are supported by a maze of ligaments arranged to offer maximum support with maximum mobility. Ligaments restrict excess foot inversion or eversion. When they are permanently damaged, the ability to maintain proper ankle stability is also impaired. Recurrent sprain is often the result. Tendons that cross the ankle on either side also aid in stabilization; on the medial side the posterior tibial tendon and on the lateral side the peroneal tendons help stability. One set pulls the foot into inversion and the other into eversion. It is through their antagonistic effort that balanced neutrality is achieved.

ankle dislocation, anterior.   Excessive forcible dorsiflexion of foot. It is caused by a fall upon the heel with the foot in the position of dorsiflexion. The symptoms are pain and disability. The signs are obvious deformity, heel shortened, forefoot lengthened, foot in position of dorsiflexion, distal ends of tibia and fibula prominent behind, malleoli possibly remaining in place or, if fracture displaced with foot, generalized swelling and tenderness. Complications may be traumatic arthritis, residual stiffness. X ray may show anterior dislocation of ankle, usually accompanied by fracture of anterior margin or articular surface; 1 or both malleoli may be avulsed.

ankle dislocation, posterior.   Foot in plantarflexion with strong forward thrust applied to leg. The symptoms are pain and disability. The signs are obvious deformity, distal ends of tibia and fibula visible and palpable beneath skin over front of ankle, distance between anterior border of tibia and heel increased markedly, inability to dorsiflex foot on leg, generalized swelling and tenderness. Complications may be traumatic arthritis and residual stiffness. X ray may show posterior dislocation of ankle, usually accompanied by fracture of 1 or both malleoli and posterior margin of tibia.

ankle dislocation, upward (compression trauma). Symptoms are pain and disability. Signs are obvious deformity, abnormal broadening of malleoli with approximation of heel to 1 or both malleoli, generalized tenderness and swelling. Complications may be traumatic arthritis and residual stiffness. X ray may show diastasis at inferior tibiofibular joint, talus pushed upward between tibia and fibula, usually considerable comminution of distal end of tibia and fracture of fibula.

ankle exostoses, talotibial. Ankle spurs, osteochondral ridges. Direct trauma; repeated forceful impingement of talus on anterior margin of tibia such as the "drive" of an athlete when cleats are fixed to the ground. Symptoms may be asymptomatic: vague complaints of lost power; inability to run, cut, or jump at full speed without pain. Signs are pinpoint tenderness directly over spur; forced dorsiflexion of foot eliciting pain localized at anterior talotibial sulcus. Complications may be avulsed spur producing loose body in ankle; traumatic arthritis. X ray may show exostosis formation usually on back or front of tibia or back of head superiorly on talus; condition varies from simple change in contour to a spur of a centimeter or longer extending along whole width of bone.

ankle fracture, abduction, 1st degree. Foot forcibly *abducted* on leg. Symptoms are pain over medial malleolar region, moderate disability. Signs are localized tenderness and swelling over medial malleolus (swelling subsequently spreads), crepitus over medial malleolus, pain elicited by eversion of foot, no deformity. Complications may be recurrent instability of ankle and nonunion of medial malleolus. X ray may show fracture of medial malleolus: roughly transverse, at or just below inferior articular surface of tibia and little or no displacement of detached portion of medial malleolus.

ankle fracture, abduction, 2nd degree. Foot forcibly abducted on leg. Symptoms are severe generalized pain and moderate to severe disability. Signs are obvious deformity with foot displaced laterally, generalized tenderness and swelling, pain elicited on inversion and eversion of foot, creptius over medial malleolar and distal fibula regions, ankle mortise possibly with spring, limited motion of ankle. Complications may be traumatic arthritis, malunion, prolonged disability.

ankle fracture, abduction, 3rd degree. Supramalleolar fracture. Foot forcibly abducted on leg. Symptoms are severe pain and disability. Signs are obvious deformity, foot displaced laterally, generalized tenderness and swelling of ankle. Complications may be traumatic arthritis, malunion, prolonged disability, residual stiffness. X ray may show transverse fracture of the lower portion of shaft of tibia plus fracture of lower fibula with diastasis of ankle joint.

ankle fracture, adduction, 1st degree. Foot forcibly adducted on leg. Pain localized at lateral malleolus and moderate disability. Signs are swelling and tenderness localized over lateral malleolus, crepitus over lateral malleolus, pain elicited on passive inversion of foot. Complications may be recurrent instability of ankle. X ray may show transverse fracture of fibula at or below articular surface of tibia, little displacement.

ankle fracture, adduction, 2nd degree. Foot forcibly adducted on leg. Generalized pain and disability. Signs are obvious deformity, foot displaced inward, ecchymosis, generalized swelling and tenderness, crepitus. Complications may be traumatic arthritis.

ankle fracture, adduction, 3rd degree. Foot forcibly adducted on leg. Symptoms are severe pain and disability. Signs are obvious deformity, foot displaced inwardly, ecchymosis, generalized tenderness and swelling, crepitus. Complications may be traumatic arthritis, malunion, prolonged disability, residual stiffness. X ray may show fibula and tibia fractured transversly in their lower 3rd and displaced medially.

ankle fracture, external rotation, 1st degree. Fibula fracture, distal portion, spiral or oblique. Leg forcibly rotated inward with foot fixed on ground; foot forcibly rotated outward on fixed leg. Symptoms are pain localized at lateral malleolar region, moderate disability. Signs are slight deformity over lateral malleolus, possible crepitus, tenderness and swelling localized to lateral aspect of lower leg. X rays show fracture line begins at front of lateral malleolus just below inferior tibiofibular articulation and passes upward and backward across the joint, emerging on posterior surface of fibula.

ankle fracture, external rotation, 2nd degree. Leg forcibly rotated inward with foot fixed on ground. Foot forcibly rotated outward on leg. Symptoms are pain becoming generalized but most severe along lateral aspect of ankle, disability, inability to bear weight. Signs are obvious deformity; crepitus laterally, sometimes medially; general tenderness and swelling; defect able to be palpated below medial malleolus; possible spring to ankle mortise. X ray may show fracture of distal fibula displaced outward as well as rotated outward; may be displaced backward; possibly accompanied by fracture of posterior margin of tibia; may show diastasis at ankle joint or an avulsion of an intermediate fragment from lateral surface of tibia (rare).

ankle fracture, lateral malleolus avulsion. Chipped ankle, ankle inversion sprain-fracture. Foot forcibly turned inward on leg while bearing weight upon it, as in placing foot upon an uneven surface while walking or running. Symptoms are severe pain on outside of ankle and some disability. Signs are acute tenderness and possible crepitus over area anterior to and below tip of lateral malleolus, marked swelling anterior to

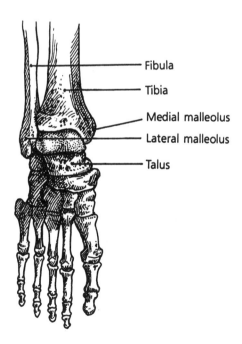

Fibula

Tibia

Medial malleolus

Lateral malleolus

Talus

Ankle joint

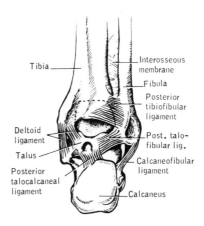

Anatomical drawing of an ankle

and below tip of lateral malleolus, marked swelling. Complications may be recurrent instability of ankle in inversion. X ray shows avulsion of tip lateral malleolus and variable displacement medially and downward; inversion stress films may show increasing talar tilt.

ankle injuries. The ankle joint is functionally a hinge joint having motion in only 1 plane, flexion, and extension. The bony structure is designed as a mortise and tendon with considerable inherent stability. The mortise is formed by the lateral malleolus, the undersurface of the tibia, and the medial malleolus. The tendon is the body of the talus, which is shaped to fit snugly into the mortise with the lateral malleolus longer than the medial malleolus. Its distal tip extends to the bottom of the talus at the level of the talocalcaneal joint. The medial malleolus is short and thick, being roughly pyramidal in shape, its base upward with the distal tip extending halfway down on the body of the talus. The distal tibia and fibula are bound together by the anterior and posterior tibiofibular ligaments, which are really thickened expansions of the interosseous membrane that fastens the 2 bones together throughout their length. The ligaments are thin fore and aft (capsule) to permit flexion and extension of the joint. Injuries to the ankle relate to the magnitude and direction of force as applied to the ankle. The way an athlete uses his ankle may also predispose him or her to inversion injuries.

Acute capsular sprains of the ankle are probably the most common single type of sports injury. The classical injury is that produced by inversion and internal rotation, which results in sprain of the lateral ligament of the ankle joint. Clinically, there appear to be 2 main types. In the 1st pain is severe, and soft tissue swelling is very pronounced, with obvious discoloration showing early. The swelling may be large, with marked limitation of movement and pain so severe that the presence of a fracture may be suspected. The 2nd and less common type of sprain has a far less well marked clinical picture. Pain varies in severity, there is little swelling, and local tenderness may be acute. The best time for accurate assessment of the degree of damage is immediately following the injury when muscle spasm is absent, pain is not severe, and swelling and hemarthosis have not developed. Rupture of the Achilles tendon occurs in very heavy and older athletes primarily. When the athlete is supported on the toes of 1 foot, the force exerted on the tendon is a multiple of the ratio of the distance from the point of support on the ball of the foot to the midpoint of the ankle and from the midpoint to the attachment of the tendon to the calcaneus. The heavy, tall athlete with long feet, such as a defensive tackle in professional football, is at the greatest risk. The tendons of the older athlete may rupture as the result of chronic strain and the gradual weakening of the tendons, which usually accompanies the aging process. Talotibial exostoses is a chronic condition that may cause pain and disability when the athlete bears weight on the leg with the foot in dorsiflexion as he drives off it. In most cases, it does not cause symptoms and occurs as a result of repeated impringement of the anterior portion of the talus against the leading edge of the tibia. As the bone builds up on both sides, the contact becomes painful, although prolonged rest with no weight bearing will relieve the symptoms. Fracture of the fibula above the joint line may be accomplished by ruptured tibiofibular and medial collateral ligaments and fracture of the medial malleolus.

ankle sprains. There are 2 types of ankle sprains. The inversion type is the most common and occurs when the foot turns inward in relation to the leg. The eversion sprain occurs when the foot turns out in relation to the leg. There are 3 degrees of severity of an ankle injury. First-degree sprain results in swelling and prolonged pain although no rupture or ankle instability is noted. Second-degree sprain involves partial rupture of supporting ligaments and mild instability on examination. Third-degree sprain causes marked instability, and a complete rupture of the supporting ligaments is present. All sprains in those categories require immediate medical attention. If ankle sprain occurs, no weight on the extremity should be tolerated until it can be examined. In considering the relation between skeletal abnormalities and ankle sprains, one must remember that the ankle is a weight-bearing joint. The heel bone directly below the ankle supports it and depending on its position determines the stability of the ankle. If the heel is turned inward, body weight is shifted to the outside and a stretch is placed on the lateral ligaments. If the heel is turned out or everted excessively, force is placed on the medial ligaments. It is therefore the position of the heel bone that determines ankle stability. Any structural foot or leg deformity that causes the heel bone to shift from its vertical position will most likely favor ankle sprains.

anserine bursitis. It is caused by repeated friction or an external blow to region of pes anserinus. The symptom is sharp pain localized to upper anteromedial side of knee. Signs are tenderness located at upper anteromedial side of knee under the unattached portion of the medial hamstring tendons, pain aggravated by flexion and extension of the knee, crepitus, occasional swelling. Complications may be chronicity.

appendicitis. A disorder producing acute abdominal pain, which requires surgical treatment. The onset is characterized by vague abdominal discomfort, which becomes progressively worse. Cramps are usually absent. The earliest symptoms are frequently located in the midabdomen. One to three hours later, the pain shifts to the right lower quadrant, during which time the individual usually becomes nauseated and vomits several times. One or two bowel movements may occur, but diarrhea is rare. The area of maximum tenderness is in the right lower quadrant of the abdomen. Later tenderness and muscle spasms appear in the same region. Usually a low fever of about 101° is present, but chills are rare. If the appendix ruptures, pain may abruptly disappear. A few hours later it usually returns but is more diffuse and is associated with signs of peritonitis. However, the infection can remain localized to the area around the appendix, forming an abscess. In the presence of that complication, a low fever usually persists, and the individual does not feel well. Nevertheless, there may be no other symptoms until the abscess ruptures at a later date, producing peritonitis, which may be overwhelming. The individual involved in sports may misinterpret the symptoms of acute appendicitis as muscle soreness or tenderness from recent athletic participation, and thus he may delay necessary medical attention.

arch sprain, static. A disorder caused by constant stress of weight superimposed on arch or repetitive vigorous exercise with long hours on feet. It occurs early in season often as a result of change from regular shoes with arch to flat athletic shoes. The symptom, pain along the arch, is promptly relieved by rest. Signs are tenderness along plantar ligament from attachment at the calcaneous to its attachment near the metarsal heads. Arch sprain is not limited to "flatfoot" individuals. Complications may be persistent disability.

arch sprain, traumatic. Acute, violent overstretching of dalcaneocuboid ligament, plantar ligament, longitudinal arch, lateral ligaments of foot, and intermetatarsal ligament. It may be caused by repeated episodes of overmotion or running in light shoes or barefooted. Symptoms are pain, difficulty in walking, and inability to run. Signs are variable degree of severity, tenderness of involved area, possible swelling, and ecchymosis. Complications may be chronicity and persistent disability.

archery and shooting injuries. Accidents can result in severe wounding. If it involves the chest or abdominal viscera, it may be fatal if prompt resuscitation and removal to hospital are not available. Recoil bruising to the shoulder is common, especially in the novice. The head may also be jolted by recoil and headache, and temporary deafness may follow repeated firing. Bowstring burns can occur if forearm protection is not worn.

arm injuries. Upper-extremity injuries caused by violent sports or recurrent overuse are common in athletics. The function of the upper arm, elbow, and forearm depends upon musculotendinous units having their origin nearest to the shoulder joint and the insertion attaching further near the wrist and hand. Contusion to the upper extremity is common in contact sports. Direct blows sustained while one is tackling and blocking can produce bleeding within muscle groups and subperiosteally along the humerus. Contusions within the muscle groups, particularly the triceps, biceps, and brachial muscles, can be painful and result in restricted motion and disability. A common site of contusion in the upper arm is over the lateral aspect of the humerus, just distal to the attachment of the deltoid and lateral to the biceps muscle. Here, either a severe single blow or repeated injuries from blocking and tackling can cause subperiosteal

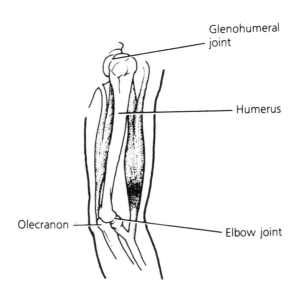

Glenohumeral joint

Humerus

Olecranon

Elbow joint

The arm.

hematoma formation with subsequent myositis ossificans (tackler's exostosis). The clinical symptoms are pain, stiffness, and associated weakness within the involved muscle groups. The muscles of the arm are subject to acute strain in excessive muscular activity, which may vary from a mild irritation of the tendon or muscle to a complete rupture. Although the arms do not have to sustain the weight-bearing stresses to which the legs are subjected, the multitude of their other functions involves more risk of accidental injury. The bones of the arm are also smaller and less strong than those of the leg, and for those reasons fractures occur more frequently in the upper limb than in the lower. That generalization holds good in relation to injuries sustained in the course of various types of athletic endeavors.

asthma. A disease of the bronchi caused by allergy. Contact with the substance to which the individual is allergic (the allergen) increases the secretion of mucus into the bronchi. Simultaneously, the muscles in the walls of the bronchi go into spasm, constricting the air passages. The narrowed bronchi, filled with excess mucus, obstruct the passage of air and cause respiratory difficulty. Asthma may be very mild, severe, or even fatal. A first attack may occur at any time and any place. Asthma is a recurring disease. The most significant sign is difficulty in breathing, particularly in expiration. The expiratory phase of respiration, which normally requires less time than inspiration, is considerably prolonged and may call for conscious effort on the part of the individual. An incessant, irritating cough is often present. Toward the end of an asthmatic attack, the individual may cough up considerable quantities of very thick mucus. Fever is usually absent, but the pulse rate may be moderately increased. The respiratory rate is usually faster than normal in spite of difficulty in breathing. The asthmatic individual should engage in athletics only under the direction of a physician.

atherosclerosis. A blocking of an artery. The obstructing material contains a high proportion of cholesterol and other fatty substances as well as other blood elements, including platelets and proteins, all of which are involved in the normal blood clotting process. Atherosclerosis often begins when one is young and takes decades to develop to a dangerous degree. It probably starts with damage to the very thin layer of cells that form the important inner wall of the artery called the endothelium. Like most of the body tissues, the endothelium weakens with age and is more prone to damage. Endothelial damage is also caused by high blood pressure and high cholesterol levels. When young, the endothelium retains the capacity to repair itself, but with time it loses that capacity, and permanent damage can occur. Then a series of complex events happens. First, the smooth muscle cells in the walls of the artery, which underlies the damaged area, are stimulated to grow and multiply. At the same time they accumulate large amounts of cholesterol and other fats. The growth of a number of other tissue elements may be stimulated, and the involved area enlarges. If it becomes large enough, it may interfere with the flow of blood within the artery. No early signs or symptoms of that obstruction will be evident for a considerable period, because the flow of blood through the artery is not significantly impaired until the cross-sectional area of the artery is reduced by more than half. That is what happens in individuals with atherosclerosis of the coronary arteries. When the blood requirements of the heart muscle are low—at rest, for example—no symptoms are present. During exercise, when the heart works harder, adequate flow of blood may not be possible in the partially blocked artery. The heart muscle becomes starved for blood, and symptoms begin. Acute events apparently are caused by sudden complete blockage of the artery, either by a clot that forms in the area already involved by the atherosclerosis, by a hemorrhage in the wall of the artery that expands the side of the involved area, or by a spasm of the artery itself. When complete blockage occurs, the results are disastrous. Death and destruction of the tissues supplied by the blocked artery occurs. If that occurs in the heart, it is called a coronary heart attack, or myocardial infarction. In the brain, it is called a stroke.

athlete's foot. A disease involving the toes and the soles of the feet but occasionally affecting the fingers, the palm of the hands, and the groin region. Fungi are the usual causes of athlete's foot, also known as epidermophytosis. In acute cases the lesions may include vesicles, fissures, and ulcers. Predisposition to fungus infection varies. Some individuals may be exposed to pathogenic fungi with no ill effects, while in other people, a mild exposure will cause a severe skin infection. Those who perspire a great deal are particularly susceptible to athlete's foot. Clean socks and alternating shoes are preventive measures usually taken by those afflicted.

athlete's heart. Reports of X rays taken among groups of athletes and control groups of nonparticipating subjects indicate that there is a significant difference in cardiac size between sporting and nonsporting subjects. In trained athletes the resting pulse is often slow, and there may even be mild hypertrophy and dilation of the heart as a consequence of the chronic increased work requirements placed on the heart. There is no evidence that such (physiological) hypertrophy is detrimental to the individual. The endurance athlete thus has a large-capacity heart with a slow "tick over." There are probably other adaptations that allow him not only to achieve a high maximum cardiac output but also to maintain a high value for prolonged periods of time. The increase in chamber size of the heart may well be complemented by an increase in blood vessel size and the diameter of the valve orifices. There are virtually no data available, however, on that feature of the athlete's heart. A cardiac output of 40 l/min through an aortic root of 2.7 diameter (Feigenbaum's figure for the average aortic root diameter) would generate a mean blood velocity of 260 cm/sec and a mean Reynolds number of 18,000. Those figures would be reduced to a mean aortic blood velocity of 117 cm/sec. A Reynolds number of 12,000 by an aortic root diameter of 4 cm would reduce somewhat the very large energy losses involved in accelerating the blood up to such high velocities and also reduce the dissipative energy losses resulting from the turbulence in the aortic flow that would seem inevitable with such high mean blood velocities and Reynolds numbers. Sustained high cardiac output would seem to require generalized enlargement of the heart and great vessels, and since cardiac output appears to be the limiting factor in defining the maximum oxygen uptake, it could well be the development of large pressure losses across the mitral valve and in the aortic root that acts as the ultimate determinant of performance.

autonomic nervous system. Although the internal organs (such as the heart, lungs, and stomach) contain sensory nerve endings and nerve fibers for conducting sensory messages to the brain and spinal cord, most of those impulses do not reach consciousness. The sensory impulses from the viscera, like those from the skin and the muscles, are translated into reflex responses without reaching the higher centers of the brain. The sensory neurons from the organs are grouped with those that come from the skin and voluntary muscles. The efferent neurons that supply the glands and the involuntary muscles are arranged very differently from those that supply the voluntary muscles. That variation in the location and arrangement of the visceral efferent neurons has led to their being classified as a part of a separate division called the autonomic nervous system. It has many special parts, including ganglia that serve as relay stations. In those ganglia, each message is transferred from the 1st neuron to a 2nd one, which then carries the impulse to the muscle or gland cell. In the case of voluntary muscle cells, each nerve fiber extends all the way from the spinal cord to the muscle with no intervening relay station. The autonomic nervous system regulates the action of the glands, the smooth muscles of hollow organs, and the heart. Those actions are all carried on automatically; and whenever any changes occur that call for a regulatory adjustment, it is done without our being conscious of it. The sympathetic part of the autonomic nervous system tends to act largely as an accelerator, particularly under conditions of stress. Stimulation of the adrenal glands, which produce hormones, including epinephrine, prepare the body to meet emergency situations in many ways. The sympathetic nerves and hormones from the adrenals reinforce each other. Dilation of the pupil and decrease in focusing ability occurs (for near objects). Increases follow in the rate and forcefulness of heart contractions. Increased blood pressure results owing partly to the more effective heart-beat and partly to constriction of small arteries in the skin and the internal organs. Dilation of the bronchial tube occurs in order to allow for more oxygen to enter. Inhibition of peristalsis and of secretory activity results so that digestion is slowed. Injuries, caused by wounds by penetrating objects or tumors, hemorrhage, spinal column dislocations or fractures, may cause damage to the sympathetic trunk. In addition to those rather obvious kinds of disorders, there are a great number of conditions in which symptoms suggest autonomic malfunction. However, the method of operation is not so well understood, and scientists do not yet entirely agree on them. Those disorders are related to the part that psychological issues may play in the functioning of the organs supplied by the autonomic nervous system.

B

back injuries. There are a few general principles relating to back problems. The 1st is that "muscle spasm" is not a diagnosis of a back disorder but a symptom or sign of many different disorders. The 2nd is that ordinarily there is little or no motion at the sacroiliac joint and that a diagnosis of sacroiliac strain is not a reasonable one. The 3rd principle emphasizes that most acute low back strains seen in athletes have a structural origin, most of which are congenital in nature. The formation of the lumbar and sacral vertebra is apparently so complex that many malformations may appear in its development in the infant and child. Those defects, unless major in nature, are not usually productive of symptoms in early life. As the individual matures, the lower part of the spine has to bear a greater weight; and as a result of increased activity, the supporting ligaments are stretched. When that happens, the spine begins to slip. Under some acute stress, such as lifting or twisting, the tolerance of that portion is exceeded, nerve root traction or pressure is exerted, and pain begins. Back pain is produced by a wide variety of disorders. Simple strain, which is one of the most common causes, can result from carrying heavy loads, working in an unaccustomed position, or sleeping in an awkward position. Normally, the vertebrae of the spinal column are separated by cushions of cartilaginous material that absorb the force from the numerous jolts to which the body is subjected. A ruptured disc is an extrusion of that semisolid cushion into the spinal canal, resulting in compression of the spinal cord or the nerves coming from the cord. The basic defect consists of degeneration and weakening of the ligaments that normally hold the cushion in place. Trauma is only the final incident in producing a ruptured disc. Unless that basic defect is present, trauma alone usually fractures the vertebrae instead of causing the disc to rupture. The nature and location of symptoms in this condition are highly characteristic. Pain begins in the lower back, radiates to one side, and passes through the buttock and down the back of the leg. The pain may also involve the outside of the leg but is rarely present in the front or inner portion of the leg. The discomfort frequently causes the individual to walk with a decided limp. Excruciating back pain, when one is moving to and from a supine position, is also characteristic. In the center of the spine, a few muscles are enclosed in a firm fibrous sheath, which forms a tight nondistensible envelope. Injuries to such muscles that result in bleeding or swelling can increase the pressure within that sheath to such a level that the circulation of blood to the muscle undergoes impairment ranging to total blockage. Consequently, the muscle dies and is replaced with nonfunctioning scar tissue, usually resulting in a permanent crippling disability of that extremity.

back, low. The lower back is composed of 5 mobile lumbar vertebrae with cartilaginous cushions (discs) between them and the fused bones of the sacrum and coccyx, which form the back of the pelvis. There are also ligaments, thick dense tough strands of connective tissue, that attach 1 bone to another. Those ligaments hold the foundation blocks of the low back, the vertebrae, sacrum, coccyx, and pelvis together. All those ligaments have some elasticity and thus provide the back with mobility. The 5 major groups of ligaments of the lower back are as follows: the interspinal ligaments, intertransverse ligaments, ligamenta flava, anterior and posterior longitudinal ligaments, and the anuli fibrosi disci intervertebralis. The muscles of the back, abdomen, and hip are responsible for both support and movement of the back. There are 4 groups of muscles essential for support of the back that can play a major role in back pain: abdominal muscles, extensor muscles, and the 2 side muscles. Those 4 groups of muscles constitute the 4 guy wires to support the back. However, the hips, by virtue of their relationship to the pelvis and thus the pelvis to the spine, can have a

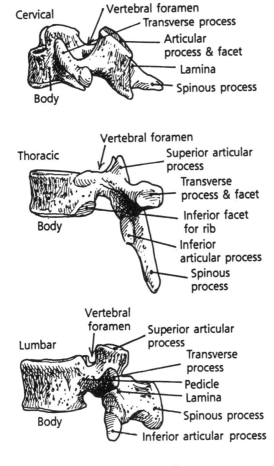

Anatomy of vertebrae

very significant effect on the back. Of the 3 hip muscle groups, the flexors (lift hips up), abductors (turn hips out), and extensors (lift hips back), the latter are the most massive and important to the back. The hip extensor muscles are a group controlling lumbar lordosis, a condition which, when excessive, is called "sway back" and is a major cause of back pain. The hip extensors, in combination with the hip flexors, are essential in the maintenance of good posture.

back, low (pain). Most athletic injuries to the low back involve either a contusion; a bruise from a direct blow; a sprain, a pulling with a stretching and tearing of the muscles or their tendons; or a strain, tearing of a ligament. In general, a strain is most painful when the back is forced in the opposite direction, and a sprain produces pain when the affected muscle is contracted. The cause of most back strains and sprains in the athlete and nonathlete alike is weak muscles, especially the abdominal muscles and hip flexors, and tension or lack of flexibility, especially in the hamstring hip extensor muscles. In general, athletes have strong extensor muscles (the back and hip), and the flexor muscles in 1 or both regions are frequently underdeveloped. Most strains and sprains develop in 1 of 2 ways. The 1st is by sudden, abrupt, violent extension contraction on an overloaded, unprepared, or undeveloped spine, especially where there is some rotation in the attempted movement. That can result in stretching a few fibers, a complete tear, or an avulsion fracture of a spinous or transverse process. The 2nd mechanism involves a chronic strain, often with associated poor posture, excessive lumbar lordosis. Here there is a continuation of the underlying disease with recurring injury to the original or adjacent sites. Through the repetition of training, many sports predispose to low back pain. Most sports involve either strong back extension movements, as opposed to strong flexion, or else external forces that produce extension. Track athletes run in forced extension. The discus thrower, shot putter, and weight lifter all propel heavy weights with the back extended. Gymnasts repeatedly dismount with a hyperextended low back as the feet hit the mat. The diver hits the water in extension with foot-entry dives.

bacteremia and septicemia. Caused by bacteria invading the bloodstream. If the organisms are destroyed while still in the bloodstream, the condition is referred to as bacteremia. In septicemia (also called blood poisoning), the organisms multiply in the blood and produce other foci of infections throughout the body. Both conditions are usually preceded by a local infection, such as an infected wound, an infected burn, or an abscess. Bacterial bloodstream invasions are characterized by chills, irregular fever, sweating, and prostration. Septicemia may be impossible to distinguish from bacteremia. Signs suggestive of septicemia are an increase in severity of chills and fever, persistence of the fever for more than 4 to 6 hours, and signs that the infection has spread to other areas. Severe headache, stiffness of the neck, and nausea and vomiting may indicate involvement of the brain or meninges. Cough and pain with breathing are suggestive of pneumonia. Prompt administration of antibiotics is important.

Baker's cyst. Posteriorly, the most common involvement in athletes is the so-called Baker's cyst. The term "Baker's cyst" has been extended to include almost any synovial hernia or bursitis involving the posterior aspect of the knee. Such inflammation may be due to actual bursitis or a structural defect in the posterior capsule that permits synovial herniation. There may be as much as a 50 percent incidence of communication between the joint space and the popliteal bursa in asymptomatic individuals. With chronic knee effusions, torn menisci, or swelling attributable to any cause within the knee, synovial fluid accumulates within the communicating bursae. Most individuals with a "Baker's cyst" complain of a mass behind the knee that may or may not be bothersome at full flexion and extension. Many individuals report periods during which the mass disappears. One type is bursitis of the semimembranosus or of the medial gastrocnemius bursa, a bursa that lies between the medial head of the gastro-

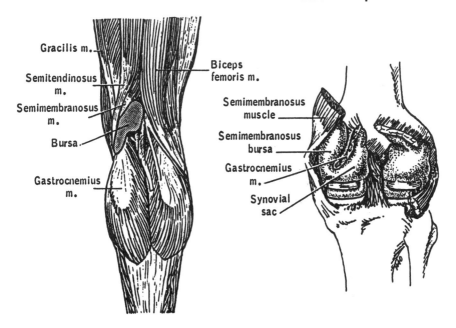

Gracilis m.

Semitendinosus m.

Semimembranosus m.

Bursa.

Gastrocnemius m.

Biceps femoris m.

Semimembranosus muscle

Semimembranosus bursa

Gastrocnemius m.

Synovial sac

Baker's cyst showing the semimembranous bursa lying between the semimembranosus and medial head of the gastrocnemius.

cnemius and semimembranous tendon. Involvement of the bursa causes expansion of its wall, usually posteriorly since there is no particular obstruction to its expansion in that direction. It presents itself as a large, soft tumor mass in the popliteal space. The appearance of the mass is usually preceded by a varying period of chronic, aching type pain in the back of the knee. Since the bursa frequently communicates with the knee, often by a valvelike arrangement, the swelling may come and go and present great difficulty to diagnosis. As a consequence of the valvelike connection with the knee joint, sufficient fluid may collect to make a sizable tumor. That fluid then concentrates to the characteristic jell contained in a synovial hernia. Later, as a result of trauma or other cause, it may be discharged into the knee, where the concentrated fluid becomes an irritative factor and causes synovitis.

barometric pressure. With decreasing barometric pressure, the partial pressure caused by oxygen falls to a point where it begins to affect performance in any activity involving endurance at an altitude of a little over 4,000 feet. It becomes increasingly difficult to support vigorous activity until the altitude exceeds 20,000 feet, at which point only very well acclimated persons do not require assistance from inhalation of oxygen. At a medium altitude of 6,000 feet to 7,000 feet, the decreased density of the air favors sprinters, jumpers, and throwers of the shot and javelin. At middle and long distances, the advantages are counterbalanced by the decreased partial pressure of oxygen. Performance in distance running events may improve with acclimatization but may not reach sea level values. Internal barometric pressures increase with the descent under water at the rate of 1 atmosphere for every 10 m. Depth in free diving is limited chiefly by breath-holding ability, which does not exceed 3 to 4 minutes even for most highly trained divers. The body is well able to stand the water pressure at depths much greater than can be reached because of the development of anoxia and hypercapnia. In scuba diving, the limiting factors are the inability of the body to tolerate hyperoxia, or excess of oxygen in the system and the increased working of breathing against the inert gas in whatever mixture is used.

barotrauma. Injury caused by pressure, specifically injury of the cartilaginous wall of the Eustachian tube and the ear drum due to the difference between atmospheric and intratympanic pressures. The middle ear and paranasal sinuses consist of numerous small chambers lined by thin mucous membranes and filled with air. Those chambers have narrow connections to the nose or throat through which air can move to equalize the pressure of the air within the chamber with that of the external atmosphere. For the middle ears, that tube enters the throat and is known as the Eustachian tube. If the pressure within the chambers is not equalized, a sense of fullness develops and hearing is diminished. Swallowing or yawning may open the Eustachian tube rather suddenly so that a "pop" is heard as the pressure is suddenly equalized. As atmospheric pressure decreases, such as during the ascent to higher altitudes, air leaves those chambers without difficulty. However, during a descent to a lower altitude, more active measures, such as swallowing or yawning, are required to open the Eustachian tube and permit the pressure to equalize. Occasionally, a cold or nasal allergy causes the mucosa around the openings of the Eustachian tube and the ducts into the nasal sinuses to swell and plug off the tubular openings. At a pressure differential of 90 millimeters (which represent a change in altitude of about 3,750 feet), the Eustachian tubes can no longer be opened by swallowing. As the pressure differential increases, the sensation of fullness in the ears and nose becomes more and more painful. Involvement of the ears can cause sensations of noise, lightheadedness, and hearing loss. If the pressure is sufficiently severe, the eardrum can be ruptured. However, pressure differential of such severity can develop only when descent is made rapidly, as occurs in unpressurized aircraft or sometimes in automobiles on steep mountain roads.

Barr Bodies. Used as a means of determining sex and are seen only in cells from the female. That can be done by scraping a few cells from the mouth mucosa or by pulling out a hair follicle. The Barr body is formed by 2nd, 3rd, or 4th X chromosomes and does not occur in the male cell. They show as dark staining bodies in the nuclei and occur in up to half the female cells. The presence of 1 per cell suggests normal femininity.

Barton fracture. A fall onto the outstretched hand. Symptoms are local pain and disability. Signs are wrist deformity, swelling, and possible crepitus. Complications may be malunion, Sudeck's syndrome, and permanent disability. X ray may show marginal fracture of distal radius with fragment plus subluxation of carpus; fragment may be palmar or dorsal.

baseball finger. Frequently in baseball, football, basketball, or volleyball, one suddenly finds one's fingers painfully jammed. Known as baseball finger, because it occurs most frequently in that sport, "jammed finger" is an affliction common to many different athletic activities. If not treated correctly, it can have chronic complications that, by preventing proper gripping, can interfere with the enjoyment of the sport. Baseball finger occurs when a hard, moving object impacts against the tip of an advertently extended finger and forces its distal or middle interphalangeal hinge joints to suddenly hyperflex backward or bend to the side. Either way, a stretch and, depending on the force, possibly a tear of the collateral ligaments of the joints result, causing swelling, immobility, and intense pain. Depending on the extent of the tear, most baseball fingers will return to normal joint function, although with more extensive tears there will be slight instability at the affected joint.

baseball injuries (elbow). There are 5 common baseball injuries of the elbow. (1) Osteochondritis (inflammation of bone and cartilage), an injury seen in the elbow of baseball players caused by repeated trauma of forced sudden extension resulting in flaking off of cartilage leading to loose bodies, cartilaginous outgrowths semiattached, and synovial thickening. Symptoms are pain and swelling and long disability because of obstruction to full extension by cartilaginous outgrowths and loose bodies. (2) Olecranon fractures, a condition that can be either of the flake type torn off the tip of the olecranon or the "hair line" type of fracture thought to be due to fatigue. (3) Spurs are situated on the inner edge of the trochlea. They are extremely painful and very small and difficult to visualize on X-ray film. (4) Anticubital swelling, occurring in baseball pitchers who, to gain a curve, forcibly supinate the wrist at the end of the throw. The condition can be disabling and is characterized by fullness over the pronator and the antecubital fossa. (5) Ossicles, either single or multiple, can form in the joint ligaments on the inner side of the ulnar nerve. They form as the result of chronic strain and probably take years to develop. Experience has called attention to the many severe injuries occurring on the elbows of young pitchers in the Babe Ruth and Little League age groups of 8 to 12 years. Those young boys with unfused epiphyses in their elbows are causing significant displacement and in many instances permanent damage to the growing epiphyses in their pitching arm by throwing too long and too hard. Many of those young, untrained players rely solely on the fast ball, and sometimes a temporarily good pitcher will pitch 5 to 7 innings, occasionally without adequate conditioning or even without warming up. Thus epicondylar, capitellum, or trochlear epiphyses become displaced, and permanent loss of function and deformity often follow.

baseball injuries (fractures and joint injuries). Fractures of the tip of the distal phalanx are frequent in poorly coordinated players. The fracture occurs almost universally in catchers who must handle fast pitches that are often deflected by the batter. Dislocation of the distal or middle finger joints occur regularly in baseball. Dislocation of the thumb metacarpophalangeal joint is common. The thumb is particularly vulnerable in baseball, and the metacarpophalangeal joint seems predisposed as a frequent site of injury. Fracture of carpus, forearm, and humerus occur occasionally in baseball. Fracture of the femur is infrequent. In knee injuries, ligament tears and meniscal injuries are much less frequent in baseball than in body contact sports, such as football. Tibial fractures are rare. Ankle injuries are 2nd only to hand injuries in the incidence of acute trauma. Moderate to severe ankle sprains are very common, and lateral or medial malleolar and bimalleolar fractures are regular occurrences. These injuries usually occur when one is sliding into a base. A spike of the shoe inadvertently catches in the turf or in the base; thus, the foot stops, while the body proceeds. That is most often the down foot in a lateral, foot first slide, resulting in an external rotation type injury.

baseball injuries. Motor power injuries. Chronic overload is caused by use of a muscle-tendon-bone unit beyond its endurance. Fatigue develops and results in muscle spasm, myositis, ischemia, of muscles, tenosynovitis, adherent tendonitis, attrition of tendons, stress fractures, and spur formation on bones. Acute overload is caused by sudden application of stress to a muscle unit, ranging from a mild tearing of a few muscle fibers to complete disruption of the unit at its weakest point or at the point of greatest stress. That type of injury is inevitable in any vigorous sport. Examples of acute overload injury occurring in baseball are as follows: (1) baseball finger, rupture of the central slip of the extensor mechanism at the middle finger joint; occurring either from a direct blow on the tip of the finger or from a direct blow across the joint. (2) triceps injury, acute strain with a swelling or hemorrhage; may result in myositis and frequently develops in incompletely conditioned pitchers. (3) Complete rupture; may occur in overambitious and undertrained players. (4) Charley horse, or acute, localized, intramuscular hemorrhage; can result either from mild to moderate muscle overload or from contusion from a direct blow. (4) Anterior compartment syndrome, generally found in vigorous early-season conditioning as an acute swelling, edema, and hemorrhage in the unyielding anterior crural compartment, which may occur and can result in necrosis of muscle and occlusion of neurovascular bundles with serious consequences unless relieved. (5) Plantaris tendon rupture, or calcaneal tendon rupture; mainly occurs with sudden spurting of speed, particularly if the athlete is incompletely conditioned or inadequately warmed up. (6) Acute arch strain; frequently occurs in training and early in the season.

baseball injuries (shoulder). The conditions affecting the shoulders of ball players are as follows: (1) Acute bursitis, resulting from trauma, treated by heat and rest. (2) Chronic bursitis; with thickening of the bursa and symptoms of crepitus and local discomfort. (3) Supraspinatus fraying; constant snubbing of the tendon against the greater tuberosity leads to fraying of the deep fibers of the tendon. The symptoms are pain in the region of the tuberosity and the anterior shoulder. (4) Bicipital tendonitis; with pain in the shoulder and tenderness of the bicipital grooves aggravated by flexing the elbow against resistance. Actual crepitus may be felt or a click if the tendon dislocates. (5) Sub-glenoid exostosis; presents a severe pain on throwing with maximal effort leading to an exostosis forming in the region of the attachment of the long head of triceps. The symptoms are local discomfort, tenderness to palpation, and pain referred to the deltoid from irritation of the circumflex nerve.

baseball injuries (soft tissue injuries). Those injuries occur in sliding and are extremely common on the hips, buttocks, and lateral thighs. In spiking injuries, the pivot man on the double play, generally the second baseman or the shortstop, is most vulnerable to this trauma, though any player attempting to make a play on a sliding base runner may be involved.

basketball injuries. The points that are most vulnerable to injury in basketball are the feet, ankles, and knees in the weight-bearing extremities and the fingers, hand, and wrists in the upper extremities. The most frequently observed injuries have been sprains in the ankles. There may be partial or complete tearing of the tibulatalar ligament. That is produced by the sudden inversion in plantar flexion of the foot with external rotation of the tibia on the talus. That injury occurs frequently because of rosin on shoes to assist in quick stops and turns. Sudden motions magnify the forces applied at the ankle joint. In severe injuries the fibulocalcaneal ligament is torn with disruption of the stability in the ankle mortise and subsequent impairment of function. Injuries in the ankles occur more frequently under the boards during the process of rebounding the ball. The next most frequent injury, commonly termed a "jammed finger," is produced by a complete disruption of the musculotendinous bone unit. Usually in a basketball injury there is no complete separation of the tendon. Any of the interphalangeal joints or the metacarpophalangeal joints may be involved. The injury is the result of a compression force caused by the basketball striking the outstretched finger or thumb. Traumatic synovitis develops with swelling, stiffness, and pain. Another injury that frequently occurs is the abrasion or "strawberry," which develops on knees or elbows as the result of falling or skidding on the hardwood floor. Abrasions may develop on any part of the body. Usually they are superficial and present no real problem. In injuries of the knee, the medial semilunar cartilage is most often damaged. In violent, twisting movements, either collateral ligament may be torn. When the force is continued, the semilunar cartilage or the cruciate ligaments may be involved. A "Charley horse" or contusion of the muscle often occurs and usually involves the quadriceps muscle. Muscle fibers are torn by a sharp blow from a blunt object, and a hematoma ensues. When the periosteum is involved, ossificans may develop. Fractures most commonly seen in basketball are those of the small bones of the hands or feet; occasionally they are accompanied by dislocations. At times a player is injured by a cerebral concussion or more serious brain damage.

Bennett fracture. A blow along the axis or dorsum of clenched thumb, elicited from striking with fist, as in boxing. Symptoms may be local pain and disability. Signs are deformity over proximal end of first metacarpal, swelling, tenderness, crepitus, increased motion at joint. Complications may be traumatic arthritis or permanent disability. X ray may show fracture dislocation of distal end of first metacarpal with fracture line extending into the metacarpal joint, large proximal fragment displaced upward and backward, small distal medial fragment remaining in position. Fracture may be incomplete with no displacement of fragment.

beta blockers. An addition to the field of chemical erogenic aids. Because beta blockers reduce the amount of circulating catecholamines, they have been used as sedatives in such areas as shooting and ski jumping (and in the performing arts by musicians and ballet dancers). Although the substances may be of some help in reducing anxiety in some somatic-type stress, there is no real evidence that their use increases performance.

bicycling injuries. In a recent year the number of Americans using bicycles was estimated at 60 million. Anually, 7,000 lives have been lost in pedal cycling accidents, and 120,000 to 15,000 disabling injuries have occurred. In 1971 the estimated total of injuries was placed at 1 million annually, including 120,000 fractures and 60,000 concussions. Nearly three-fourths of the deaths are in the 5-to-14-year-old groups, and 90 percent of those youngsters are boys. The great majority of the deaths are due to collisions with motor vehicles and involve errors on the part of the cyclist, such as failure to yield the right of way, improper turning, etc. In addition to the severe injuries to bicyclists, there are other hazards of cycling. An uncommon overuse injury experienced by bicyclists is "handle bar palsy," a neuropathy secondary to trauma of the deep palmar branch of the ulnar nerve. There is usually weakness and wasting in the intrinsic muscles of the hand without sensory involvement. Cyclists may experience that injury from pressure on handlebars. Riders have complained of the complex features of the bicycles, such as the brakes and gears. Difficulty in controlling those features was directly related to many injuries. There has been reported an increasing incidence of craniofacial trauma related to bicycles with small front wheels, low-set front axles, long narrow seats, and high, wide handlebars. Two types of facial injuries have occurred: fractures of the mandible, usually bilateral, from falls on the chin, and maxillofacial and nasal injuries, usually unilateral, resulting from falls on the side of the face.

blisters. Common nuisances in sports, produced by localized pressure and friction. They are frequently seen on the hands and fingers in bowling, rowing, racket, stick, club, and fencing sports and on the feet in all running sports. Blisters can often be traced to new or poorly fitted shoes, quick stops and turns, sock seams, wrinkled socks. New athletic shoes should be worn for several weeks before use during athletic activity. In addition, taping, protective equipment, heat, and constant sweat within athletics contribute to blister formation. In blister development an accumulation of serum occurs between intradermal layers after friction has separated the layers. Before development, a "hot spot" will be noted at the site of irritation. Without proper care, infection can develop a mild irritation into a distinct disability with serious complications. The associated pain varies with intensity, often inhibiting performance in a given activity by producing a "favoring" away from the irritation, which easily predisposes sprains and strains through changes in normal biomechanics.

blood doping. This is a method used to increase the athlete's hemoglobin and his oxygen-carrying capacity. Blood is withdrawn (up to 3 pints) and stored to be reinfused at a later date. In the interval the athlete responds to the blood loss by providing fresh red cells and in 3 to 4 weeks has restored the loss. The stored blood is then reinfused, thus raising the total hemoglobin level. A certain loss occurs in storage. Transfusion of packed cells raises blood viscosity and may partly embarrass the circulation. There exists the possibility of introduction of infection and of technical mistakes and the confusion of specimens.

blood pressure.   Since the pressure inside the blood vessels varies with the condition of the heart and arteries as well as with other factors, the measurement of blood pressure together with careful interpretation may provide a valuable guide in the evaluation of a person's wellness. The pressure decreases as the blood flows from arteries into capillaries and finally into veins. Ordinarily, measurements are made of arterial pressure only. The instrument used is called a sphygmomanometer. The 2 measurements made are of: (1) the systolic pressure, which occurs during heart muscle contraction and averages around 120, expressed in millimeters of mercury, and (2) the diastolic pressure, which occurs during relaxation of the heart muscle and averages around 80 millimeters of mercury. Chronic lower-than-normal blood pressure is called hypotension. Many apparently healthy persons have systolic blood pressure below 110. The sudden lowering of blood pressure is an important symptom of shock. It may occur also in certain chronic diseases as well as in heart block. Hypertension is high blood pressure, which occurs temporarily as a result of stress, excitement, or exertion. Although importance has been placed on the systolic blood pressure in many cases, the diastolic pressure is the more important. The condition of the small arteries may have more effect on the diastolic pressure. The determination of what constitutes hypertension should be left to a physician, as a blood pressure that is normal for one individual may be low for another and too high for a third. It is difficult to give any hard and fast rules as to what levels of blood pressure might be considered dangerous for participation in any sport. Chronic elevation of blood pressure (say up to 110 diastolic) has been shown statistically to increase the chances of myocardial infarction and stroke by a factor of 2 or 3. Those increased risks are operative all the time and may be accentuated by some forms of exercise. Any sport in which there is powerful prolonged isometric (nonaerobic) exercise, such as weight-lifting and perhaps wrestling, produces marked rises in blood pressure which, if the pressure is already raised, may be undesirable. Sports where temporary loss of mental faculties or physical control because of hypertension could be lethal, such as underwater diving or parachuting, would need to be stricter in criteria than others.

blood transport.   The blood transport of oxygen depends upon the maximum cardiac output, the oxygen-transporting properties of the blood, and the maximum arteriovenous oxygen difference. The effectiveness of a given cardiac output is also influenced by its relative distribution between the active muscles, skin, and viscera. Peak heart rates of 250/min and more may be encountered briefly in such events as skiing, where there is a combination of stress and intense isometric exertion. However, the maximum rate that can be sustained by a young person over several minutes is appreciably lower, averaging 195/min. It may be even less (about 185/min) in well-trained endurance athletes. The resting heart rate of the endurance athlete may be as low as 36 to 42/min. The maximum stroke volume depends on body posture and the type of exercise performed. The large stroke volume of an athlete is achieved without marked changes of myocardial contractility, i.e., the gain of stroke output is achieved at the expense of not only a more complete emptying of the ventricle but also some expansion of the end-diastolic volume. The hemoglobin level of the blood is sometimes low in athletes, thus restricting the potential carriage of oxygen per liter of blood. Increases in circulating haptoglobins suggest that the most important cause of the problem is an enhanced destruction of red cells, either through pressure trauma or secondary to the increased rate of blood flow. The maximum arterio-venous oxygen difference is about 160 ml/l in the endurance athlete, compared with 140/ml/l in a sedentary individual. The difference is due to a rather complete extraction of oxygen from the mixed venous blood of the athlete.

body temperature abnormalities.   Abnormalities of body temperature may be due to exposure to extremes of ambient temperature with which the thermoregulatory mechanisms are unable to cope or to defects in thermal regulation. The popularity of the so-called adventure runs during training for marathons in temperate climates increases the risk of sudden accidental exposure of healthy runners to low temperatures at a time when body cooling may be accelerated by wet clothes and vasodilation and prolonged by lack of access to shelter. The clinical manifestations of "hypothermia" need to be recognized because of deterioration in judgment and strength of the exposed person, which occurs with great rapidity and may lead to death if preventive measures are not rapidly instituted. With rectal temperatures below 30.2°C, clouding of consciousness and sometimes a restless stupor occur. Slurring of speech, ataxia, and involuntary movements are common. Pallor, cyanosis and edema of the skin of the face, slow cerebration, and a croaky voice may suggest the presence of hypothyroidism. The pupils are abnormally dilated or may be pinpoint and react sluggishly to light. Muscle tone is increased, and the individual may show a generalized rigidity and neck stiffness. Shivering is characteristically absent at this stage. During hypothermia, deep tendon reflexes are sluggish, and delayed relaxation of the ankle jerk, like that seen in myxedema, has been observed. The most common cardiovascular abnormalities are hypotension without compensatory tachycardia, slow arterial fibrillation, or sinus bradycardia. The increasing participation in outdoor activities has lead to recognition that many deaths that are attributed to "exposure" are most likely due to hypothermia. Victims often wear unsuitable clothing, lacking windproof outer garments. Such clothing, when wet, in many cases may provide less insulation than that ordinarily worn in cities on warm sunny days. Many accident victims are also handicapped in the maintenance of body temperature by self-administered or prescribed medication. Hypothermia, once it occurs, can lead to loss of circulatory reflexes with orthostatic hypotension. Clinically, hypothermia is thought to be present if the central body temperature is below 35°C. Between that level and down to 32.2°C, normal thermoregulatory activity occurs and, provided consciousness is not impaired or other physical disability supervenes, that does not interfere with appropriate exercise and behavioral efforts at temperature conservation, which are usually successful in restoring body temperature to normal.

body temperature, normal.   The normal temperature range, as obtained by the usual thermometers, may extend from 97° to 100°F. Temperature of the body varies with the time of day. Usually it is lower in the early morning, since the muscles have been relaxed and no food has been taken for several hours. Temperature usually is higher in late afternoon and evening because one has been physically active and has had food. Normal temperature also varies with the part of the body. Skin temperature, as obtained in the armpit (axilla), is lower than mouth temperature. If it were possible to place a thermometer inside the liver, it is believed that it would register a degree or more higher than the rectal temperature. The temperature within a muscle might be even higher.

body temperature regulation.   Normal body temperature maintenance depends upon a balance between heat production from activity and gain or loss from the environment. That involves many organ systems including a neural regulatory mechanism within the hypothalamus. Heat in that instance is infrared energy, and there are 3 main mechanisms of losing heat to the environment to keep body temperature down. The 1st is radiation, a direct loss to the environment, which accounts for 66 percent of heat loss when one is at rest. Convection relies upon air movement to carry heat away and accounts for approximately 15 percent of heat loss when one is resting. The remaining 19 percent is lost via evaporation through the lungs and skin. As environmental temperature rises to near body temperature, heat loss by radiation and convection decreases and evaporative cooling is relied upon. Evaporative cooling is less effective when environmental relative humidity increases. Strenuous physical activity or even passive existence in extremes of heat generated by muscular activity may exceed the body's cooling capacity. Evaporative cooling depends upon the temperature, movement, and humidity of surrounding air and clothing permeability. Sweat cools only if it evaporates; sweat wiped or dripped from the body carries with it little heat, while accounting for a significant fluid loss, which may compound the problem. The cooling capacity of sweating is, therefore, dependent upon atmospheric humidity and pressure. Cutaneous abnormalities, ichthyosis, ectodermal dysplasia, scarring from burns, and scleroderma interfere with sweating and predispose to heat stroke. Restrictive or excessive clothing may interfere with evaporation and impede heat loss. Atropine, scopolamine, probanthine, cogentin, and certain major tranquilizers and general anesthetics may also inhibit sweating.

bone. The hardest substance in the body, composed of inorganic calcium salts and organic materials. Bones are living organisms, which not only form the skeleton but also have the function of supporting various vital organs, producing blood cells, and storing and releasing minerals to various parts of the body, etc. Bone is composed of 2 components. The bone matrix is a protein substance upon which calcium salts are deposited to form the bone. The other component is an intercellular substance, which fills the microscopic spaces within the hardened calcium and acts as a sort of cement to hold the entire structure together. In addition to being formed of 2 components, bone also has 2 basic characteristics, which might be called "hard" and "soft." The deep interior or core of any bone is relatively soft when compared with the exterior, which is hard. The soft interior is known as the cancellous portion of the bone, while the hard exterior is known as the cortical portion. The proportion of hardness and softness varies among the bones of the body. The large structural bones tend to have a greater degree of hardness, whereas certain smaller bones (the bones of the spinal column, for instance) tend to be on the softer side. The bones of the body are alive, and portions of the body's bones are constantly dissolving, and new bone is being produced to replace it. There are 2 major types of bone, flat and long. Additionally there is 1 specialized type of bone, the sesamoid, which is found within the tendon. A good example of the latter is the patella, situated within the quadriceps patellar tendon mechanism. Bones of the skeleton come into contact with one another at joints, where they are moved by the action of muscles. The skeleton thus is a rigid framework for the attachment of muscles and protection of organs and flexible framework to allow the parts of the body to move by muscular contraction. The skeletal framework allows an erect posture against the pull of gravity and gives recognizable form to the body. Bones are just as much living tissue as muscle and skin. A rich blood supply constantly provides the oxygen and nutrients bones need. Each bone also has an extensive nerve supply primarily from the periosteum. Each bone is composed of a protein framework that allows it growth and remodeling. Calcium and phosphorus are deposited into that framework to make the bone hard and strong. The processes of bone growth and fracture healing have several things in common. When a bone is broken, a hematoma forms around the broken ends. The hematoma organizes into soft callus, which functions as the cartilage model. The soft callus becomes impregnated with calcium and other minerals, increasing in hardness; the hard callus gradually becomes bone, producing union.

bone deformation, plastic. Healthy growing bone has the ability to bend rather than break when stressful forces are applied. Failure may be microscopic and within the bone and thus not evident as a gross fracture, because a definite fracture line may not be evident as a gross fracture. Because a definite fracture line may not be evident on X ray, the condition may be overlooked. That process is termed plastic deformation of bone. If the bending of the bone is unrecognized, it can become a permanent deformity with loss of function. If plastic deformation is recognized early, it can be corrected.

bone fracture. A rupture of living connective tissue, whose repair is achieved by cellular growth, the same as repair in all living tissues. The time taken for union of a fracture depends on a great number of variable factors. Small bones, such as the metatarsals or metacarpals, can be united in about 4 weeks, as there is seldom any displacement. When it comes to fractures of the larger weight-bearing bones, such as the tibia or the femur, then it is difficult to forecast a specific time. Simple spiral fractures, where there is a large area of bone contact between the fragments, will unite rapidly and without much trouble. Where the fracture is transverse, comminuted, displaced, or complicated by damage to the overlying skin, to nerves, or to blood vessels, it may be impossible to give an approximate estimate. Such fractures seen in sporting activities are usually due to the application of violence to the injured limb. The violence can be direct, where the force causing the break is applied directly to the limb. It can be indirect, where the force causing the break is not applied directly to the injured bone but at a distance. A fall on the outstretched hand may break the forearm, the head of the radius, or the collarbone by transmitted force. The nature of the force can determine the type of injury. Fractures caused by direct violence may be comminuted or displaced by the force applied, or the overlying tissues may be traumatized or even breached, exposing the fractured bones. When a fracture is exposed to the external environment by a wound of the skin and tissues overlying it, the fracture is said to be compound. Such a fracture is liable to be contaminated by dirt and debris and subsequently becomes infected. When the skin overlying a fracture is intact, it is said to be simple.

bone fracture, greenstick. Bending forces applied to a bone at each end are concentrated as a tension force in the diaphysis. When that occurs rapidly and with sufficient force in adult bone, there is a complete fracture. In younger persons, with growing diaphysis, there may be only an apparent partial fracture, with some of the cortex remaining intact on the compressive side. That results in a greenstick fracture, so named because of its similarity to the partial disruption that occurs in a growing tree branch. Greenstick fractures are usually obvious because of an accompanying deformity. The fractured bone cortex is open, which allows hemorrhage into the adjacent soft tissues and further increases the pain and deformity. The greenstick fracture has an inherent "springiness," that is, a tendency to return to the deformed position if the pressure of the corrective force is released.

bone fracture, torus. When a longitudinal force is applied along the shaft of the bone, it may be dissipated and concentrated at the distal end, or metaphysis. That longitudinal compressive force results in the outward buckling of the new, thin cortex of the metaphysis. That bulge in the bone gives it the appearance of the base of a Roman column, and because of this columnlike protuberance, it is called a "torus" fracture, derived from the Latin word *torus,* meaning "protuberance." The most common torus fracture is of the distal radius. A torus fracture frequently is overlooked and dismissed as a simple sprain because of minimal symptoms, lack of deformity, and juxtaposition to a major point. Symptoms are minimal because the cortex remains intact and there is little bleeding from the fracture site into soft tissues. Such a fracture rarely produces a significant deformity and heals rapidly.

bone, growing. Bones must grow not only in width but also in length. Bony tissue, the majority of the tissue for such bones as the humerus and femur, is a rigid tissue that cannot expand within its matrix. The growth of bony tissue must take place on its surface. Surface growth can easily occur on the sides of the bones, increasing their width. However, the ends of the bones usually are covered with articular cartilage, and surface growth in length cannot occur here. For a bone to grow in length, there must be a tissue that can grow by expansion of its matrix, such as cartilage. Growth is accompanied by remodeling and maturation, which further alters the structure of the bone. A typical growing bone can be divided into 4 areas. Each has its unique biomechanical characteristics and reacts differently to stress. The end of the bone is called the epiphysis, containing the articular surface composed of cartilage. That surface grows in a hemispherical manner, increasing not only in width but also in length. The majority of joint ligaments attach here. Linear growth of the bone occurs in the physis or epiphyseal plate. The epiphyseal plate is composed of cartilage with a matrix that can expand. The cartilage is stimulated to grow primarily by growth hormone; that stimulus decreases at sexual maturity. The epiphyseal plate cartilage is replaced by bone through a process called endochondral ossification. The blood supply to the growing cells in the epiphyseal plate enters through the epiphysis itself. The cartilage in the epiphyseal plate allows expansion and growth, but its biomechanical characteristics are such that it is less resistant than bony tissue to tensile and sheer force. Remodeling of the initial growth process occurs in the metaphysis. The central and most mature part of the bone is the diaphysis. The area has achieved maximum strength and is usually a rigid cylinder in form. Bone growth on the outer surface of the cortex, coupled with remodeling on the inner cortex, allows the bone to increase in width. The cortex is usually thickest in the diaphysis. That area has the most resistance to stress.

bone, pathologic fractures. Growing bones may have areas in which there was a defect in development. That imperfection, either a nest of fiber cells or a fluid-filled cyst, serves as a weak point that can fail with relatively minor trauma. Stress as minimal as that involved in throwing a baseball can result in a fracture. An injury out of proportion to the violence of the force applied should be promptly checked for a pathologic condition; i.e., a malignant bone tumor may first become evident because of a pathologic fracture.

bone, stress fractures. The result of repetitive stresses concentrated at a specific area of the bone. They are usually the result of "patterned motion," the same motion repeated over and over at a specific site, resulting in a gradual failure of the bone. Stress fractures are usually manifested by local pain accentuated by participation in the inciting activity and relieved by rest. The 1st signs appear on X rays 2 to 3 weeks after the initial symptoms and are seen as periosteal new bone formation. That is a result of the small hemorrhages beneath the periosteum that lift it away from the bone and stimulate callus formation. Stress fractures usually occur at the beginning of a training period and are associated with some type of repetitive activity. Failure to recognize a stress fracture and stop the inciting activity can result in the development of a complete fracture. A complete fracture in the femoral neck can be very serious. Stress fractures are seen at a variety of sites, but they are most common in the tibia, fibula, metatarsals, and calcaneus. Fatigue fracture of the fibula is seen in soccer players and affects the lower 3rd of the bone, where torsional strain is applied when one turns rapidly. Ballet dancers and runners may also develop such fractures in the tibia.

boutonniere deformity (buttonhole deformity). Trauma to the dorsal aspect of the middle phalanx of finger, excessive forcible flexion of proximal interphalangeal joint. Symptoms are local pain and disability. Signs are flexion deformity of proximal interphalangeal joint with inability of extension, local tenderness, swelling.

bowler's hip. Pain and inflammation that seem to be centered deep inside the hip. It gets its name because it is so frequently found among bowlers, but it can occur quite easily in any sport that includes extensive and recurrent hip extension coupled with twisting motions of the lower back. Bowler's hip is an inflammation of the iliopsoas tendon and its bursae, where they attach the iliopsoas muscle to the lesser trochanter, which is on the inner part of the femur just below the hip joint. The basic bowling motion is a long, forward stride in which the leg opposite the bowling arm is suddenly extended, with the hip and knee sharply flexed, as the ball is released. That motion, when performed again and again, tends to fatigue the iliopsoas muscle, especially when the movement ends with a twisting of the back. As the abductor muscles convey applied stresses to their tendons, the tired and recurrently overstrained iliopsoas passes the stress to its connecting tissues at the femur and progressive pain and inflammation result. It is not a serious ailment but is annoying for the chronic pain it produces deep in the hip during athletic activities that require such hip extension.

bowler's thumb.　Injury almost always limited to bowlers. They grip quite heavy balls between the thumb and first 2 fingers, all of which are inserted into holes made for that purpose. Most bowlers like to put a little "English" on the ball as they release it. In many cases it is necessary in order for the ball to strike the pins at a desirable angle rather than straight on. Putting English on the ball means inwardly twisting or pronating the wrist as the ball is released. In bowling, because the thumb is imprisoned in the ball's thumbhole until release, that natural thumb flexion is prevented. As the ball is released, the 2 fingers begin to slip out of their holes but the thumb stays in its hole until the last possible moment so as to maintain control over the ball's spin. When the ball is finally released, the wrist is in extreme pronation. Free of the thumbhole, the thumb, which has been straining to remain in extension while it was in the hole, suddenly and belatedly flexes in toward the palm. That flexion occurs later than it would if the individual was pronating the wrist without gripping the base. The repeated abduction and extension strain, followed by the sudden adduction and flexion of the thumb, tends to fatigue the muscles around it aiding in those motions. That fatigue is transferred to the connecting tendons, especially to those of the opponent muscle at the thumb's base, and inflammation, often becoming chronic, follows.

boxer's knuckles.　Soft-tissue injuries to the knuckle are fairly common, especially in boxers. The condition is often described as boxer's knuckle when in fact it may be more than 1 pathology. A traumatic bursa may form over the metacarpal head, which can become chronically inflamed. The other form is distraction of the intermetacarpal ligament. That can be a source of quite considerable deformity. The habit of bandaging the hands before a bout (where the tapes are applied to the outstretched extended hand around the base of the fingers) leads to the condition. In extension, the intermetacarpal ligaments are relatively slack, allowing abduction of the fingers. As the hand goes into flexion, the slack is taken up in bringing the fingers into apposition. Any material inserted between the fingers will, under such circumstances, tend to cause distraction of the intermetacarpal ligaments.

boxing injuries.　The most common boxing injuries are as follows: (1) nose bleeding; (2) deflected septum, a cartilage injury that is relatively common and may cause considerable nasal obstruction; (3) abrasion, common on the face and skull; (4) laceration, which occurs in many fights; (5) hematoma, the common "black eye"; (6) concussion, usually caused by a direct blow to the jaw, an accumulation of the effects of blows to the head, or by the head striking the floor of the ring; most boxers regain consciousness by the count of 10 and can be assisted to their corners; (7) fractures and sprains, the most common being that of the index metacarpal. Fracture of the shaft usually occurs within the proximal third of the bone. The Bennett type of fracture, at the base of the thumb metacarpal, involves a crude dislocation of the carpometacarpal joint. The most common joint to be damaged is the thumb metacarpal joint. There may be extensive damage to the capsule with possible rupture of a collateral ligament, or a chip of bone may be avulsed. The more common and more serious injuries are cuts in the skin around the eyes. Deep cuts are usually opened in the first instance by a blow from the opponent's head, but in later bouts the damaged area may be split by a punch. Ribs are frequently bruised, sometimes fractures by body punching, and occasionally a rib may be separated at the costo-sternal junction. The hazards greatest to the professional boxer or to the athlete with a prolonged career are the injuries centered around the head. The "punch-drunk" syndrome has been observed most often in fighters of the sluggish type, who are usually poor boxers and take considerable punishment in seeking a knockout blow. It is also found common in 2nd-rate fighters used for training purposes. The early symptoms are mental confusion and slight unsteadiness of gait. Progressively, the individual may develop leg dragging, hesitant speech, hand tremors, head noddings, expressionless facial characteristics of parkinsonism, vertigo, deafness, and finally marked mental deterioration. It has been estimated that nearly 50 percent of veteran fighters develop some form of the condition. One study indicated that 60 percent of the fighters studied, working 5 years or more, became punch-drunk or developed mental and emotional changes that were obvious to those who knew them personally. Following a knockout blow, the head (brain) may be more seriously damaged by a 2nd injury as it strikes the floor of the ring.

brain injury. In any head injury it is the brain damage that matters most. It is well recognized that a fatal brain injury may occur without blemish to the scalp or a skull fracture. The simplest form of brain injury is concussion, the essential feature of which is its reversibility, with complete recovery usually occurring within a few seconds or minutes. Electroencephalogram studies have confirmed that most changes in rhythm do not persist for more than 4 minutes. In more severe cases there may be brain laceration or contusion, particularly if the skull is fractured. Secondary complicating factors, such as hemorrhage, cerebral edema, and late infection, may ensure. Since cerebral edema is aggravated by a fall in oxygen level, a good airway must always be preserved in unconscious persons. There is usually a loss of consciousness, and confusion, irritability, headache, nausea, vomiting, photophobia, and double vision are often present. Serious signs are increasing confusion, dilated or irregular pupils, rapid and feeble pulse, rapid respiration, weakness and sensory disturbances in the limbs, including ataxia. Skull fractures are classified as simple or compound, linear, comminuted, or depressed. Usually a boggy swelling is found over the fracture. Blows to the nasal or frontal region may injure the delicate cribriform plate with resulting rhinorrhea. A black eye appearing some hours later with little or no damage to the skin around the eye and with a flame-shaped subconjunctival hemorrhage indicates a fractured anterior fossa. Blood in the ear that does not clot because of admixture with cerebrospinal fluid indicates a middle or posterior fossa fracture.

brain syndrome, chronic (punch-drunk syndrome, chronic cerebral injury). Presumably, repeated head trauma (as in boxing) that leads to a form of chronic neurophysiological disorder characterized by emotional and/or mental impairment and/or motor deficit. Symptoms are mental confusion, tinnitus, giddiness, euphoria, and personality changes. Signs are gradual and progressive onset, which may be associated with confabulation hallucinations, lack of associated movements, unsteadiness in gait, or masked facial expression.

breast injuries. In the female athlete running and running games cause the breast to suffer in 2 ways. (1) Severe chafing of the nipple may produce severe soreness and is common in joggers and called "jogger's nipple." (2) "Bouncing breast syndrome," also produced by running and running games. It can produce severe breast pain owing to an inflammatory response of the suspensory ligaments and may go on to an interstitial form of mastitis. Both problems are obviated by wearing a well-fitting supporting brassiere.

bronchitis. An infection of the major air passages to the lungs. It is rarely disabling but can progress to pneumonia. The disease frequently comes on during or after a cold, causing the disorder to be called a "chest cold" or "cold in the chest." However, a cold is a viral infection. Although the trachea and bronchi may be infected by the same virus, bronchitis is usually a bacterial infection that supervenes during the viral infection. Bronchitis can also occur without a preceding viral infection. The predominant symptoms of bronchitis are a persistent, irritating cough that may be dry but frequently becomes productive after 1 or 2 days. The sputum is usually green or yellow and is thick and tenacious. Slight pain may be associated with the coughing, and the individual may notice early fatigability. However, one usually does not appear severely ill and has only a slight fever or none at all. If the infection involves the larynx (voice box), he or she may be hoarse. A few wheezes and rales may be heard throughout the chest, but they tend to disappear with coughing.

bronchial asthma. A disease characterized by increased responsiveness of the trachea and bronchi to various stimuli, manifested by a widespread narrowing of the airways that changes in severity either spontaneously or as a result of therapy. Individuals exhibit episodes of shortness of breath and wheezing and symptoms-free intervals. The development of asthma is influenced by many factors, including genetic elements, infections, stress, and exercise. Those stimuli produce bronchospasm and increased mucus production. Sensitivity of the airways to those factors varies day to day.

bronchitis, chronic. A disease that is a chronic or recurring productive cough. Pathological abnormalities can be found in individuals without cough or sputum. Those abnormalities include: hypertrophy of mucous glands, hypersecretion of mucus and ulceration and damage of structures within the bronchial and bronchiolar walls as well as scarring of those walls. At times total obliteration and destruction of small air passages occur. Damage to the surface epithelium of the large bronchi is more common than damage to the deeper part of the bronchial wall. Damaged surface epithelium is replaced by metaplastic squamous epithelium, and at times bronchial polyps are found. Recurrent infection is common, resulting from bacterial proliferation in mucus. Bacteria growing in intraluminal mucus attract white blood cells, which migrate between bronchial epithelial cells and produce pus. With infection, cellular mucus is transformed into yellow or green mucopus. The structural abnormalities resulting from bronchitis may be local or scattered. Scarring develops in small bronchi, and narrowing occurs, leading to airways obstruction. In addition to undergoing scar formation, bronchioles are weakened and dilate, and some are totally destroyed. Severe damage in the bronchioles accompanied by peribronchiolar extension of infection may lead to damage of the microcirculation of the bronchial and pulmonary arterial systems and eventually to the development of pulmonary emphysema.

bunions. Abnormal enlargements in the heads of the metatarsal bones, where they meet the phalanges of the toes. A bunion is actually an abnormality at the metatarsal head. It usually occurs at the big toe but may also develop in the little toe as well. Through constant strain at those sites, because of either fallen-arch pressure or too tight shoes, the heads of the metatarsal bones become enlarged. In the joint of the big toes, that expansion eventually produces a bone spur, which grows over the inner aspect of the metatarsal head. Simultaneously, the big toe itself deviates outward, often pushing the adjoining toe upward. A bursa is formed around the bony spur, and if excessive pressure from tight shoes is applied, it becomes inflamed, swollen, and very painful. The bunion of the little toe, often called a "bunionette" comes about in a similar manner.

burnout syndrome. A stress syndrome occurring in both athletes and their trainers. Symptoms include feelings of guilt about taking time off from work, also anxiety, depression, sleeplessness, sexual dysfunction, general fatigue.

burns. In sports car racing many accidents occur in which there are all types of burns. The severity of a burn depends upon the size of the area it covers, the depth to which it extends, and its location on the body. Few individuals survive burns involving more than 50 percent of the body surface. In contrast, few burns covering less than 20 percent of the body prove fatal if given proper care. Burns of the face and neck, hands, armpits, and crotch are frequently more incapacitating because specialized organs and complex anatomical structures are involved or the areas are difficult to keep clean. Burns are classified as 1st-, 2nd-, or 3rd-degree according to the depth to which damage extends. First-degree burns are superficial, do not kill any of the tissues, and produce only redness of the skin. Second-degree burns cause death of the upper portion of the skin, resulting in blisters. Third-degree burns produce death of the full thickness of the skin and may extend deeply into the underlying tissues. Such burns, if more than 1 inch in diameter, do not heal unless covered by skin grafts and can produce extensive deforming scars.

bursitis. An inflammatory reaction within a bursa, which may vary in degree from a very mild irritative synovitis with discomfort to suppurative bursitis with actual abscess formation. A bursa is specifically designed to facilitate motion between continuous layers of the body, and the athlete with his violence of motion is particularly prone to bursal injury resulting from repetitive movement that causes tissue friction or from direct blow. Athlete bursitis can usually be classified as acute or chronic, usually caused by trauma. Acute traumatic bursitis occurs in those bursae subject to direct injury. A typical example is prepatellar bursitis, where the bursal sac becomes distended, often with a blood effusion. Chronic traumatic bursitis is caused by repeated insults to the bursa, the bursal wall becomes thickened, and the sac volume increases so that the bursa extends far beyond its usual confines. Acute bursitis with infection is seen in the athlete who sustains a penetrating injury. The prepatellar bursa lies anteriorly between the skin and the outer surface of the patella. That location makes it particularly susceptible to direct trauma. In acute prepatellar bursitis there is a tender, erythematous area of swelling over the patella; with knee flexion, increased skin tension directly over the bursa produces pain. Direct pressure over the bursa is also painful. The deep infrapatellar bursa is positioned beneath and behind the patellar tendon and in front of the infrapatellar fat pad that lies on the anterior surface of the tibia. Those neighboring structures make direct injury to the bursa difficult. Infrapatellar bursitis may be an overuse syndrome caused by friction between the patellar tendon and bone. The superficial infrapatellar bursa rests between the skin, and the anterior surface of the infrapatellar tendon, when inflamed because of direct trauma, may be clinically indistinguishable from Osgood-Schlatter disease. The bursa anterior to the Achilles tendon at the heel or the one in the region of the attachment of the Achilles tendon to the os calcis can become inflamed. The athlete complains of pain in that area. Frequently there is swelling. Examination reveals tenderness in the heel distal or anterior to the insertion of the Achilles tendon, depending on which

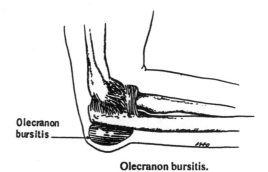

Olecranon bursitis.
Olecranon bursitis.

bursa is inflamed. There may be a fluctuant mass, indicating fluid within the bursal space. Falling on, or being hit upon, the greater trochanter of the femur may cause inflammation of the greater trochanteric bursa. Such an injury is followed by pain and occasionally by swelling. There are many bursae around the knee, all of which are prone to inflammation, either following direct trauma or through overuse. The bursa becomes swollen to protect contiguous moving parts. The athlete complains of pain in one of the areas of the bursa. Examination reveals localized tenderness and usually swelling.

C

calcaneus fracture, margin avulsion. Forced plantarflexion of foot. Symptoms are local pain and disability. Signs are tenderness and swelling localized over the lateral aspect of foot near the calcaneocuboid joint, pain elicited on plantarflexion, and forced eversion of foot. Complication may be persistent disability.

calcaneus fracture, sustentaculum tali. Forced eversion of foot. Symptoms are sharp pain on inner side of foot, moderate disability. Signs produced by motions at ankle are relatively asymptomatic and unimpaired; variable amount of swelling over inner surface of calcaneus appears to be slightly displaced outward; foot tends to be held in pronation. Complication may be painful flatfoot.

calcaneus fracture, tuberosity avulsion. Sudden violent strain on Achilles tendon, as in fall upon ball of foot, or from muscular action, as in jumping. Symptoms are pain, inability to bear weight, and some disability. Signs are swelling and tenderness around calcaneal tuberosity and posterior to malleoli on either side of Achilles tendon, no swelling or tenderness in anterior portion of foot, separated fragment palpable in space between Achilles tendon and posterior surface of tibia, pain elicited by plantarflexion of foot against resistance.

calcific tendinitis. Deposits of calcium in the form of calcium apatite are quite often observed in the tendons of the rotator cuff of the glenohumeral joint but may also be seen in other sites, such as the common extensor origin at the elbow. The abrupt deposition of those salts is accompanied by an acute inflammatory reaction in the capsule and synovial membrane of the joint and causes intense pain, muscle spasm, and limitation of joint movement. Deposits may also slowly accumulate over a period of years, presumably in areas of degenerate tendon, and cause little or no discomfort. It is not unusual for acute calcific tendonitis to be spontaneously relieved by the deposit of calcareous material rupturing into the joint cavity of subacromial bursae.

calf sprain. Sudden violent stress, as in body weight forcibly throwing foot into extreme dorsiflexion; excessive forcible use in poorly conditioned person. Symptoms are severe pain in deep muscle, especially on dorsiflexion of foot, and disability. Signs are graded by degree of severity: inability to walk on tiptoe; possible palpable defect; swelling, edema, tenderness localized; ecchymosis; muscle spasm; diffuse inflammation; active contraction eliciting bunching instead of flattening. Complications are proneness to recurrence, thrombophlebitis, and prolonged disability.

callosities. Localized areas of hyperplasia of the horny layer of the epidermis as a result of pressure and friction. Plantar callosities, probably more than any other type, can become disabling in track when they produce a subcallus blister. Divers also present some special problems from board friction because the constant immersion in pool water and showers leaches natural skin oils from the keratinized plaque. That causes the area to dry, crack, and split, often to the degree of bleeding and secondary infection. Callus formation is nature's response to chronic irritation. Once a callus becomes thick, it in itself can become a chronic irritant (as a keratinized plaque) and produce a subcallus blister in the deeper tissues. Once it develops, treatment is the same as that for a superficial blister, but callosities can be prevented by having the player periodically use a fine emery board to prevent undue callus buildup.

calluses. A chronic injury, which usually occurs on the feet and may also be seen on the hands, is callus from repeated minor stresses. A callosity is an area of thickened skin overlying a bony prominence. The presence of a callus usually indicates abnormal pressure between a shoe and a bony protrusion. In that condition the MP joint is hyperextended, pushing the head of the metatarsal into the sole of the foot. Abnormal pressure can develop under the metatarsal head or at the flexed IP joint of the corresponding toe. Common areas for callosities are beneath the metatarsal heads, on the lateral border of the foot at the 5th metatarsal head, on the medial border of the foot at the 1st metatarsal head, and along the medial border of the great toe. Further investigation usually reveals either an abnormal bony prominence or some anatomical variance, such as a hammer toe or a bunion.

canal collapse (ear). Owing to relaxation of soft-tissue support, the medial end of the chondral cartilage may drop forward to narrow the lateral end of the external canal. The resulting slit can easily be opened with a speculum, but normal cerumen passage is inhibited, leading to infection and possible otitis externa.

canoeing, rowing and sailing injuries. Muscular strains and injuries are quite common to the abdomen, back, and arms. Shoulder pericapsulitis and painful arc syndrome owing to supraspinatus tendinitis and bicipital tendinitis occur. Wrist tenosynovitis of the dorsal extensor or De Quervains types occur. Skin abrasions and blisters are common. Hazards are encountered from the waters in which rowing takes place, especially if they are polluted. Infection with bacteria and with other organisms such as schistosoma can occur in some countries. Injuries, particularly to the hands and fingers, may be inflicted by rope handling, sail handling, and by various bits of apparatus, such as winches and winch handles. A life jacket should always be used in case of head injury combined with falling into the water; otherwise drowning will inevitably follow.

capillaries. Blood is distributed by arterioles to capillaries. Those vessels have very thin walls of flat pavement or squamous-type endothelium. Through the thin walls, the sole purpose of the circulatory system is achieved, i.e., only from capillaries can blood give up food and oxygen to the tissues and take in carbon dioxide, waste, and other products. The capillary walls are semipermeable. They allow small molecules in solution (such as glucose, amino acids, fatty acids, glycerol, minerals, vitamins, and urea) to pass through it. Large molecules, such as plasma proteins, cannot pass through in significant amounts. Blood is delivered to the capillaries under hydrostatic pressure. That is a force tending to push water and solutes through the capillary wall into the tissue fluids.

capsular injuries. Injury of a sheath enclosure around an organ or structure. A sudden unexpected force, either in the normal plane of movement or acting in an abnormal plane, can result in capsular tears. At the same time damage to the synovial membrane can occur. Tearing of the fibers of the capsule leads to hemorrhage and tenderness locally, whereas damage to the synovium leads to an effusion in the joint and sometimes hemarthrosis. Provided the stability of the joint is retained, those lesions respond very well to measures indicated in the general outlines of treatment, such as ice, pressure, muscle reeducation, and, after initial rest, a graduated exercise program.

carbohydrates. Carbohydrates are composed of 3 elements (carbon, hydrogen, and oxygen) arranged into molecules each containing 6 carbon atoms, called sugars. Slight changes in the arrangement of the atoms of the sugar molecules produce a variety of different sugars. Among the common ones are glucose, fructose, and galactose. Glucose is the sugar the body metabolizes directly as an energy source. Other sugars must be converted to glucose in the liver before the body can use them. Carbohydrates are often divided into 2 main classes, simple and complex. Simple carbohydrates or sugars include the single-sugar molecules like glucose or 2 sugar molecules hooked together, such as honey or table sugar. Complex carbohydrates are formed when many sugar molecules are joined together. Grains, fruits, and many vegetables are good sources. Unlike simple carbohydrates, the food sources of complex carbohydrates are excellent sources of vitamins, minerals, and fiber; their calories are not "empty." Simple carbohydrates are rapidly absorbed from the gastrointestinal tract and induce vigorous production of insulin by the pancreas. If too much simple sugar is consumed, the finely tuned insulin mechanisms may be overwhelmed. High blood sugar levels or even diabetes conditions may result. Sometimes the opposite happens; too much insulin is produced, and the blood sugar falls too low, a condition called hypoglycemia. Complex carbohydrates, absorbed much more slowly, are better handled by the body. Glycogen, the storage form of carbohydrate found in muscle and liver cells, is a series of glucose molecules hooked closely together. When glucose is needed, glycogen is broken down to supply it. Adequate stores of glycogen are those vitally necessary for muscular activity and normal function of the organs.

cardiac cycle. The cardiac cycle is the sequence of events in the heart during 1 heartbeat. When the heart is resting (in diastole), the valves between each auricle and ventricle (the auriculoventricular (AV) valves) and those guarding the entrance to the aorta (the aortic valves) and the pulmonary artery (the pulmonary valve) are closed. Venous blood slowly drains from the upper part of the body (from the head and neck region), via the superior vena cava into the right auricle, and from the lower part of the body, trunk, and limbs, via the inferior vena cava, into the right auricle. At the same time the left auricle is filling with freshly oxygenated blood draining back to it from the lungs via the pulmonary veins. The pressure gradually rises in the 2 auricles. A point comes in the cycle when the pressure in the auricles is greater than that in the ventricles and the AV valves are pushed open. The ventricles now begin filling with blood. About this time systole commences. The walls of the auricle begin to contract. That serves to push most of the remaining contents down into the ventricles. They are still relaxed, though now "overfilled" and stretched. Ventricular systole can now begin. As the ventricular muscle contracts, a moment comes in the cycle when the pressure in the ventricle is greater than that in the auricle and the AV valves are snapped shut. Because of the "guy-ropes," the chordae tendineae attached by papillary muscles to the wall of the ventricles, the walls cannot be everted, or pushed inside out. The ventricles are now closed cavities; all valves are shut. Since the ventricular walls are still contracting, pressure within the 2 ventricles continues to rise. A moment is reached when the pressure in the left ventricle is greater than that in the aorta, and the pressure in the right ventricle is greater than that in the aorta, and the pressure in the right ventricle is greater than that of the pulmonary artery. The semilunar valves (guarding the entrance to those vessels) are thrust open, and blood is forcibly ejected into them, to the systemic circulation from the left ventricle and to the pulmonary circulation from the right ventricle. The ventricles now relax, and the heart goes into its resting phase, diastole. The total cycle of events takes about 8 seconds when the heart is beating at a rate of 75 times per minute.

cardiac dyspnea. Undue shortness of breath with exercise caused by heart disease. It may occasionally occur at night and awaken the individual with a sense of suffocation, causing him or her to sit up or move out into fresh air to obtain relief. Examination usually discloses a rapid heart rate, rapid respiration, and anxiety. Auscultation of the chest may reveal rales or crackling sounds indicating the presence of fluid in the lungs.

cardiac enlargement. Some degree of cardiac enlargement, with displacement of the apex beat of the heart beyond the midclavicular line, is common in athletes and is a result of physiological hypertrophy. It is common to feel a "left ventricular impulse" consistent with the large stroke volume consequent of a slow heart rate. However, anything more than moderate hypertrophy and any evidence of right ventricular hypertrophy would need a medical specialist's opinion.

cardiac hypertrophy. In contrast to skeletal muscles, cardiac muscle does not have an adaptive increase in respiratory capacity in response to endurance training. The heart, like the skeletal muscle, also hypertrophies in response to strenuous endurance exercise, so that endurance-trained athletes have heavier (larger) hearts than do sedentary controls of similar body weight. An echocardiographic study of college swimmers, runners, wrestlers, and controls showed that swimmers and runners had statistically significantly larger left ventricular internal dimensions and volumes. The swimmers, runners, and wrestlers had statistically significantly increased left ventricular masses, but only the wrestlers had an increase in wall thickness. Those results show that endurance (isotonic) athletes develop cardiac hypertrophy of a volume-load type in contrast to isometric athletes (wrestlers), who develop hypertrophy of a pressure-overload type. The increase in left ventricular size is important in the development of increased work capacity because there is good correlation between heart size and maximal cardiac output.

cardiac output. About 5,000 ml blood per minute leaves the right ventricle to pass through the lungs; the left ventricle thrusts the same volume of blood into the systemic circulation. At the heart rate of 72 beats per minute, that means each ventricle ejects about 70 ml blood per beat. In exercise the cardiac output can be increased up to 30 liters per minute. That is achieved partly by an increase in heart rate and partly by an increase in stroke volume, i.e., in the amount ejected with 1 "beat." The increased venous return stretches cardiac muscle. The greater the degree of stretch, the more forcibly does the heart muscle contract in the next systole. The stroke volume, therefore, increases. In addition, stimulation of the stretch receptors in the great veins leads to reflex quickening of the heart rate. In any 1 cardiac cycle, the same volume of blood must leave the left ventricle for the systemic circulation as leaves the right ventricle for the pulmonary artery. A moment's reflection will show that it must be so. If the left ventricle ejected 1 ml per beat less than the right, within 15 minutes (at a heart rate of 72 per minute), there would be about a liter of blood dammed back in the pulmonary circulation. That would quickly lead to congestion and to edema of the lungs. Tissue fluid would be forced out into the alveoli with inevitable blockage of respiratory function. If the right ventricle, on the other hand, ejected 1 ml less per beat than the left, blood would soon be dammed back in such organs as the liver. Edema fluid would begin to collect in the peritoneal cavity and in the ankles, as the right heart failed to cope with the venous return.

cardiorespiratory changes at rest and during exercise. The size of the heart increases as a result of aerobic activities because of increases in volume. In some instances there is hypertrophy of the ventricle wall. That is in no way a hazard to health. Physical training augments the total capacity for maximum exercise. There is an increase in the maximum attainable cardiac output because of increased stroke volume. There is also an increase in the capacity of the muscles to extract oxygen from the blood, which is related to an increase in the number of muscle mitochondria. More frequent and longer training periods will, in general, increase physical fitness. Frequency, intensity, and duration of aerobic exercises are important factors in bringing about lower heart rates both at rest and during submaximum exercises. There are also some inherent benefits for general fitness. But there are exceptions. With interval training, maximum oxygen consumption is not appreciably increased by unrestricted frequency or duration of training. The effects are as good from 2 or 3 training periods a week for 7 weeks as from 4 periods a week for 13 weeks. Multiple daily training sessions are not more effective than single sessions and may be even counterproductive; thus they are not recommended. The most important factor affecting gains in endurance appears to be "intensity" of training rather than frequency or duration. Capability for work is to a large extent influenced by genetic factors. A superior training program cannot reach its maximum effect unless there is a genetic potential for developing superior physical fitness.

cardiovascular capacities. The efficiency of the heart depends on its ability to increase its output substantially during any period of exercise. It does so by increasing its size, both in the thickness of its muscle wall and in the volume of its chambers. The former effect produces a permanent slight enlargement of the heart; dilation of the chambers is lost when training stops. Limiting factors in the enlargement of the heart are the dimensions of the chest, its fixation to the arteries and veins that leave and enter it, and the cross-sectional diameter of the aorta, which does not enlarge with exercise. Diseased (swollen or enlarged) hearts may become much larger than superior athlete's hearts, but they are inefficient because of swelling and the weak myocardium and its poor circulation. An increase in the number of capillaries in the lung and in the muscles facilitates the exchange of oxygen and carbon dioxide. Those changes occur in response to intense aerobic exercise. Other adaptive mechanisms (relating to cardiovascular capacities) are increases in the total hemoglobin of the blood and increases in plasma volume. Hemoglobin increases under the stress of vigorous exercise, especially when it is combined with decreased barometric pressure, as at moderate altitudes. The limiting factor appears to be the decreasing viscosity of the blood. Plasma volume increases in response to heat stress but diminishes slightly at moderate altitudes. The advantage of increased plasma volume is to maintain adequate return to the heart and increase heat dissipation under conditions of elevated air temperature and increased relative humidity. The limiting factor is in the ability of the heart to handle the increased volume.

cardiovascular or circulatory system. All cells are bathed by tissue fluid. It is from that fluid that oxygen and food material diffuse into each cell, and carbon dioxide and waste products spread out of the cells. The cardiovascular or circulatory system is the chief transport system of the body. Its specialized tissue, blood, takes in oxygen in the lungs, collects foodstuffs after their absorption from the gut, conveys those materials to the tissues, picks up waste elements, and transports them for filtering to the kidneys. The organs of the system include the heart, a muscular "pump," which drives blood round a closed system of tubes, and the blood vessels. Those that carry blood away from the heart are called arteries; those that take blood back to the heart are called veins. The small, thin-walled vessels in the tissues (where the exchanges of gases, food, and waste products between blood and tissue fluids take place) are called capillaries.

carpal navicular fracture (scaphoid fracture). Trauma indirectly transmitted upward from the hand, usually caused by a fall onto a pronated hand. Symptoms are pain on the radial side of the wrist and disability. Signs are acute tenderness and a swelling of the wrist, limitation of wrist motion in dorsiflexion and radial deviation, or weakness of grip. Complications may be nonunion and traumatic arthritis.

carpal tunnel syndrome. A nerve compression syndrome featuring median nerve entrapment at the carpal tunnel resulting in symptoms in the hand and fingers, often extending up the arm to the elbow. The cause may be either an increase of structural volume within the tunnel or any condition that tends to narrow the tunnel. The history will often indicate an old scaphoid fracture, peri-lunate dislocation, or tendinitis at the wrist. Frequently, the history tells of a fall stopped abruptly by the palm of the hand when the wrist was sharply dorsiflexed or of overstress in people who strongly manipulate their wrists, such as in javelin throwing, tennis, hockey, or batting. A syndrome may also be produced by radial or ulnar arterial impairment since those arteries also pass beneath the transverse carpal ligament. Such symptoms may be aggravated by pressure of a sphygmomanometer cuff during blood pressure evaluation. There is a history of pain, numbness, and tingling, which worsens at night and with wrist compression, in the first 2 or 3 digits and the area proximal to the wrist. Weakness is exhibited by a history of dropping light objects and difficulty in holding a pen or pencil while one is writing. Venous engorgement and a bulge may be seen in the flexor mass in the distal wrist, which is characteristic of tenosynovitis or hypertrophied muscles. The 1st sign is swelling of the volar wrist. Later thenar atrophy and sensation impairment are found in the thumb, forefinger, middle finger, and medial half of the ring finger. Compression or percussion of the carpal ligament usually initiates or increases pain.

carpometacarpal, first dislocation. Dislocated thumb. Sudden violence forcing a metacarpal upward and backward, as in striking with a fist. Symptoms are local pain and disability. Signs are local swelling, deformity at base of 1st metacarpal in region of anatomical snuff box; thumb shortened, held in moderate adduction; tenderness. Complications may be chronicity. X ray may show dorsal displacement of the first metacarpal bone at carpometacarpal joint.

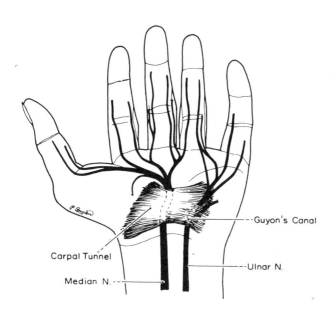

Guyon's Canal

Carpal Tunnel

Ulnar N.

Median N.

carpometacarpal subluxation. Excessive forcible motion of wrist in any direction; spontaneous reduction. Symptoms are local pain and some disability. Signs are tenderness on pressure over area, swelling, and/or abnormal mobility. Complications may be abnormal motion and weakness.

cauliflower ear. Normally associated with boxing or wrestling. The condition is the result of untreated or poorly treated hematoma. The clinical picture progresses from (1) trauma to the ear, causing persistent throbbing pain, which lasts long after the athletic event; (2) possible fibrocartilage fracture; (3) swelling, local heat, tenderness followed by the development of a hematoma after several hours, initially between cartilage and overlying skin, visible to the naked eye; (4) tissue hardening and the development of early fibrous tissue in about 14 days; and (5) the resulting keloid mass, development of new cartilage, and permanent deformity of the external ear characterized by skin wrinkling, thickening, and contraction at the site of injury.

cartilages. The word *cartilage* comes from the Latin word for "gristle," a tough, dense, rubbery tissue. In the human body cartilage exists in 2 forms. The first and more common form exists as translucent membranous covering on the ends of bones, where they rub against each other at the joints. It secretes a lubricating fluid and serves as 1 of several lubricating mechanisms in the body's joints. It is not in that form that cartilage comes into play in relation to ailments. Cartilage also exists in the form of flat, rubbery, crescent-shaped discs within the knee joint. Their function is to help ease the articulation of the joint surfaces. Although they are often called the "cartilages" of the knee, their proper name in medical terminology is "meniscus" in the singular and "menisci" in the plural. They are capable of being fragmented or ripped away from their connections in the knee during a sudden, abnormal motion of the knee. When that occurs, the fragment then floats loose in the knee and usually lodges between the 2 articulating surfaces, causing friction, inflammation, pain, and interference with joint motion.

celiac plexus syndrome (solar plexus syndrome). Direct trauma (hit or blow) to abdomen in epigastric area over celiac plexus ganglion; thought to be a reflex dilation of splanchnic blood vessels and lessened circulating blood volume to the head. Symptoms are inability to take a breath, fainting, and local pain.

cellulitis. A bacterial infection of the skin and underlying tissues that is produced by organisms that do not cause obstruction of blood vessels. Such infections do not tend to remain localized, and the bacteria may spread to other areas more easily. The site of the infection is usually red, swollen, hot, and tender and is usually sharply demarcated from the surrounding tissues. Fever of varying severity is usually present. Since the blood vessels remain open, the infections can be successfully treated with antibiotics.

cerebral concussion, acute, 1st degree (mild cerebral concussion). A common result of a direct blow to head or helmet, producing clinical syndrome characterized by immediate and transient impairment of neural function. Variable symptoms are temporary memory impairment, mental confusion, unsteadiness, tinnitus, and dizziness. There may be no signs, appearances, or brief periods of mental confusion. Complications may be insidious cerebral hemorrhage, vulnerability to subsequent head trauma, postconcussion syndrome, and perhaps posttraumatic epilepsy.

cerebral concussion, acute, 2nd degree (moderate cerebral concussion). A strong direct blow to the head or helmet, producing clinical syndrome characterized by immediate and transient impairment of neural function. Symptoms may be transitory unconsciousness with retrograde amnesia, variable symptoms of mental confusion, tinnitus, and headaches. Signs are appearance of transitory unconscious state and subsequent mental confusion. Complications may be insidious cerebral hemorrhage, vulnerability to subsequent head trauma, postconcussion syndrome, and perhaps post-traumatic epilepsy.

cerebral concussion, 3rd degree (severe cerebral concussion). A major direct blow to the head or helmet, producing a clinical syndrome characterized by immediate and perhaps protracted impairment of neural functions. The symptoms are unconscious-ness for prolonged intervals with extended periods of retrograde amnesia plus varia-ble symptoms but of greater duration than those experienced in mild or moderate types and possible convulsions. The signs are the appearance of prolonged uncon-scious states and subsequent mental confusion. Complications may be insidious cerebral hemorrhage, vulnerability to subsequent head trauma, postconcussion syn-drome, and perhaps posttraumatic epilepsy.

cervical (spinal) disk degeneration. The degeneration of 1 or more of the cervical disks, the ones that run along the neck portion of the spine, is a common occurrence. It is often associated with arthritic changes in the neck, so that there develops a com-bination of bony spurs plus disk protrusions that creates pressure on the spinal cord and nerve roots. When the cervical disks are involved, the symptoms are confined to the upper extremities. They usually consist of pain centered in the neck and radiating down through the shoulders and arms to the hands. If the nerve compression is exces-sive, the individual will develop weakness and atrophy of the forearm and hand mus-cles and loss of sensation in the fingers and hand. Basically, the same course of events for the lumbar region of the spine is followed as in the cervical region but for a few significant differences. One is that the neck is not subjected to the same stresses, loads, or forces to which the lumbar spine is so that cervical disk protrusions are not very large. Another is that the portion of the spinal cord that lies within the cervical region of the spinal cord is much larger and contains many more nerves. Conse-quently, in some respects damage to that area can be much more serious than to the lumbar region because it involves the entire spinal cord. Except for those individuals who have sudden injuries to the neck, such as cervical sprain, whiplash, or a specific trauma that may lead to early or premature degeneration, cervical disk problems are more common in older people than in younger.

cervical strain. A problem frequently seen that is caused by the athlete receiving some type of jolt that produces either acute flexion or acute extension of the neck. In cervical spine injuries compression, hyperextension, and a combination of flexion and rotation are the movements that cause spinal injuries. Compression injuries occur in diving into shallow water, performing trampoline exercises, high jumping, and pole vaulting. Hyperextension injuries have occurred in football when one is tackled from behind or when the chin is in collision with a knee or the ground. Wrestling also has a proportion of lateral rotational injuries to the neck. All cervical injuries produce local pain sometimes with radiation to the upper limbs, while weakness may be present in both the arms and legs after cord damage. Because the entire nerve supply to the body passes down the neck, that area is uniquely vulnerable to spinal cord trauma, which may lead to complete paralysis, or paraplegia. Low neck pain in the athlete may be due to structural abnormality of the cervical spine, which may lead to asymmetry and poor mobility which, in turn, predispose to ligamentous strains in the neck. Occa-sionally, an extra rudimentary rib or band of fibrous tissue may be present and press upon some of the soft-tissue structures including the nerves as they leave the cervical spine to make up the brachial plexus supplying the arm. Symptoms may be felt as a tingling or discomfort in the upper limb rather than as a neck pain and may be repro-duced by gentle traction downward on the arm.

cervical spine sprain—jammed neck or neck sprain. Forceful, abnormal range of motion of neck. The symptoms are a variable degree of severity of pain, strength, and function loss. The signs are tenderness or palpation over involved area, muscle spasm variable with severity of ligamentous injury, and limited motion.

charley horse. A term used to describe a muscle hematoma and originally used to describe the outcome of an impact injury to the quadriceps femoris when it was in contraction. The result is a hematoma caused by the rupture of a few fibers. The term has also been used in hamstring injuries of similar origin. Occasionally such injuries go on to an ossifying myositis.

chest pain (on exertion). Chest pains on exertion need not be angina, and many runners suffer transient chest pains. A burning retrosternal raw pain after severe exertion in cold weather is presumably due to tracheitis and for some reason (despite similar ventilation rates) tends not to occur with increasing fitness and, presumably, adaptation to the low relative humidity of the cold air. A spontaneous pneumothorax may occur on exertion and will produce a sudden pleuritic pain associated with breathlessness, the degree of which depends on the size of the pneumothorax. A pneumothorax may occur with sudden trauma to the chest. Angina is unlikely to occur but would tend to appear at repeatable levels of exertion.

Cheyne-Stokes respiration. Above 13,000 feet, almost everyone has Cheyne-Stokes breathing. It is not rare at altitudes as low as 8,000 feet. The pattern of respiration begins with a few shallow breaths, increases in depth to very deep, sighing respirations, and then falls off rapidly. Respiration can cease entirely for a few seconds, then the shallow breaths resume, and the pattern is repeated. That type of irregular breathing is so common at high altitudes that it is usually not considered abnormal. Cheyne-Stokes breathing may be present on some occasions and not on others. It may be a sign of a serious disorder if it occurs for the 1st time during an illness after a significant injury. During the period when breathing has stopped, the person often becomes restless and sleep may be broken. Occasionally the individual awakens with a rather distressing sense of suffocation.

chills (sickness types). A chill is a feeling of chilliness accompanied by shivering, which is produced by small showers of bacteria or viruses entering the blood stream. Such a chill accompanies infections and is frequently the first indication of the presence of such disorders. In contrast to the chill commonly resulting from exposure to cold or sunburn, a chill resulting from infection is much more severe, progressing to violent, uncontrollable shaking involving the entire body. The teeth chatter, the lips and nails are purple, the skin is pale and cold, and the victim feels miserable. The feeling of coldness persists in spite of blankets or heating pads until the chill has run its course, usually 5 to 15 minutes. A chill is usually followed in a very short time by a fever that may reach high levels. There is no specific treatment other than caring for the underlying infection. Pneumonia, meningitis, and "strep throat" are frequently introduced with a single shaking chill. Malaria, infections of the liver and bile ducts or kidneys, and generalized bacterial infections are characterized by recurrent chills.

chondromalacia patellae. Common in adolescent girls but may be found in cyclists and, occasionally, in those involved in sports such as hockey when a blow to the knee has been an aggravating factor. The articular cartilage loses its normal smooth, glistening appearance. In 1 or more areas it becomes edematous, dull, and soft so that at operation, it is easily indented. Fine, irregular fissures or a small erupting area (like a blister) is found at surgery.

cigarette smoking. Tobacco smoke is a complex mixture containing several thousand distinct chemical compounds. The physiological consequences of smoking are myriad. Acute inhalation of cigarette smoke may increase airways resistance and elevate blood carboxyhemoglobin because of the high concentration of carbon monoxide in cigarette smoke. Chronic cigarette smoking may result in permanent reduction of ventilatory and gas exchange capacity. The effects on the circulatory system range from acute blood pressure and pulse rate elevation to promotion of degenerative cardiovascular disease.

clavicle injuries. The tip of the shoulder, near the lateral aspect of the clavicle, is a common site of extremely painful tendon contusions to the trapezius. The acromioclavicular joint is relatively weak and inflexible, yet must bear constant stress in contact sports. Those who expose the joint to excessive and repeated trauma risk contusion, sprain, and separation. Posttraumatic arthritis is a typical consequence. Any force that tends to spring the clavicle from its attachments to the scapula is bound to cause severe sprain to the acromioclavicular, coronoid, and trapezoid ligaments unless the clavicle fractures beforehand. The acromioclavicular joint serves as a roof for the head of the humerus. It is one of the weakest joints in the body though assisted by the strong coracoclavicular ligament. The ends of the joint are bound loosely so the scapula can raise the glenoid fossa. During shoulder injury the scapula often rotates around the coracoid, which acts as a fulcrum. The intrinsically weak superior and inferior acromioclavicular ligaments give way, and the joint dislocates. In other instances a downward force of great intensity lowers the clavicle onto the 1st rib, which acts as a fulcrum, tearing the acromioclavicular and coracoacromial ligaments, resulting in complete acromioclavicular separation. Continued force can fracture the clavicle. Incomplete luxation can tear the intra-articular meniscus and lead to degenerative arthritis of the joint.

coccyx. A small, triangular bone composed of 4 (occasionally 3 to 5) fused vertebrae. On occasions, the first coccygeal vertebra is a separate bone. The anterior surface of the coccyx is concave, and the posterior surface is convex. The upper surface of the first coccygeal vertebra has an oval articular facet, which articulates with the facet on the apex of the sacrum. Projecting upward, from the posteriolateral corners of that articular surface, are 2 cornua, which articulate with the cornua of the lower end of the sacrum. On either side of the upper end of the coccyx, a rudimentary transverse process projects laterally. The position, anatomically, of the coccyx renders it prone to injury in various athletic pursuits.

coccyx fracture (fractured tailbone). A result of a direct blow, such as a fall on the buttocks. Symptoms are local pain and disability. Signs are tenderness, swelling, ecchymosis. Rectal examination may elicit false motion of click; displacement is palpable. Complications may lead to coccygodynia.

cold environment. In a cold environment muscle viscosity increases and joints stiffen, impairing performance considerably. With minimal clothing, as in running or swimming costume, energy stores must be used at an increased rate available for running or swimming. Swimmers in marathon events frequently have to give up because of hypothermia. The combination of cold air temperature and high wind velocity will induce hypothermia and frostbite rapidly in the individual who is not well protected.

cold exhaustion. When rectal temperature falls below 95°F (35°C), cerebral and muscular function is being impaired. Oral or axillary temperature gives little indication of core temperature. Temperature reduction is the multiple effect of a decreasing core temperature, exhausted glycogen stores, and a reduced blood-sugar level. Physical findings vary with oral temperature; low 90s, shivering; high 80s, dilated pupils, decreased motor function, bradycardia; low 80s, hyperventilation, stupor, coma, arrhythmias. The warning signs before syncope are muscle weakness and cramps, followed quickly by locomotor dysfunction, as witnessed by awkwardness, a slowed pace, and poor coordination or stumbling. The individual becomes talkative with slurred speech and excitable. Rapid recovery can be made at that stage if corrective action is taken. If ignored, the state progresses into apathy or anxiety symptoms and finally into collapse within 1 to 2 hours. In mountain climbing cold exhaustion usually occurs as a combined response to falling blood sugar and decreased body temperature; cerebral function begins to fail if the rectal temperature drops below 95°F (35°C). At that stage the intramuscular reserves of glycogen have been exhausted by (1) battling high winds, (2) attempting to match the climbing pace of fitter colleagues, and (3) the added metabolic demands of shivering and other attempts to sustain body temperature (nonshivering thermogenesis). The earliest signs of difficulty are a slowing of pace, unsteadiness, clumsiness, muscle weakness or cramps, and stumbling. If shelter and food are sought at that stage, recovery is rapid. However, if such symptoms are ignored, the body has increasing difficulty in sustaining heat balance. Mental symptoms appear, such as anxiety, irritability, apathy, or loss of purpose, and collapse occurs within 1 to 2 hours.

colles fracture. Wrist hyperextension fracture. Indirect trauma, usually a fall onto outstretched, pronated hand. Symptoms are local pain, numbness in fingers, and limited supination-pronation. Signs are local swelling, ecchymosis, "silver fork" deformity with radial shortening, tenderness on palpation over distal radius. Complications may involve injury of median nerve, variable loss of function of hand, wrist, and malunion.

Colorado tick fever. A viral disease that is transmitted by the wood tick, occurring in all of the western states and far more common than Rocky Mountain spotted fever. Infections usually occur in spring and early summer, when ticks are active. Four to six days after exposure, chills and fever appear along with headache and generalized aching. Photophobia (sensitivity of the eyes to sunlight) may be present. The attack lasts about 2 days and is followed by a disappearance of fever and symptoms and then by recurrent attacks with similar symptoms. The possibility of tick infection has been associated with hiking and mountain climbing.

common cold. A large number of viruses cause upper respiratory infection (colds), but the identities of many of the viruses remain unknown. In addition, secondary bacterial infection and allergy to the virus, or bacteria, cause many of the symptoms. Some generalized viral infections often mimic a cold during their initial states. The virus is spread by personal contact. Chilling and exposure may play a role in contracting the infection, primarily by increasing the susceptibility to infection. However, in the absence of the causative viruses, chilling and exposure alone do not produce colds. The symptoms of a cold are familiar. A sense of dryness, a slight soreness, or a tickling in the throat usually appears first and is followed after a few hours by nasal stuffiness, sneezing, and a thin, watery nasal discharge. After 48 hours, when the disease is full-blown, the eyes are often red and watery, the voice husky, and the nose obstructed. A fairly abundant nasal discharge is present, and taste and smell are diminished. A cough is commonly present, which is dry at first but later may be productive of a moderate amount of mucoid material. Fever is usually absent but may be as high as 102°F. The throat may be sore but exudates are not present, and the lymph nodes around the neck and jaw are not enlarged. The treatment for a cold consists of rest and measures to alleviate the symptoms.

concussions. Concussions are immediate, temporary, posttraumatic alterations in consciousness that may last from a few seconds to 24 hours and may be accompanied by amnesia or other symptoms. The minimal concussion is the most common sports head injury, described as the "threshold" brain injury. Athletes with minimal (Grade I) concussions are confused, disoriented, or dazed, but they have no amnesia or associated symptoms. The impact alters their level of consciousness by stunning cortical projections of the reticular activating system. Athletes with mild (Grade II) concussions are stunned and have posttraumatic amnesia (i.e., they cannot recall all the events occurring after the impact). The amnesia may begin at the moment of impact or 5 to 10 minutes later. Athletes describe the injury as being "dinged" or having their "bells rung." There may be associated symptoms such as headache, vertigo, or unsteady gait. They may develop into the postconcussion syndrome, which is characterized by difficulty in concentrating, irritability, and recurring headaches. Athletes with moderate (Grade III) concussions are stunned and have both post-traumatic amnesia and retrograde amnesia (i.e., they cannot recall events and information before the impact). They also may develop associated symptoms and the postconcussion syndrome. After severe mechanical impact to the brain, consciousness is lost. Athletes with classical severe (Grade IV) concussions develop flaccid uncon-sciousness at the moment of impact. They usually begin to recover within a few minutes, becoming first stuporous, then confused, and then they awake with somewhat automatic behavior and are finally lucid. They have sustained an impact that physiologically disconnects the cortex from the brain stem reticular formation. Both posttraumatic and retrograde amnesia are present, and associated symptoms, such as headache, vertigo, etc., frequently develop. Amnesia after a blow to the head indicates physiologic brain injury; the timing and duration of the amnesia indicates the severity of concussion.

conjunctivitis. Common in athletes because, when perspiring, they tend to rub the sweat from their eyes with fingers that are not always clean. It may also occur secondary to the occurrence of small foreign bodies, especially dust and dirt from playing surfaces. Conjunctivitis is an inflammation of the delicate membrane that covers the surface of the eye and the under surface of the eyelids. The inflammation is most frequently started by irritation from a foreign body. Infection follows and is normally the result of bacterial or viral growth. "Pink eye" (a fairly common type of conjunctivitis) is produced by the bacteria that were the most common cause of pneumonia in preantibiotic days. The individual characteristically feels as if he or she has something in the eye, even if the foreign body has been removed. Movement of the eye aggravates the irritation. The eye appears red, and the blood vessels on the surface are engorged. The flow of tears is increased, and exudate may be crusted on the margins of the eyelids and the eyelashes. The exudate may almost seal the lids together during a night's sleep. If the disease shows no evidence of clearing after 6 to 10 days of therapy, the individual should see a physician immediately. He or she may have a serious form of conjunctivitis, which, if not given medical attention, could cause blindness.

contact dermatitis (Dermatitis Venenata). A highly pruritic lesion with many external causes. Because it is caused by contact with chemical, animal, or vegetable substance, it usually occurs on exposed surfaces of the skin. The skin is edematous and erythematous, and it has firm vesicles that can burst and crust over. The diagnosis is not difficult, but the cause is not always apparent. Contact dermatitis is noncontagious. When a person has been exposed to the oil of the poison ivy plant, it may penetrate the individual's clothing. The oil will not dry if the fabric is nylon. Touching the contaminated clothing can cause dermatitis when there has been no direct contact with the plant.

contusion (to body and/or head). A direct blow against the integument, causing bruising of the skin or underlying tissues. That results in capillary rupture and an infiltration type of bleeding followed by edema and inflammatory reaction. The result is local swelling, which may be superficial or deep depending upon the nature of the object striking the blow and the location involved. A few contusions merit special attention because they cause problems out of proportion to their apparent severity and may be underrated. Most notable is the quadriceps contusion or "charley horse." The injury is common in football, wrestling, hockey, and soccer and is usually the result of being kicked or "kneed" in the thigh. That contusion usually is anterior at midthigh level, but it occasionally is anterolateral or anteromedial. The more severe contusions of the quadriceps are immediately disabling and result in severe pain. There is almost immediate swelling, frequently of a spectacular magnitude. Quadriceps dysfunction may occur to the extent that continued athletic activity is impossible. Because of the immediate disability, the injuries usually receive medical attention. The greater potential problem lies within the quadriceps contusion that is not so spectacular (the contusion that allows continued participation) but after a period of rest becomes disabling because of pain and quadriceps spasm. The injury is almost always regarded as "just a bruise," and the athlete is told to "run it out" or to "run through the pain." The injury frequently is subjected to vigorous and painful massage to "work out the cramp," and the athlete is encouraged to do squatting exercises to stretch the muscle and sometimes painful weight lifting to "keep it strong." However, the problem is far more serious when bone formation is seen on X ray and myositis ossificans has developed. It is inevitable that the disability will last for months. In more severe head injuries, the brain may be contused or lacerated, particularly if the skull is fractured and bone fragments are driven in (as in penetrating wounds). That damage may also occur in closed injuries without a skull fracture or with linear fractures with no displacement of the fragments. The brain is bruised or torn by violent impact against the skull, especially against the sharp edges of the sphenoidal ridge, the bony prominence of the anterior fossa, and the free edge of the tentorium. In simple contusions the meninges are turned with the blood vessels traversing them, subarachnoid hemorrhage is profuse, and clots are found in the sulci and brain. If death does not occur, the bleeding stops, the clots becoming organized or liquified with accompanying edema. Recovery of consciousness may not take place for hours or days and may be followed by a period of drowsiness and confusion before the individual is fully oriented and rational. Severe headache is common in the acute stage, particularly where there has been subarachnoid hemorrhage. Giddiness is also normal and is characterized by a momentary feeling of unsteadiness that occurs with sudden change of posture. In many cases severe neurological defects (which are apparent when the individual regains consciousness) clear up almost completely in a matter of days or weeks. In some cases the individual is left with some degree of intellectual defect, varying from slight impairment of memory and concentration to profound dementia.

conus medullaris contusion. Direct blow to spine with structural alteration of the lower spinal cord characterized by extravasation of blood cells and tissue necrosis with edema. Symptoms are numbness over the buttocks with bladder and bowel dysfunction and, later, spastic gait. Signs are partial or permanent impairment of neural function; lower extremity and sacral hyperesthesia or hyperalgesia; weakness, spasticity, hyperreflexia of lower extremities. X ray may show associated fracture; myeologram may show partial or complete block.

convulsions. Often a sign of disease of the nervous system. Commonly occur during infections involving the brain or following brain injuries. However, convulsions also occur during the course of diseases that affect the brain only indirectly. Convulsions associated with renal failure are not at all uncommon. Occasionally, a person suffers a single convulsion for which no cause can be determined and which never recurs. Epilepsy is a condition in which a person suffers repeated convulsions over a long period of time. Sometimes a cause of the episodes can be found, but more often the etiology remains undetermined. The onset of a convulsion is usually sudden and may be marked by an outcry of some kind. The individual characteristically loses consciousness and falls to the ground, his or her body twisting and writhing and all 4 limbs twitching and jerking. The jaw may be involved also, and the individual's tongue can be badly injured by biting. There may be profuse salivation, resulting in drooling and frothing or defecation or uncontrollable voiding. In any single convulsive episode, all or none of those features may be present. Sometimes the individual exhibits only a slight twitching of the extremities. A person who is unconscious from a head injury may exhibit only a series of jerking movements, which gradually increases in intensity and then subside. The convulsion usually lasts only 1 or 2 minutes but can persist for 5 minutes or longer. A period of unconsciousness follows, lasting from a few minutes to several hours. It may be a very deep coma in which the individual is almost completely unresponsive even to painful stimuli.

coordination. The ability to integrate separate abilities into a complex task. Well-coordinated movement, usually involving the large muscles, requires perfect timing between the nervous and muscular systems, as seen in bowling, gymnastics, badminton, throwing, jumping hurdles, handball, tennis, ice hockey, baseball, golf, or soccer.

core temperature (body). Increasing surface temperature reflects the effects of a progressively rising and dangerous core temperature, the increase in subcutaneous circulation, and the amount of perspiration. An increasing core temperature increases oxygen consumption in inactive tissues and diverts a large proportion of the circulation to skin vessels even when optimal cardiac output is maintained. That results in a reduced supply to active muscle tissue. Because of the demand for heat dissipation, prolonged exertion during hot weather causes a progressive reduction of central blood volume. As the core temperature increases, peripheral vein capacity increases and the formation of tissue fluid increases during the early minutes of activity. In a hot, dry climate, expired water losses also increase. Sweating contributes greatly to a fall in blood volume and may under severe conditions amount to as much as 1 to 2 liters per hour. If a player's pulse rate does not reduce during rest periods, that is evidence that body heat is accumulating. Rectal temperature should be checked for verification.

corneal abrasions and lacerations. In the typical athlete protective reflexes tend to prevent extensive corneal abrasions, but even minor lesions are quite painful, resulting in blurred vision, photophobia, excessive lacrimation and usually requiring some hospitalization. The injuries are usually the result of scratches from a fingernail, a ball, or a piece of equipment in close contact sports and always present a threat of possible visual impairment. The clinical picture is one of an extremely red eye, pain, photophobia, and excessive lacrimation. Lacerations of the eyeball from sharp or pointed objects result in eye pain and visual impairment. On examination, the cornea will appear cut, present an irregular corneal reflex, possibly exhibit a tear-shaped pupil with a small ebony tip at the apex of the tear, or the iris may exhibit a hole from perforation. Injuries to the cornea may set up a general inflammation of the membrane, but more frequently they cause loss of substance of the cornea and thus cause corneal ulcers. Those ulcers heal quickly if small and not infected. They present little pain and leave only a temporary opacity proportionate to their extent. An injury causing bending of the cornea may exhibit a number of fine gray streaks (striate keratitis), more or less perpendicular to the corneal injury, noticed from a few hours to a week or more after the trauma.

corns. Round or cone-shaped localized callosities of skin that possess a horny core. The typical corn is one of a circumscribed area of hypertrophied skin, resembling a small shell containing a harder core, which presses on nerves of the foot in the weight-bearing position. The cause of corns can usually be attributed to atypical bone formation or position, to external pressure, or to repeated trauma. There are 2 types, soft and hard corns. Soft corns form in areas where skin touches skin, such as between the toes, in an area where heat is poorly released, perspiration has difficulty in evaporating, and an adjacent bone puts pressure on the skin. Hard corns are firm, rigid, and dense. They arise over prominent protuberances on parts of the foot where sport shoes exert considerable pressure and/or friction. Examples are the lateral side of the small toes and the top of the middle toe.

cramps. The muscles of the body extend outward in layers from the bones to the frame to just beneath the skin. They are composed of pliant, fibrous tissues through which tiny blood vessels, capillaries, and nerve endings flow. The capillaries feed the muscles, that is, supply them with oxygen and nutrients; the nerves are there to inner-vate them, that is, enable them to contract and relax in response to voluntary or invol-untary impulses from the brain. As muscles are being used, they expand energy. In other words, every time a muscle contracts, its fibers require energy to sustain the contraction. So a muscle is constantly using up energy. The necessary energy is pro-vided by both the fresh oxygen and sugars fed into the muscle by the blood vessels. As the oxygen is used up in the muscle tissues, it manufactures a by-product called lactic acid. Under normal conditions, part of the lactic acid is carried off as waste while new oxygen is being supplied, so that 2 substances exist in a kind of natural balance in the muscle tissue. But when the muscles are overused, an excessive amount of lactic acid is produced because of insufficient oxygen supply. The muscles enter into a condition known as "oxygen debt." It is when the muscles go into oxygen debt that cramps usually occur. Cramps are basically nothing more than a form of muscle spasm. As muscles or groups of muscles become starved for oxygen, they react by going into uncontrollable spasms. When the oxygen debt reaches a certain intolerable level, the nerves become alerted and send panic sensory messages to the brain. Back come equally panicky motor-messages, and the muscles themselves go into panic. There are basically 2 kinds of cramps relating to the weekend athlete—runner's cramps and swimmer's cramps.

cranial concussion. A syndrome in which there is an immediate impairment of neural function following a blow to the head. It may result in disturbances of consciousness, memory faults, visual disorders, or equilibrium problems. It is the most common injury to the brain following a cranial blow. Concussion is defined as an essentially transient state that is caused by head injury, has an instant onset, and manifests widespread purely paralytic (flaccid) symptoms without neurologic evidence of gross brain injury. It is always followed by a degree of transient unconsciousness and amnesia from the actual moment of the accident. The degree of posttraumatic amnesia appears to be a guide to the severity of the concussion. Headache is often the sole posttraumatic complaint, but shallow breathing, pallor, feeble pulse, reduced reflexes, and other signs of surgical shock may result. Pure concussion is rare. Most head injuries are accompanied by some degree of brain injury with a reaction similar to injury found in other tissues. Edema and congestion occur and are coupled with a moderate rise in cerebral venous pressure, although the cerebrospinal fluid may be clear. Unconscious-ness may be prolonged, memory loss more pronounced, and reflex change and even convulsions may be manifest.

craniocerebral hematoma, epidural. Head trauma producing ruptured middle men-ingeal artery or torn dural sinus; may occur with or without skull fracture at middle meningeal groove in temporal region or at lambdoidal suture at lateral sinus in the oc-cipital region. Symptoms usually include loss of consciousness. The injury may be followed by a period of mental clarity, usually of hours, rarely of days, then relapse, loss of consciousness, possibly contralateral paresis or paralysis. Signs are possible scalp contusion, ipsilateral pupillary dilation with bilateral pyramidal tract signs (ten-torial or temporal lobe pressure cone), possible contralateral hemiparesis, slow pulse, rising blood pressure. Complications could lead to death, especially if hematoma is not decomposed immediately.

crepitus. There are several types of crepitus that characterize a specific type of lesion. They are bone crepitus, traumatic pulmonary emphysematous crepitus, joint crepitus, and tendosynovitis crepitations. Bone fractures elicit an audible grating when the ends of the broken fragments rub against each other during movement. The crepitation from an epiphyseal separation resembles that of a broken bone but is softer in character than bone crepitus from a fracture. Crepitus may be felt when the fingers are placed with mild pressure over the affected area. Joint crepitus may be tested by placing a hand over the joint while passively moving the joint with the other hand. Crepitus may also be felt over an effused joint following inflammation of the tendon sheath.

cricket injuries. In cricket vary according to the level at which the game is played. Factors include: (1) the standard of the pitch, (2) the standard of equipment used, and (3) the relative fitness of participants. The first 2 are apt to produce direct impact injuries while the 3rd may produce "indirect" problems owing to poor preparation by the player. At county and international level the incidence of injury depends on whether the match is played over 1, 3, or 5 days. As the pitch wears, injury can increase dramatically when there is fast bowling on an uneven pitch. Common impact or direct injuries are fractures and dislocations of the fingers. Rib fractures and contusions to the thoracic cage and head and facial injuries occur. Fractures of the ulnar or forearm owing to a fast rising ball are fairly common. Injury to the feet occurs when the ball is bowled low to the batsman. As cricket tends to be a unilateral game, then problems caused by prolonged 1-sided joint stress in the form of osteoarthrosis of hip, knee, and ankle can occur. Gross arthritic changes in the hands of cricket keepers are common. In summary, hazards are encountered by (1) running both between the wicket and in the outfield; stress injuries to lower limbs and feet and injuries to ankle and knee are common; (2) bowling and throwing; shoulder, elbow, back, foot, and ankle injuries may occur; (3) Impact injury; a hard ball is used in cricket and injuries to a batsman's head, face, teeth, chest, genitals, hands, and legs are possible, especially when he faces a fast bowler on an uneven pitch. The areas are protected by a helmet and mask, leg pads and gloves, and a "genital" box. Injuries to fingers are common in fielding, especially when the ball is not cleanly caught and fingers can be badly stubbed to produce fractures and dislocations. Mallet deformity is common. Environmental hazards such as sunburn, exposure to cold, insects, and snake bites and bowel upsets when one is playing in tropical areas are all associated hazards.

cuboid syndrome. The term describes pain felt on the lateral aspect of the foot over the outer 2 metatarsals. Pain can be elicited by pressure over the peroneal groove and tends to occur in the pronated foot. Fracture of the cuboid, metatarsal bone, calcaneonavicular bar, and peroneal tendinitis must be excluded. With the foot pronated, the midtarsal joint is unstable, the peroneas longus acts at a greater mechanical advantage and can subluxate the cuboid dorsally on the lateral side. This depresses the medial aspect, which can lock the cuboid in a displaced situation, and manipulations to correct it may be needed.

D

dancer's knee. Known medically as patellar chrondromalacia (a softening of the articular cartilage on the undersurface of the kneecap). It occurs most frequently in young women, especially those who take up ballet dancing as a form of exercise. The reason is most probably the fact that a woman's pelvic girdle is wider than a man's. Therefore the thigh bones meet the knees at a more acute angle, forcing the knee inward and causing them to be slightly knock-kneed. This natural knock-kneed configuration causes an unequal pull on the kneecap when the knee is bent. One side of the kneecap (the inside) gets pulled higher than the outside by the quadriceps muscles each time the knee is bent and straightened. The underside of the kneecap articulates with the front of the knee joint. To do so, it has a layer of articular cartilage, the hard, rubbery, glistening substance attached to the bone. As the kneecap is pulled unequally, its articulation becomes irregular and the articular cartilage may become inflamed. It usually reacts by softening, which produces further inflammation and deep-knee pain. A piece of the cartilage may even tear off and float free within the joint, causing locking and other instabilities.

darts injuries. This English game is usually played in public houses or drinking areas. The dart is sharp and pointed and has 4 fins or feathers to direct its flight. It is thrown against a cork dartboard, which is divided by wires into scoring areas of differing values. Hazards include strains to the shoulder and elbow from prolonged playing and penetrating injuries from the darts, which can sometimes ricochet off the metal partitions on a dartboard to transfix bystanders and other players. An occasional serious eye injury may result from a wayward dart.

dehydration. Dehydration from any cause will result in a reduction of total plasma volume, stroke volume, and cardiac output, elevation of heart rate during submaximum exercise, a reduction of liver glycogen, losses of electrolytes (especially sodium and chloride but also potassium, calcium, and magnesium), and compromised thermoregulation. Dehydration will also adversely affect athletic performance because of reduced muscle strength, endurance time, and mental acuity. Maximum oxygen uptake is usually not changed. Dehydration is ubiquitous at high altitudes. Contributing to the loss of fluids is faster and deeper breathing of cold air. Air is warmed and moistened as it passes through the mouth, nose, and other major passages so that it has a relative humidity approaching 100 percent and the same temperature as the body when it reaches the lungs. The greatest respiratory efforts required at high altitudes increase the amount of water required to moisten the air. Cold air with a high relative humidity, when warmed to body temperature, becomes relatively dry. As a result, the cold air found at higher altitudes requires more water to provide a relative humidity near 100 percent in the lungs. Mouth breathing during which almost all of the moisture in expired air is lost, sweating with exertion, and unavailability of water for drinking also contribute to fluid shortage at higher altitudes. The dehydration is further aggravated by loss or dulling of the sensation of thirst that accompanies the loss of appetite, nausea, and occasionally vomiting occurring with acute mountain sickness. People must consciously push themselves to drink fluids, even if they are not thirsty when at high altitudes. At sea level an average individual requires about 2 liters of fluid per day. At high altitudes, particularly above 15,000 to 16,000 feet, requirements often exceed 4 liters per day.

dental pain. Dental disease in athletes may affect their performance. Pain in the teeth on taking sweet foods is usually due to decay and may be relieved by the insertion of a filling. Pain on thermal changes in the mouth indicates inflammation of the pulp, which is usually reversible by treatment but may require removal of the pulp for relief of the pain. A tooth that is tender on biting may be so because pressure is transmitted to the pulp through dentin weakened by decay or, in an apparently intact tooth, because of inflammation of the periodontal ligament. Those changes are often reversible without extraction of the tooth. An apical abscess results from death of the pulp and suppuration in the bone surrounding the root, producing a swelling of the gum overlying the root and, if neglected, possible infection and swelling of the face. Tenderness of the gum behind the last standing molar tooth in the lower jaw indicates inflammation of the gingival tissues (gingivitis) or a buried or partially erupted wisdom tooth.

dermatitis, contact. Caused by contact of skin with irritants, such as tape, tincture of benzoin compound, penicillin, mercury applications, and other substances. Symptoms are variable degrees of pruritis and burning pain. Signs of the acute type are exposed portion of skin first affected with consequent edema, erythema, vesicles, bullae and rupture of vesicles and bullae, producing denudation, oozing, crusting, and/or scaling. Signs for the subacute type are papules, thickening of skin, excoriations, and crusting. For the chronic type: lichenification, dryness, hyperpigmentation, and fissures. Complications may be secondary infection with systemic manifestations.

diet. A well-balanced diet should include carbohydrates, fats, proteins, vitamins, mineral salts, and water. Carbohydrates are essential to the body for the provision of energy. They are present in 3 forms: (1) monosaccharides, the simplest form of carbohydrate. Monosaccharides are absorbed directly into the bloodstream from the alimentary canal and need no digestion. Glucose is the main monosaccharide present in the body. Small quantities of other monosaccharides are absorbed from the alimentary canal, but they are converted into glucose in the liver. (2) Disaccharides are composed of 2 units of monosaccharides joined together. The most common disaccharides present in the diet are sucrose, or ordinary sugar and lactose. Disaccharides are broken down in the alimentary canal into their constituent monosaccharides, which are then absorbed. (3) Polysaccharides (starches) are complex carbohydrates composed of several units of monosaccharides. Polysaccharides are also broken down, in the alimentary canal, into their constituent monosaccharides. Polysaccharides are present in potatoes, root vegetables, cereals, and bread. Fats are essential to the body for the protection of certain vital organs, such as the kidney and the eye, and for the absorption of the vitamins that are fat soluble. Fats can also be uesd for the provision of energy when there is a shortage of carbohydrates. Fats are broken down in the alimentary canal into fatty acids and glycerol. The fatty acids and glycerol are then absorbed from the intestine into the lymphatic vessels and pass via the thoracic duct into the bloodstream. Fats are present in the diet in 2 forms, animal fat and vegetable fat. Animal fats are present in butter, milk, cream, cheese, eggs, and fatty meat. Vegetable fats are present in olive oil, nut oils, and some margarines.

Proteins are a major building block of the human body. They are essential ingredients for the maintenance and repair of most of the body tissues that are not the results of calcification processes (i.e., bones, teeth, and cartilage). Those include all of the muscles, nerves, glands, and organs. The body can make proteins, but most of them come from diet. Protein also plays an important part in the developing and maintaining of musculoskeletal strength, flexibility, neuromuscular conditioning, and stamina. They also may play a major role in retarding the aging process. Proteins are generally the most difficult of foods to digest, in that they usually take longer (up to 4 hours) and require more of the digestive system and liver (more bile and HCL) to break them down, into molecules that can be absorbed into the bloodstream. Consequently, they may ferment in the stomach when they are mixed with other foods that digest more quickly (some vegetables take as little as 15 minutes). Vitamins also play an important part in the digestive process. Many foods will not digest properly if certain enzymes are not present. Vitamins and proteins combine to form holoenzymes (complete enzymes, i.e., apoenzymes and coenzymes) and are essential for optimal health and fitness.

Vitamin deficiencies may contribute to a wide variety of disorders, sicknesses, and diseases. The body does not store and cannot manufacture vitamins in adequate amounts. Therefore, they must be taken on a regular basis as part of the diet. Mineral salts supply the many needed elements that make up the cells of a body. They are important for maintaining chemical balance and "wellness" of the cells. They may also play a vital role in longevity. Pure (unpolluted) drinking and cooking water are very important parts of a nutritional diet. The human organism is made up of approximately 92 percent water. The clear, odorless, tasteless liquid is an important transport mechanism and cleansing agent for many processes within the body. It is a basic ingredient of life, and one cannot exist without it.

digestive system. The organs that are concerned with the digestion and absorption of foods eaten and with the elimination of the undigested and unabsorbed residues. Digestion involves the mechanical and chemical breakdown of food into forms that can be absorbed by the body and used for growth, repair of tissues, and the provision of energy. The digestive system is composed of the alimentary canal, which extends from the mouth to the anus, and certain accessory organs. That canal, which is about 30 feet in length, is composed of the mouth, the pharynx, the esophagus, the stomach, the small intestine, the large intestine, and both the ascending and descending colons. The accessory organs are the 3 pairs of salivary glands, the pancreas, the liver, and the biliary apparatus.

disk rupture, cervical. A blow to the head along the longitudinal axis, as in spearing, lifting, straining, twisting, with mechanical disadvantage. Symptoms include pain in neck, arms, and/or fingers, especially on tilting head backward or to involved side; accentuation of pain on coughing; sneezing; or straining. The individual may have weakness in upper extremities, but bladder or bowel impairment is rare. Signs are pain radiating to the neck, shoulder, arm, forearm, or hand elicited by biceps or triceps reflex and—if midline disk with cord compression—possibly tetraparesis or tetraplegia with complete sensory loss and hyperreflexia and hypertonia with pyramidal tract signs. Complications could be compression of nerve root (pinched nerve) with paralysis of specific muscles of upper extremity, possibly compression of spinal cord with paresis, paralysis of extremities and bladder, bowel incontinence, and sensory loss to the level of lesion.

disk rupture, lumbar. Lifting, straining, twisting with mechanical disadvantage or often for no apparent cause. Symptoms can be a pain in the back or in sciatic distribution, especially on bending to the side of the lesion; pain accentuated by coughing, sneezing, or straining; numbness in calf or foot; weakness in muscle of toe, in foot on dorsiflexion, or possibly in quadriceps. Signs are limitation of motion, pain elicited by foot dorsiflexion with knee extended, tilt of spine away from side of lesion, positive straight leg-raising test, sensory loss in lumbrosacral dermatomes; loss of diminution of Achilles or patellar reflexes; weakness in foot dorsiflexion. Complications may be compression of nerve root with intractable pain, foot drop, bladder-bowel incontinence.

dislocation. Defined as an actual displacement of the opposing contiguous surfaces making up a joint. That, of necessity, presumes loss of function of some of the ligament structures of the joint, since the ligaments are designed to prevent displacement or abnormal motion. In acute sprain, when the ligament finally tears, the joint subluxates either by a slipping of the bone ends on themselves or by a separation of the bone ends. If the force continues until the joint is actually disrupted, there is a dislocation. It may be spontaneously reduced, or the bones may lock in the dislocated position; in either instance there is a loss of function of the ligament.

diuretics. Dehydration by the use of diuretics has been a common practice among boxers, wrestlers, and weight lifters. The rapid loss of weight just before competition is thought to gain advantage for athletes by qualifying them to compete in the lowest possible weight class. But a number of studies document that performance is decreased with dehydration and the loss of fluid and electrolytes.

E

ear, hematoma, acute (early cauliflower ear). Contusion or repeated friction of auricle, as in wrestling and boxing, characterized by intra-auricular hemorrhage and edema. Symptoms are moderate to severe pain. Signs are swelling, discoloration, and local fluctuation. Complications may lead to deformity (cauliflower ear) if untreated; infection may occur after aspiration (rare).

ear injuries and disorders. Bruises of the ear produce bleeding between the cartilage framework and the thin overlying skin. Left untreated, these hematomas remain as masses of unsightly scars, the familiar "cauliflower ear." In warm weather or when people swim a great deal, the ear canal tends to remain damp. That allows infection to occur, which feels worse if the outer cartilage of the ear is tugged on. Sometimes fluid drains from the ear. The eardrum creates a seal between the canal and the middle ear. The middle ear normally contains air and is connected to the back of the pharynx (throat) by the Eustachian tube and may become infected following colds, causing swelling and blockage of the Eustachian tube. The major symptoms are deep ear pain with a full feeling and decreased hearing, with occasional fever. If the infection is allowed to progress, the eardrum may burst and drain infected material. Injury to the internal ear does not happen frequently, with the possible exception of the ruptured eardrum.

Obstruction of the external auditory canal by wax or foreign bodies may interfere with the conduction of sound waves to the tympanic membrane. Inflammation and scarring of the tympanic membrane or the joints between the ossicles may prevent normal vibration and amplification of sound waves. Otosclerosis is a type of deafness in adults usually between 18 and 40, more frequently in women. Bone changes prevent normal vibration of the third ossicle (stapes). There seems to be a hereditary predisposition to the disease. There are many other causes of deafness and many other kinds of deafness. Injuries to the internal ear, the acoustic nerve, or of the parts of the brain that conduct or interpret auditory messages may cause deafness. Such injuries may be due to infections such as measles, mumps, syphilis, or meningitis. In some cases alcohol, quinine, arsenic, or mercury compounds are damaging to these organs.

The history of a blow across the side of the head with pain, slight hemorrhage from the ear, and a feeling of fullness in the ear should be medically checked. The ear is more seriously threatened by pressure damage, or barotrauma. The ear consists of an eardrum attached to the hearing apparatus with air at equal pressure on each side of the drum. Externally lies the atmosphere; internally the Eustachian tube leads to the back of the nasopharynx. Normally, any change in pressure, such as moving in an elevator or landing in an airplane, is rapidly equalized by chewing, swallowing, yawning, or similar actions by which the Eustachian mechanism matches the external air pressure on the eardrum. Under some circumstances the free exchange of air is impaired with pressure differences liable to cause injury, or barotrauma. In outer-ear barotrauma, a tightly worn diving hood, for example, causes artificial restriction of air movement and pressure in the outer ear. That may cause discomfort and blood blistering in the ear canal. In otitic barotrauma (the squeeze), the outside air pressure rises, as in an airplane descent, and if the Eustachian tube does not allow equalization of pressure, earache results. If the pressure increases, small hemorrhages occur in the middle ear and the drum may burst. Ruptures of the drum usually heal spontaneously, but in the young athlete, if there is any question at all as to damage of the drum or inner or middle ear, a medical examination should be made. The most dangerous sequel could be infection.

ear, otitis externa, acute (external ear dermatitis). Bacterial infection, allergy, swimming in contaminated water, loss of local natural resistance to infection from prolonged and repeated swimming. Symptoms are burning pruritis, acute pain, tinnitus, or impaired hearing.

eczema. An unpleasant disease that may be found in all age groups and in both sexes. However, it is more common in the very young and in the elderly. Eczema may affect any and all parts of the skin surface. It is a noncontagious disorder that may manifest itself in redness (erythema), blisters (vesicles), and pimplelike (papular) lesions. There also may be scaling and crusting of the skin surfaces. Eczema may be a manifestation of an allergy to certain foods, detergents, soaps, and other chemicals. Psychological and emotional disturbances may precipitate or aggravate an attack of eczema, just as they bring on bouts of asthma and other allergic responses. There may be a hereditary predisposition to allergic disorders; therefore some individuals must give more than the average attention to diet as well as to proper physical and mental hygiene.

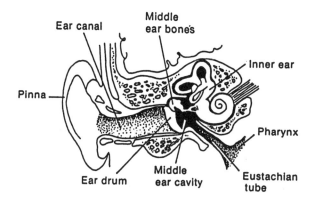

Ear.

elastic arteries. Elastic fibers are circularly arranged in the walls of arteries as a series of concentric lamellae. In systole, when the ventricles are contracting and the aortic and pulmonary semilunar valves are pushed open, blood is forcibly ejected into the aorta and the pulmonary artery. The walls of those vessels are stretched to accommodate much of the cardiac output. In that way they act as reservoirs for blood. The walls "store" energy from the contraction of the heart. In diastole, when the ventricles are relaxing and the pressure within the heart falls, the aortic and pulmonary semilunar valves are pushed shut by the back pressure of the blood in those vessels. The walls of both arteries then recoil to their original state. That recoil of the elastic tissue serves to push blood onward when the heart itself is resting. In that way both the aorta and the pulmonary artery act as subsidiary pumps, their walls expending the energy previously stored from the heart's contraction.

elbow dislocation, anterior. Caused by a direct blow to a point of the flexed elbow, as in a fall. Symptoms are severe pain and disability. Signs are elbow fixed in a near-complete extension; rounded condyles of the humerus palpable at point of elbow, olecranon absent from normal position or local swelling and tenderness. Complications may be nerve, vascular injury; traumatic myositis ossificans; residual partial disability. X ray shows olecranon resting on anterior surface of lower humerus; radial head is anterior to and above external humeral condyle.

elbow dislocation, posterior. Caused by forcible hyperextension at elbow or a fall onto outstretched hand with elbow extended and forearm supinated. Symptoms are severe pain and disability. Signs are elbow fixed in moderate flexion; olecranon prominent and higher than normal; fullness in cubital fossa over front of elbow. X ray shows oclecranon and radius displaced posteriorly with humerus distal.

elbow injuries. The elbow is a hinge joint between the humerus and the ulna with a further strut, the radius, meeting the front of the humerus adjacent to the ulna and permitting the forearm to rotate as well as hinge. The arrangement allows all the complexity of throwing and turning movements that could not have been made possible by means of 1 simple hinge. The extensor muscles that raise the wrist and hand into extension originate from the lateral epicondyl on the outer side of the humerus in a common bulk before separating gradually into component muscles and tendons to the wrist and hand. Inflammation in the region of the lateral epicondyle at the origin of the supinator muscle is a common problem. It is frequently seen in tennis players and thought to be caused by overuse of an inadequately conditioned muscle group. The weekend athlete will complain of pain over the lateral epicondyle of the humerus when he or she is shaking hands, twisting a doorknob, or performing any activity that requires gripping. Examination usually reveals tenderness that often extends distally over the radial head in the extensor-supinator muscle mass. Resistance applied to the wrist extension will re-create the pain at the elbow. Lateral epicondylitis in a tennis player is thought to be produced by 1 or a combination of conditions: too large or too small a racket grip, racket strings either too tight or too loose, or an improper stroke, particularly the backhand. Probably factors creating the condition are too much tennis too early in the season or playing too much tennis in 1 day when one is not conditioned for it.

Inflammation of the flexor pronator group of muscles at their origin on the medial epicondyle of the humerus is much less frequent than lateral epicondylitis. Symptoms and physical findings are similar, the only real difference from lateral epicondylitis is that the medial epicondyle lies immediately in front of the ulnar nerve. Occasionally the inflammation may be extensive enough to irritate the ulnar nerve, with the athlete complaining of paresthesias in the ulnar nerve area. The elbow is a very stable joint powered by a strong bicep in flexion and the strong triceps in extension. Therefore, sprains and strains are uncommon injuries, even in the most violent of sports. When

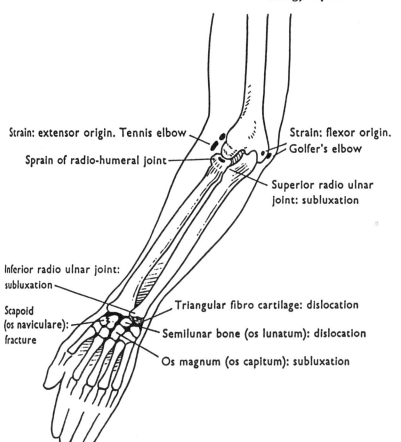

Strain: extensor origin. Tennis elbow

Sprain of radio-humeral joint

Strain: flexor origin. Golfer's elbow

Superior radio ulnar joint: subluxation

Inferior radio ulnar joint: subluxation

Scapoid (os naviculare): fracture

Triangular fibro cartilage: dislocation

Semilunar bone (os lunatum): dislocation

Os magnum (os capitum): subluxation

Elbow and wrist injuries.

they do occur, the symptoms and findings are usually similar to those of other joint injuries, depending on whether they are 1st, 2nd, or 3rd degree. Treatment depends on severity of the sprain.

electrolyte loss during exercise. Sweat is hypotonic in comparison with other body fluids. Excessive sweating may cause an exercising individual to lose significant amounts of electrolytes, especially sodium and chloride. The concentration of sodium in sweat, ranges from 50 to 80 mEq/l, and the concentration of chloride ranges from 30 to 60 mEq/l. The concentration of potassium, calcium, and magnesium in sweat seldom exceeds 5 mEq/l. Physical conditioning and acclimation to exercise in heat reduce the loss of salt in sweat, but the sweating rate is higher among conditioned or acclimated people.

energy expenditure. During optimal health function of individual body parts depends upon total body function, and vice versa. For that to continue, a relatively constant cellular environment must be maintained and body fluid compositions kept constant. Muscle metabolism varies greatly from rest to maximal exercise. Muscles use about 100 times as much energy during peak activity as is used in rest. Nerve cells are always highly active metabolically, regardless of whether a person is asleep or is engaged in demanding mental gymnastics. The widely varying needs of muscles during rest and effort must be accommodated. The resting metabolic rate for a 75-kg person is about 7 MJ (1,700 kcal) per 24 hours, or equivalent to the energy expended in walking 35 km to 50 km. Carbohydrates and fats are the main substrates for muscle metabolism, but protein breakdown also occurs during extended or strenuous physical activity. Increasing work rates during certain athletic performances lead to greater carbohydrate utilization. An important effect of physical training is the capacity of the body to oxidize fat for energy and decrease the use of glycogen for that purpose. The glycogen-conserving mechanism improves physical performance in many situations, but that is particularly seen in long-distance events. Training improves physical performance because the number and size of skeletal muscle mitochondria are increased, and mitochondrial enzymes are favorably modified. There is also increased capillary density per unit of muscle tissue, which reduces the distance nutrients have to travel between capillaries and muscle cells. Maintenance of constant body weight depends upon balanced energy intake and expenditure, even though energy expenditure may vary widely. If it is less than calorie intake, and particularly if it is below a certain level, the surplus intake usually leads to obesity. In that condition satiety is reached only after larger amounts of energy have been taken in than have been utilized.

energy source. The energy sources for muscular work have been traditionally divided into anaerobic and aerobic. The primary process supplying the free energy necessary to do work has been identified as the splitting of the higher energy phosphate bonds, adenosine triphosphate (ATP), adenosine diphosphate (ADP), phosphocreatine (PC), in general the high-energy phosphates. Those compounds are found in varying concentrations in all living cells and particularly in those, like muscle fibers, that are differentiated for contraction. They are the special form of chemical energy in which the energy (set free by the oxidation of the substrate or by anaerobic glycolysis) is stored so that it can be released to the tissues upon demand. The amount of energy set free by the oxidation of 1 mole of glucose is about 690 kcal. However, only 400 kcal-mole glucose is captured in the form of high-energy phosphates and therefore available to perform work. When oxidative resynthesis of the high-energy phosphates is limited or blocked (such as in hypoxia or anoxia), the energy necessary for the process may be derived from another energy-yielding process, that is, anaerobic glycolysis. When a series of nerve impulses reaches muscle fiber, the splitting of ATP into ADP and inorganic phosphate (P_1) occurs together with the liberation of energy. Actin and myosin utilize the energy (set free by the ATP splitting) and combine into actomyosin (that process being the basis of muscle contractions). Actomyosin, on the other hand, when activated with calcium ions, acquires an ATP activity. In the presence of oxygen, the energy required for the resynthesis of PC is drawn from oxidative reaction without any lactic acid formation.

environmental stress. Symptoms of altitude sickness may appear at elevations of only 4,500 feet. At 7,500 feet they are common. At 10,000 feet they are felt by almost everyone during the first week of acclimation. They include headaches, anorexia, fatigue, and vague muscle aches. In most people they are completely gone after the 1st week. In persons who are more seriously affected and in higher altitudes (15,000 feet to 29,000 feet), altitude sickness may become subacute or chronic. Pulmonary edema occurs in some individuals as the result of prolonged (several days) exposure to high altitude. It is most apt to occur in those who are lifted suddenly to a high altitude and least likely to occur in experienced climbers who make their way up slowly in stages. Owing to excessive salt loss under conditions of high ambient temperature, heat cramps may be prevented effectively by loading the system with salt before exposure.

Heat exhaustion is primarily due to loss of body water with resultant decreases in venous return to the heart or collapse. Peripheral vasodilation and pooling of blood in the lower extremities caused by standing for long periods also contribute to that condition. Failure of the body to be able to dissipate heat at a rate faster than it is being stored is due to the ambient temperature and humidity. The continuing high rate of heat production and absorption is responsible for heat stroke. The critical period comes when sweating ceases, as a result of the onset of hydromeiosis, causing the body to lose its chief cooling mechanism. Prolonged exposure of the human body to very cold temperatures without adequate protection will produce hypothermia and, if not counteracted by rewarming, possible death. The relative humidity of the air is a negligible factor, but if clothing is wet through or if the individual is in the water, hypothermia will come on more rapidly. The effect of the air movement around the body is of paramount importance. Frostbite results from cooling of the skin and subcutaneous tissues to the point where the circulation becomes (frozen) virtually zero. If not rapidly corrected, the skin loses its viability.

epithelium.   Forms a protective covering for the body and all its organs, being the main tissue of the outer layer of the skin. It forms the lining of the intestinal tract, the respiratory and urinary passages, the blood vessels, the uterus, and other body cavities. Epithelium has many forms and purposes. The cells, of which it is composed, vary accordingly. As an example, the cells of some kinds of epithelium produce secretions, such as mucus, digestive juices, perspiration, and other substances. The digestive tract is lined with a special kind of epithelium whose cells not only produce secretions but also are designed to absorb digested foods. The air we breathe passes over another form of epithelium that lines the respiratory tract. That lining secretes mucus and has tiny hairlike projections, called cilia. Together, the mucus and cilia help trap bits of dust and other foreign particles that could otherwise reach the lungs and damage them. Some organs, such as the urinary bladder, must vary a great deal in size during the course of their work. And for that purpose, there is a special wrinkled, crepelike type of epithelium that is capable of great expansion but will return to its original form once the tension is removed (such as when the bladder is emptied). Certain areas of the epithelium (those that form the outer layers of the skin) are capable of modifying themselves for greater strength whenever they are subjected to unusual weak and tear (the growth of calluses is an example). Epithelium will repair itself very quickly if it is injured. Sometimes, however, particularly after repeated injury, abnormal growths will occur, which are given the general name of tumors.

erysipelas.   A debilitating condition more common in basketball elbow blows than in other sports trauma. It can attack an athlete who has low resistance and has received a head injury. A bright red lesion (St. Anthony's fire) appears in the infected skin, peaking 4 to 8 days after injury and infection. Upon suspicion of erysipelas, immediate referral to a physician should be made. While the infection is active, the athlete's vision and timing are impaired (up to 3 months) to some degree, some balding may occur, and associated apathy and listlessness are common. It usually takes an athlete about 6 weeks to recover his or her full competition strength, but symptoms begin to ebb after 3 weeks.

exercise.   The exercising athlete is performing work; the endurance athlete, the runner, the swimmer, or the cross-country skier must work to accelerate and then maintain his or her pace. The weight lifter or football player also performs work, even if no motion occurs. Power, the rate at which work is performed, is the usual measure of work capacity. The mechanic efficiency of work is the proportion of energy input that is transformed to external work. Power demands in athletics vary with the type of activity and the rate at which it is performed. The hyperpnea of exercise is paralleled by the increased oxygen demand of the respiratory muscles themselves. Human work, including athletics, is always accomplished by muscle contraction, which is powered by the high-energy phosphate bonds of adenosine triphosphate (ATP). The ATP stored within a muscle will meet energy requirements only transiently, for less than 1 second. Regeneration of ATP by creatine phosphate is another short-term, limited ATP source. Sustained exercise, with continued demand for ATP, ultimately requires the utilization of body stores. Fuels available for exercise include fats and carbohydrates. Protein utilization requires muscle and parenchymal tissue breakdown and does not occur with ordinary endurance exercise. Body stores are primarily in the form of fat. The carbohydrate is stored principally as muscle glycogen, 350 g, and hepatic glycogen, 40 g to 90 g. Those fuel supplies vary with diet and exercise patterns. Muscle cells convert fats and carbohydrates to ATP through both aerobic and anaerobic processes. During exercise the muscles utilize muscle glycogen and blood-borne glucose as carbohydrate fuel. Skeletal muscles are a mixture of 2 fiber types, which vary in their capacity to sustain aerobic metabolism. The fuels utilized during exercise vary with the intensity and duration of the activity. Initially, before circulatory compensation occurs, stored ATP and regenerative ATP (derived from creatine phosphates) drive muscle contractions. Anaerobic glycolysis is also important initially but declines unless the work load is high. In the early phases of sustained exercise, muscle glycogen is the principal energy source. Subsequently, uptake of blood-borne glucose and free fatty acids increases. As muscle glycogen supplies are depleted during the first hour of exercise, blood-borne glucose becomes the major source of carbohydrates. With continued exercise, glucose utilization may decline, while free fatty acid utilization continues to increase and becomes the predominant energy source. Heavy exercise increases the demand for muscle glycogen.

extensor digitorus longus tenosynovitis (toe). The excessive forcible use of toe extensors, as in running early in the season and in tight-fitting shoes. Symptoms are pain over dorsum of foot and toes, especially on movement. Signs are tenderness, swelling, and crepitus over dorsum of foot and toes; pain elicited by active extension and passive flexion of toes; and active dorsiflexion and passive plantarflexion of ankle. Complications may be persistent disability and recurrence.

extensor hallucis longus tenosynovitis. Possibly caused by excessive forcible use of great toe extensor, as in running early in season or tight-fitting shoes. Symptoms are pain over foot and great toes, especially on movement. Signs are tenderness over dorsum of great toes, pain elicited by active extension, possible flexion of great toes, and active dorsiflexion and passive plantarflexion of ankle. Complications may be persistent disability and recurrence.

external barotrauma. During a diving descent below 30 feet, when the ear is protected by ear plugs or a hood, a negative pressure develops that causes the drum to bulge outward, usually without discomfort or rupture. Capillaries within the external canal may break to form small blisters in the skin of the exterior canal, which presents a roughened surface. Individuals so afflicted should avoid scuba diving.

exostoses (ear infections). A factor predisposing to otitis externa is the presence of exostoses (which grow in susceptible people) in response to the irritation of cold water on the skin of the outer ear canal. Exostoses are not related to otitis externa and are not caused by infection, but since they prevent water from draining out, they make the skin susceptible to infection. The bony swelling continues to grow while there is continued exposure to cold water. The temperature that qualifies as cold is that found in seawater and outdoor unheated swimming pools in temperate climates. They are often seen in swimmers, especially saltwater swimmers, who are often predisposed to otitis externa. The superior aspect of the canal just lateral to the pars flaccida of the drum is a favorite site of those benign bony tumors of the exterior canal. They are neither the cause nor the effect of the otitis directly. They are usually asymptomatic and rarely cause complete canal blockage, but they do encourage otitis externa because they interfere with cerumen passage and inhibit water within the ear from draining. Ear plugs may help in prevention and in avoiding continued growth, but surgical removal may be necessary.

eye defects. Myopia (nearsightedness) is a defect of development, where the eyeball is too long, or the bending of the light rays is too sharp, so that the focal point is in front of the retina. Objects at a distance appear blurred and may appear clear only if brought very near to the eye. Another visual defect is astigmatism, caused by irregularity in the curvature of the cornea or the lens. The surfaces do not bend the light rays the same amount, resulting in blurred vision with severe eyestrain. Astigmatism often is found in combination with hyperopia or myopia. Strabismus, or cross-eyedness, means that the muscles of the eyeballs do not coordinate together so that the 2 eyes are looking in different directions. There are several different kinds of strabismus (in another sense it means squint), but the cross-eyed type in which the eyeball is pulled inward (medially) is fairly common and appears in early life. Some of the symptoms of eyestrain include inflammation and infection of structures in the eyelids, as, for example, sty formation, in which oil glands on the lid's edge become infected; excessive tear formation (lacrimation); pain in the eyes; headaches and other nervous disturbances; digestive disturbances; and loss of appetite with malnutrition.

eye, globe injury. Penetrating wound, nonpenetrating contusion. Symptoms are severe pain, sensation of hot liquid escaping from eye, imparing vision, and photophobia. Signs may vary according to extent of injury including evidence of trauma, hyphema, escape of intraocular fluid, shallowness or absence of anterior chamber, tear and prolapse of iris, dislocation of lens, detached retina, optic nerve injury. Complications could lead to infection, iridocyclitis, ophthalmitis, glaucoma, or blindness.

eye infections. Inflammation of the membrane that lines the eyelids and covers the front of the eyeball is called conjunctivitis. It may be acute or chronic and may be caused by a variety of irritants and pathogens. "Pink-eye" is an acute conjunctivitis that is highly contagious and is caused by cocci or bacilli in most cases. Sometimes

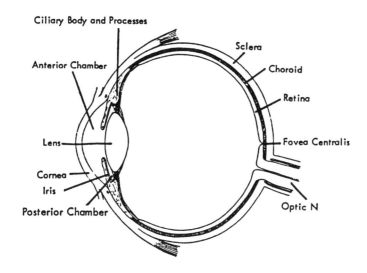

Sagittal Section of Eye.

irritants, such as wind and excessive glare, for example, from snow, may cause an inflammation that then may bring about a susceptibility to bacterial infection. Trachoma, sometimes referred to as granular conjunctivitis, is caused by a virus and is highly contagious, particularly in the early stages. That disease is characterized by the formation of granules on the lids, which may cause such serious irritation of the cornea that blindness can result. The iris, the choroid coat, the ciliary body, and other parts of the eyeball may become infected by a number of different organisms. Such disorders are likely to be very serious, but fortunately they are not very common.

eye injuries. The eyeball is well protected by the structures of the hard bony orbit and is suspended within the socket, cushioned by fat. The blink reflex, the eyelashes, and forcible close of the eyelids all provide further protection. The head will also move rapidly and reflexively if a speeding object is approaching, while the eyeball, if struck, will move within the orbit. Thus eye injuries are not so frequent as bruising and lacerations around the orbit. The eye is involved in about 2 percent of all sports injuries. Although a serious injury may not be apparent at the time of an accident, a search should be made in all cases of trauma to the eye, frontal, nasal, and temporal regions. Body contact team games frequently involve direct or glancing blows to the eyes and orbits. Those direct blows may be from the ball itself or from collision of heads, elbows, hands, or feet. Individual sports can also be a cause for serious eye injuries from rackets and balls, such as tennis, squash, or racketball. The smaller the ball the faster it travels, and the greater the risk of serious injury. Foreign bodies may blow or be thrown into the eyes in many sports whether team or individual. Mud and grit can be thrown up into the eyes from motorcycling, playing football, riding, from the surface of tennis courts and golf course sand bunkers. Severe concussive blows to the orbital region usually cause bruising and edema of the eyelids. Foreign bodies or trivial injuries to the conjunctiva may cause a subconjunctival hemorrhage. Such injuries may be caused by lightly touching the eye with a finger or perhaps a score card. Corneal abrasions occur in sports, such as water polo, wrestling, and boxing, that involve a close physical contact. They are due to fingers catching the eye and the athlete experiencing a sudden sharp pain in the eye. After a few minutes the eye becomes very red and photophobic, and it waters a great deal. Concussion injuries to the eyes, such as with a football or tennis ball, can cause hemorrhage into the anterior chamber of the eye (between the cornea and iris). The hemorrhage comes from damage to small vessels on the iris and could be potentially serious. Any moderately sharp object or a small ball of high velocity may cause penetration of the globe. A broken racket, a fall in skiing, or a hard-hit racquetball can cause rupture of the globe. Immediate loss of vision in the eye, pain, and redness follows. There is usually prolapse of the iris through the wound and hyphema. A concussion injury to the eye gives rise to retinal hemorrhages, ruptures in the choroid, retinal breaks (tears and disinsertions), and sudden failure of vision.

eye muscles. Certain muscles are inside the eyeball itself and therefore are described as intrinsic, while others are attached to bones of the eye orbit as well as to the sclera and are called extrinsic muscles. The intrinsic muscles are found in 2 circular structures: (1) The iris, the colored or pigmented part of the eye, which has a central opening called the pupil. The size of the pupil is governed by the action of 2 sets of muscles, one of which is arranged in a circular fashion, while the other extends in a radial manner resembling the spokes of a wheel. (2) The ciliary body, which is shaped somewhat like a flattened ring with a hole that is the size of the outer edge of the iris. That muscle alters the shape of the lens. The purpose of the iris is to regulate the amount of light entering the eye. If a strong light is flashed in the eye, the circular muscle fibers of the iris, which form a sphincter, contract and thus reduce the size of the pupil. On the other hand, if the light is very dim, the radial involuntary iris muscles, which are attached at the outer edge, contract, and the opening is pulled outward and thus enlarged. This pupillary enlargement is known as dilation. The pupil changes size according to whether one is looking at a near object or a distant one. A near object causes the pupil to become smaller; a far view will cause it to enlarge. The muscle of the ciliary body is similar in direction and method of action to the radial muscle of the iris. When the ciliary muscle contracts, it removes the tension of the suspensory ligament of the lens. The elastic lens then recoils and becomes thicker in much the same way that a rubber band would thicken if it were pulled and released. That action changes the focus of the lens and thus adjusts the eye for either long views or close-ups. The 6 extrinsic muscles connected with each eye are ribbonlike and extend forward from the apex of the orbit behind the eyeball. One end of each muscle is attached to the bone of the skull, while the other end is attached to the white (sclera) of the eye. Those muscles pull on the eyeball in a coordinated fashion, causing the 2 eyes to move together in order to center on 1 visual field. Located within the orbit is another muscle, which is attached to the upper eyelid. When that muscle contracts, it keeps the eye open.

eye, periorbital hematoma (black eye).   Direct blow to periorbital rim of surrounding structure, resulting in subcutaneous hemorrhage. Symptoms are local pain and possibly impaired vision. Signs are tenderness, swelling, or eccymosis of eyelids. Complications are occasionally associated with subcutaneous emphysema in presence of orbital fractures and conjunctivitis in severely swollen eyes.

eye, retinal detachment.   Choroidal hemorrhage, neoplasm, myopic degeneration, chorioretinitis. Symptoms are pain, sensation of flashing lights with trauma, impaired vision, and/or later appearance of dark cloud in visual field. Complications could be blindness and secondary glaucoma.

F

fabella fracture. Direct blow or violent contraction of gastrocnemius muscle. Symptoms are pain on posterolateral aspect of knee, especially on contraction of gastrocnemiums. Signs are tenderness over affected area, with possible disability.

facial injuries. Minor facial injuries, such as cuts and bruises, are frequent in contact sports. However, the more serious injuries, especially to the eye, must be readily recognized and referred to appropriate specialists. Injury from foreign bodies is frequent in football games on dusty grounds and in the winter months, when small pieces of grit and mud can lodge in a player's eye. Corneal abrasion can be caused by a finger in the eye during wrestling or water polo. Often the player feels that a foreign body is lodged in the eye. Anterior chamber hemorrhage can be caused by a ball or stick or a clash of heads at soccer or football games. Blood is seen in the anterior chamber obscuring the pupil and iris; later a fluid level is formed. The hemorrhage usually absorbs (heals) in 7 days. A penetrating injury can occur from a flying missile or broken racket. There may be immediate loss of vision and prolapse of the iris. Repeated or severe trauma to the orbit and temporal region can cause choroid or vitreous injuries, lens prolapse, retinal edema, and retinal detachment. The latter serious condition frequently begins with a small retinal break (dialysis), which appears in the periphery (usually temporal). However, retinal detachment may not occur for many weeks, and it is important to diagnose the dialysis before that happens. After ophthalmic surgery, the athlete is usually advised to give up contact sports, especially boxing, wrestling, and judo. Hematomas of the auricle (cauliflower ear) are caused by shearing forces. The smaller peripheral hematoma is due to small vessel bleeding, but the larger hematomas are produced by rupture of the auricular artery or vein, and the whole ear may be involved.

fainting. A common disorder that is often related to sports and usually is not a sign of any serious disease. It can follow strong emotion or pain and sometimes appears to occur almost spontaneously. Even when fainting is the result of disease, it is rarely a sign of a disease involving the nervous system. Fainting occurs following the dilatation of numerous peripheral blood vessels, particularly those in the muscles. As the blood fills those vessels, the blood supply to the brain is reduced, resulting in unconsciousness. The episode of unconsciousness is usually preceded by a period of a few seconds to several minutes in which the person feels weak. Weakness is often accompanied by restlessness and occasionally by nausea. The individual frequently breaks out in a "cold sweat," in which the body is covered with perspiration but the skin feels cold and clammy. The individual may appear quite pale, and the pulse is usually rapid. Those signs and symptoms are similar to those of shock. However, in fainting the physiological derangements are not so severe as they are in shock, and there is rarely any underlying illness that could be expected to produce shock. Unconsciousness rarely lasts for more than a few minutes. As soon as the individual feels well, he or she can be on his or her way again. A single episode of fainting is rarely significant. Repeated episodes can be indicative of a serious underlying disease.

fat pad, infrapatellar, contusion (fat pad pinch). Direct trauma or impingement of pad; usually associated with other knee joint derangements. Symptoms are sharp twinges of pain during pendulum extension and upon complete flexion of knee and a history of discomfort. Signs are tenderness at patellar ligament just below inferior pole of patella, pain-free passive extension of knee, knee instability upon weight bearing, and/or mild effusion. Complications may be traumatic arthritis, calcification, ossification, or fibrosis.

femur fracture, greater trochanter. Fall onto trochanter. Violent abducting muscular action. Symptoms are pain localized in trochanteric region upon shifting of body weight and disability. Signs are tenderness and swelling localized in trochanteric region, loose fragment, which may be palpated, pain elicited by rotation and active abduction of leg. Complications could be persistent weakness in abduction of leg.

femur fracture, intercondylar (T fracture of femur). Direct blow, as from fall onto foot or knee. Symptoms are local pain and disability. Signs are hemarthrosis (excess fluid in knee joint), marked swelling in lower half of thigh, variable amounts of visible deformity and shortening of extremity, tenderness in supracondylar region extending around femur, marked broadening of the lower end of femur visible and palpable, and/or condyles that can be squeezed together. Complications may be severe and permanent disability if reduction is not successful, chronic synovitis, or injury to popliteal vessels and nerves.

femur fracture, lateral condyle. Direct blow to lateral side of knee, fall from height onto feet, or forcible adduction torsion action. Symptoms are pain, history of severe trauma, and disability. Signs are hemarthrosis (excess fluid in knee joint), swelling, not shortening, false motion toward side of lesion if caused by avulsed lateral collateral ligament; and localized tenderness. Complications may be traumatic arthritis.

femur fracture, lesser trochanter. Excessive forcible hyperextension and abduction of hip; sudden violent strain on iliopsoas muscle. Symptoms are pain in upper and inner aspects of thigh and disability. Signs are weakness of iliopsoas muscle, tenderness and swelling in upper position, or pain elicited on hyperextension of hip. Complications may be prolonged disability.

femur fracture, medial condyle. Direct blow on medial side of knee, fall from height onto feet, forcible abduction torsion of leg. Symptoms are history of severe trauma, local pain, and disability. Signs are hemarthrosis (excess fluid in knee joint), swelling, not shortening, false motion only toward side of lesion if due to pushing up of condyle or away from side of lesion if medial collateral ligament avulsed, local tenderness, or locked knee. Complications may be traumatic arthritis.

femur fracture, neck (intracapsular femur fracture). Direct blow or fall from height. Symptoms are pain over front of hip upon leg motion, disability, inability to bear weight. Signs are leg in position of external rotation, shortening of extremity, swelling, ecchymosis, or trochanter elevated. Complications are nonunion, aseptic necrosis of femoral head and shock.

femur fracture, posterior condyle. Fall from height. Symptoms are pain over posterior aspect of knee upon movement, limited motion of knee, disability. Signs are tenderness localized to posterior aspect of knee and swelling. Complications could be persistent disability, stiffness of knee, traumatic arthritis, or vascular necrosis of fractured fragment.

femur fracture, shaft. Direct blow or fall from height. Symptoms are pain and disability. Signs are shortening of extremity, tenderness, angular deformity, false motion, swelling, or crepitus. Complications could be severe shock, delayed union, malunion, nonunion, damage to femoral or popliteal vessels and sciatic or peroneal nerves, and/or fat emboli.

femur fracture, trochanteric (extracapsular femur fracture). Direct blow or fall from height. Symptoms are pain in hip on movement of extremity, disability, inability to bear weight. Signs are swelling, shortening of extremity, leg fixed in position of external rotation, trochanter elevated, tenderness, false motion, or crepitus. Complications could be nonunion, malunion, coxa vara deformity, and/or shock.

femur fracture—separation, proximal epiphysis. Forcible torsion action, direct blow, stepping into hole when running, attempting to save self from falling after tripping. Symptoms are pain in hip, knee or along inner side of thigh followed by complete inability to bear weight actively. Signs are swelling in Scarpa's triangle, slight shortening, thigh fixed in position of external rotation and slight adduction, active movement of hip impossible, passive movements eliciting soft cartilaginous crepitus. Complications are chronic pain, traumatic arthritis, or disability.

fever. A condition in which the body temperature is higher than normal. Usually the presence of fever is due to an infection, though there can be many other causes, such as malignancies, brain injuries, toxic reactions, reactions to vaccines, and diseases involving the central nervous system. Sometimes emotional bouts can bring on a fever. It is usually preceded by chill, a violent attack on shivering, and a sensation of cold that such measures as blankets and hot water bottles seem unable to relieve. At the same time heat is being generated and stored in the body; and when the chill subsides, the body temperature is elevated. During a fever there is an increase in metabolism that is usually proportional to the amount of fever. In addition to the use of available sugar and fat there is an increase in the use of protein, and during the first week or so of a fever there is definite evidence of destruction of body protein. When a fever ends, sometimes the drop in temperature to normal occurs very rapidly. That sudden fall in temperature is called the crisis and usually is accompanied by symptoms indicating rapid heat loss: profuse perspiration, muscular relaxation, and dilated blood vessels in the skin. A gradual drop in temperature, on the other hand, is known as lysis. The body (especially the brain) cannot endure temperatures beyond about 112° level because at that point tissues are irreversibly damaged and death occurs.

fibula fracture, head. Direct blow, excessive forcible varus strain on knee. Symptoms are pain localized over fibular head and disability. Signs are tenderness and swelling about the fibular head. It may show abduction stress instability. Complications may involve peroneal nerve, biceps of the femoris tendon, or lateral collateral ligament.

fibula fracture, neck. Direct blow; excessive forcible torsion action. Symptoms are localized pain to lateral aspect of leg just below knee or disability. Signs are tenderness and swelling localized over lateral aspect of leg just below the knee, muscle spasm, or crepitus on palpation of upper fibular. Complications could be peroneal nerve injury.

fibula fracture, shaft. Direct blow to lateral side of leg; indirect leverage action. Symptoms are pain on weight bearing and disability. Signs are tenderness localized over site of fracture, false motion, crepitus usually not demonstrable, pain elicited by pressing tibia and fibula together or by rotating ankle while knee is flexed.

finger dislocation, interphalangeal.   Forcible hyperextension, direct blow to interphalangeal capsule and ligaments. Symptoms are pain and disability. Signs are deformity, swelling, limitations of motion, or instability. Complications are chronic instability and limited motion.

finger fractures.   Fracture of the epiphyseal plate of the proximal phalanx just distal to the collateral ligaments of the metacarpophalangeal joint is a common injury in sports. It results in an angular deformity, which frequently is accompanied by a possible less obvious rotational malformation. Those fractures are usually easy to reduce, but it is important to assess the rotation of the finger after the reduction. The so-called baseball or mallet finger occurs when a ball hits the tip of an extended finger, causing sudden hyperflexion injury. In the adult that frequently results in avulsion of a piece of bone with the extender tendon from the distal phalanx. Surgical repair may be indicated if there is a large amount of articular surface with this piece of bone.

finger fracture, distal phalanx.   Direct violence, crushing blow. Symptoms are a throbbing pain. The signs are swelling, tenderness, cyanosis of finger tip. Complications are bone necrosis caused by pressure, nonunion, rotary or angular deformity.

finger fracture, middle phalanx.   Direct blow, indirect force. Symptoms are pain and disability. Signs are deformity, swelling, stiffness, and crepitus. Complications are permanent deformity and stiffness.

finger fracture, proximal phalanx.   Direct blow, as in being stepped upon by cleats, may be from hyperextension, hyperflexion, or torsion forces. Symptoms are pain and disability. Signs are tenderness, swelling, or crepitus. Complications are malunion of oblique type fracture.

finger sprain, proximal interphalangeal (jammed finger).   Telescoping blow to finger. Symptoms are pain and disability. Signs are local tenderness, swelling, weakness, or variable degree of severity of joint instability. Complications are permanent deformity and stiffness.

flail chest.   If a number of ribs are broken in several places, a sizable plate of chest wall can become loosened, destroying the rigid integrity of the chest wall. Such injuries require immediate treatment, since respiratory function is usually severly impaired. The bellows action of the diaphragm and chest walls pulls air into the lungs during the inspiration by creating a negative pressure within the rigid thoracic cage. Multiple rib fractures can produce a mobile section of chest wall that moves back and forth during respiration, i.e., a flail chest. When the chest is expanded, the negative pressure pulls the loosened portion of the chest wall inward rather than pulling air into the lung. If the area of flail chest is large, ventilation may be so impaired that death ensues. If the damaged area is smaller, severe respiratory insufficiency results. Flail chest should be differentiated from a simple broken rib, which produces pain with breathing but does not interfere with the movement of air.

flatfoot.   A common disorder in which the arch of the foot, the normally raised portion of the sole, breaks down so that the entire sole rests on the ground. That condition may be congenital, in which case it usually gives little trouble. However, flatfoot can result from a progressive weakening of the muscles that support the arch, and usually that condition is accompanied by a great deal of pain. Incorrect and/or minimal use of the muscles that support the arch (especially lack of exercise) are thought to bring about flatfoot.

flexibility. Can be defined as the full range of possible movement in a joint (as in the hip joint) or series of joints (as where the vertical column is involved). All athletes need a moderate degree of flexibility to provide fluid motion and to avoid soft tissue injuries. For some, superior flexibility is essential to performance. A hurdler must have excellent hip extension and flexion flexibility, a gymnast needs back flexibility for tumbling, and the diver who cannot execute a deep pike position will never achieve outstanding success. Flexibility depends in part on the structure and alignment of bones and joints and in part on the amount of muscle and fat tissue that may restrict movement. However, the major determinant of flexibility is the condition of the muscles, ligaments, and tendons that join 2 bones. Therefore, flexibility can be improved by sports or exercises requiring substantial movement and stretching. To maintain good flexibility, stretching and movement must be performed on a regular basis.

fluid loss. Fluids are lost from the body in several ways. The "sensible loss" excreted by the kidneys ranges from 1 to 2 liters per day. The "insensible loss" of perspiration and evaporation through the lungs (to moisten air that is inhaled) amounts to approximately 1 liter daily in temperate climates and at low altitudes. An average adult requires 2 to 3 (2.1 to 3.2 qts) liters of fluid daily to replace those losses. Fluid depletion (dehydration) can result from normal losses in the presence of inadequate fluid intake or, conversely, increased loss with no increase in intake. Inability to ingest fluids may result from protracted vomiting or unconsciousness. Water shortages also reduce fluid intake. Increased fluid losses occur in a number of ways. In hot weather, or with a high fever, several liters (2+ qts) of water may be lost each day through perspiration. At high altitudes 2 to 4 quarts of fluid may be lost daily through the lungs. Severe vomiting or prolonged diarrhea also leads to fluid depletion. Deaths attributable to cholera result from severe dehydration caused by massive diarrheal fluid loss through the intestines. Salt (sodium and chlorine) and other chemical substances including potassium and bicarbonate (electrolyte) are vital constituents of body fluids. As with water, a balance between intake and loss must be maintained. The average adult's daily salt requirement is 5 g. In desert climates, where large amounts of salt are lost through perspiration, needs may climb as high as 15 g per day. The kidneys are very sensitive to change in the body's fluid balance and react immediately to conserve or eliminate water as circumstances may require. The urine volume over a 24-hour period provides the best indication of the balance between fluid intake and loss. A urine volume of less than one-half liter (500 cc) is indicative of fluid depletion; an increased volume, 2 liters (2.1 qts) or more, is a sign of excessive fluid intake.

fluid needs. The weight loss over a marathon run may exceed 5 percent of body weight, not only in top-level competitors, but also in middle-age men or women who cover the 42 km course over 5 or more hours. On a short-term basis, 1.5–2.0 kg of weight loss is covered by (a) catabolism (about 0.2 kg), (b) water produced in catabolism (about 0.3 kg), and (c) water liberated by usage of body glycogen stores (up to 1.6 kg). For that reason, the body probably tolerates a weight loss of up to 3 percent with no symptoms except thirst. However, larger losses are associated with progressively higher rectal temperatures, the danger zone of 40°C being reached with a 5 percent weight loss. Many marathon runners incur very large water deficits. The athlete who is left to follow his or her personal inclination rarely drinks sufficient fluid to maintain a water balance, either during an endurance contest or immediately afterward. The maximum possible fluid intake of an active person is still debated but is probably about 200 ml (one 8-oz glass) of fluid every 15 minutes. The early demand for sweating can be curbed by applying ice or cold water to the clothing. It is more effective to wet the thighs than the trunk, since the former have a greater surface area, are the main source of heat production, and are exposed to greater relative air movement during running.

folliculitis. Ranges from simple pimple or furuncle, which is isolated or multiple, to the coalescence of a group of furuncles producing the carbuncle. The organisms are a particular menace to the athlete, who, when the skin is soaked with sweat, may rub a lesion with the hands or clothing. They then have a means of spreading to establish new sites of infection. By personal contact and through clothing, equipment, or lockers that become contaminated, the infections can spread rapidly through a team. In the majority of the cases, the offending organisms are staphyloccoci. The hemolytic staphylococcus aureus, particularly the so-called coagulase-positive strain, is difficult to eradicate from the individual and appear to be highly contagious.

foot biomechanics. The main function of the foot is to serve as a mobile adapter, allowing itself to absorb kinetic energy and the entire body to adapt to the weight-bearing surface, and to serve as a rigid level for propulsion. The subtalar joint rotates around an axis, which allows supinatory and pronatory motion of the foot. That axis is directed 41° from the transverse plane and 17° from the sagittal plane. Normally when the foot first strikes the ground during walking or running, the heel contacts just to the outside or in a mildly inverted position. The heel wear pattern on the running shoe will give some indication where the heel is contacting the ground. Immediately, thereafter, while the ball of the foot begins to descend toward the ground, the heel bone rotates outward as the foot pronates. That pronation, or flattening out of the foot, is necessary when the entire foot meets the ground to allow for greater mobility in the rear part of the foot for adapting to varying or uneven terrain. After this time and continuing until toe-off, the heel bone rotates in the opposite direction (inverts) as the foot supinates. That allows the foot to become a rigid lever from which to propel. The phase of gait when the foot is actively resupinating is vitally important so that the foot may propel as a rigid lever with the greatest efficiency. Mechanical or structural pathology will invariably disturb the delicate balance. The most common abnormalities, such as forefoot varus, subtalar varus, and tibial varus, may not allow the foot to become rigid or resupinate when it should. The foot under those abnormal states will remain pronated or highly unstable and mobile during the later stages of gait and cause muscles to fatigue in their attempts to stabilize an unstable foot. The muscles of the foot, leg, and thigh work longer and harder than normal, and that often results in the more common overuse complaints of endurance athletes. Even without acute overuse symptoms, a runner propelling from an unstable foot is losing both energy and valuable seconds if he or she is participating in a race.

foot contusion, plantar (bone bruise). Direct trauma to plantar aspect of heel or ball of foot, as by repeated pounding on hard surface, by stepping on hard, small object or incorrectly placed spike or loose cleat, or by a wrinkle in the sock. Symptoms are persistent pain localized in site of trauma; or varying disability. Signs are local tenderness, palpable nodule at site of trauma, boggy softening of subcutaneous tissues. Complications may be circulatory, nerve, and lymph involvement as well as periosteal changes, calcification, proneness to recurrence.

foot injuries. The bony skeleton of the foot is composed of 26 bones. The talus articulates with the tibia and fibula to make up the ankle joint. The inferior surface of the talus articulates with the calcaneus, making up the subtalar joint, which contributes to the inversion and eversion foot movements. The head of the talus articulates with the navicular bone on the medial side of the foot, and the calcaneus (anterior process) articulates with the cuboid bone on the lateral side of the foot. The combination of movements of the 3 articulations—talocalcaneal, talonavicular, and calcaneocuboid—results in the complex foot movement of eversion and inversion, pronation and supination. The remaining bones of the foot are the 3 cuneiforms, 5 metatarsals, and the phalanges, 3 for each of the lateral 4 toes and 2 phalanges for the great toe. The bones of the foot are arranged structurally to form 2 arches, the longitudinal arch and the transverse arch. The arch of the foot provides an elastic, springy connection so that the jar of weight bearing is dissipated to a large extent before it reaches the long bones of the leg and thigh. The arch also has the function of improving locomotion by adding speed and agility to the gait.

Fractures of the various bones of the feet are relatively common in athletes. They vary widely in severity and in ways in which they are produced. The phalanges of the toes may be broken either as a result of an unexpected contact between the unprotected foot and a hard object, or as the result of crushing when something heavy is dropped or falls on that area. Metatarsal fractures are not uncommon. Fractures of the neck of the bone, often multiple, are produced by indirect violence. The metatarsal shafts and bases are fractured by direct violence, the 1st and 5th bones being most exposed to injury. The os calcis is one of the more common sites of fractures in the lower limb. Those injuries are due to direct violence almost invariably associated with a fall from a height on the hells, the knees and hips being extended on impact. Acute foot strain is frequently found in athletes with high, arched feet or those with flat, rigid feet. Often the condition occurs suddenly with some strenuous exercise. As a result of strain, the spring ligament, the tendons of the tibialis posticus, flexor hallucis longus, and the peronei are particularly liable to be involved. Contusion of the foot is a frequent occurrence and may be caused by any sort of direct trauma, such as being stepped on or being struck by another player. Contusion of the dorsum of the foot may be quite distressing because of the extremely sensitive nature of the area. The complications of contusion may be more important than the contusion itself. The blow may cause damage to a nerve, causing intractable pain over the dorsum of the foot, to the blood vessels with phlebitis or hemorrhage, to the tendons with resulting tenosynovitis, and to the periosteum or the joint. Several foot deformities are sources of potential problems. The cavus foot has an excessively high longitudinal arch, restricting subtalar motion, which limits the foot's ability to absorb the forces encountered during heel strikes. The opposite deformity to the cavus foot is flatfoot or pronated foot, in which the longitudinal arch is flattened. The hindfoot may be valgus or twisted. Flatfeet are classified as flexible or rigid, with flexible flatfoot the most common and usually asymptomatic in the milder forms. The rigid flatfoot is a much more difficult problem and may prohibit such activities as long-distance running. Deformities of the toes are also common, such as Morton's foot. Clawing of the toes is hyperextension of the MP joint and flexion of the IP joints, usually resulting from some subtle muscle imbalance in the foot. Painful callosities often develop on the dorsum of the IP joints from pressure against the shoe and under the metatarsal heads, where they press against the sole of the shoe.

football ankle. Disorder consists of a traumatic *osteitis,* which is sometimes confused with chronic sprain. There is general ankle pain, minimal swelling, and soreness, which is aggravated by kicking the ball. Roentgenography shows new bone formation on the margins of the inferior articular surface of the *tibia,* but the joint surfaces are not involved, as in osteoarthrosis. Conservative care with rest and graduated active exercise will usually correct the problem. If not, the spurs must be removed surgically.

forearm injuries. Injuries consist of bruises, muscle tears, and fractures. Tenosynovitis, which may cause considerable trouble in management, affects most often the extensor group in the forearm in racket players and in oarsmen. It can also be seen in canoeists. The features are typical. Pain is experienced over the dorsum of the forearm, there is palpable and visible swelling, and crepitus may be felt around the long extensor tendons. To some extent, it seems that it is associated with hypertrophy of the bellies of the abductor longus and extensor brevis muscles of the thumb, where they lie over the long extensor.

forefoot valgus. A deformity of the distal portion of the foot where the plantar aspect of the ball of the foot is everted, with the subtalar joint in the neutral position

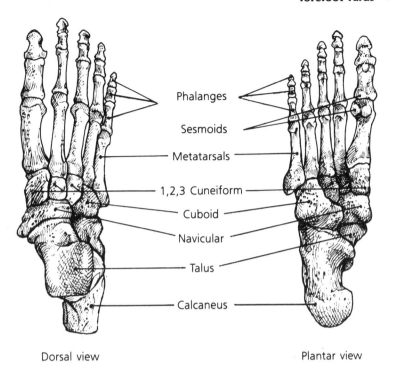

Phalanges

Sesmoids

Metatarsals

1,2,3 Cuneiform

Cuboid

Navicular

Talus

Calcaneus

Dorsal view   Plantar view

Bony skeleton of the foot.

and the midtarsal joint fully pronated. In many cases the first ray is plantar fixed. That is believed to be an acquired condition, resulting in a dynamic imbalance of the intrinsic muscles of the foot. The lack of balance could result from the activity of the peroneus longus muscles or the retrograde buckling of the hallux. The anterior tibial muscles are very weak in runners with that type of foot deformity. In the rigid type of forefoot valgus, the calcaneus strikes the floor during the gait cycle in an apparent normal position. But in about 15 percent of the gait cycle, when the ball of the foot contacts the supporting cycle, the first ray (the tibial sesamoid) assumes more of the vertical stress than is normal. The 4th and 5th metatarsal heads are not yet in contact with the floor, and the foot brings them into contact with the supporting surface. It does so by inverting at the midtarsal joint and supinating at the subtalar joint. Owing to excessive external rotation of the leg, there is excessive stress upon the tensor fascia lata muscle. Runners with rigid forefoot valgus tend to run in an unstable manner and are subject to inversion sprains. Rigid forefoot valgus types function with the foot in a supinated position during the stance phase of gait, and the runner propels off the lateral portion of the foot and digits. There is, therefore, excessive stress on the outside of the leg with chronic ankle sprains and chronic tensor fascia lata soreness. Clinically, there is very deep, nucleated callous tissue under the tibial sesamoid area and under the 4th and 5th metatarsal heads. The lesser digits are dorsally dislocated with hammer toe formation. There is a history of bursitis or periostitis of the calcaneal area.

forefoot varus.   A foot condition, probably the next most common foot type, after subtalar varus, among distance runners. In such an injury the forefoot is in a varus position. It is a fixed, congenital osseous deformity in which the plantar surface of the foot is inverted relative to the plantar plane of the rear foot when the subtalar joint rests in its neutral position and the forefoot is pronated to its maximum. Therefore, when the subtalar is in a neutral position, the forefoot is inverted and the plantar aspect faces the midline of the body. That is thought to be an ontogenetic, inherited, structural condition, caused by the lack of valgus rotation of the head and neck of the talus, relative to the body of the talus. That type of foot appears in a compensated, uncompensated, partially compensated, or supinated position. The forefoot varus is measured relative to a posterior perpendicular bisection of the calcaneus. The calcaneus is held in the neutral position to prevent unlocking of the midtarsal joint. There is compensated forefoot varus when there is enough subtalar joint pronation to allow calcaneal eversion equal to or in excess of the degree of forefoot varus. The uncompensated forefoot varus is a condition in which the subtalar joint does not allow the medial aspect of the foot to reach the transverse plane. Forefoot supinatus is a forefoot varus in which a fixed positional osseous deformity is present. It is a secondary foot deformity that occurs after long-term pronatory forces have been at work on the foot and the calcareus everts beyond the perpendicular. That is due to a shortening of the span of the anterior tibial musculature. Partially compensated forefoot varus allows subtalar pronation but not enough for the forefoot to reach the transverse plane. Therefore, the foot stays inverted until heel lift.

fractures. A break in the continuity of a bone or a separation of a bone into 2 or more parts. A great amount of soft-tissue damage may accompany such an injury. Fractures are classified as open or closed. An open fracture is one in which there is a break in the skin that is contiguous with the fracture. The bone is either protruding from the wound or exposed through a wound channel, such as one produced by an arrow, a javelin, a bullet, or other missile. A closed fracture is not complicated by a break in the skin, but there is usually soft-tissue damage beneath the intact skin. Intra-articular fractures are not uncommon in sports. They involve the articular surface of joints and the associated articular cartilage. Osteoarthrosis results if reduction is not accurate. Fracture dislocations often involve joint impaction and fragmentation. They usually represent great instability and require operative repair. Hairline fractures, where a true fracture line is not clear, may develop in the weight-bearing bones after injury and trauma. They will usually not be evident in films taken immediately after injury. Often 7 to 10 days must elapse before they can be visualized. On occasion, they are seen only by overlying periosteal elevation and callus formation, and not by a readily detected fracture line. Calcification begins in a callus from 1 to 4 weeks and is usually complete in 6 weeks, depending upon the size of the displacement. The callus may show little early evidence of calcium deposit when there is slight fragment displacement or none at all. In compound fractures, callus formation tends to be slow and irregular. Callus is not seen within joint capsules, such as in the necks of the femur, nor is it seen following fractures of the vertebral bodies, skull, or ilia. When fractures involve joints, the prognosis is guarded because it is difficult if not impossible to accurately judge how much damage is done to soft tissues or what effect fracture repair will have on function.

Frieberg's disease. An osteochondritis of the metatarsal head, usually before the epiphysis closes, similar to Perthes' disease at the hip. Freiberg's disease should be suspected when an athlete complains of pain underneath the 2nd metatarsal head. It normally occurs in the younger athlete. Examination reveals tenderness over the 2nd metatarsal head, with or without thickening of the skin. Movements of the 2nd metatarsal phalangeal joint are usually painful and restricted. X rays of the foot show an abnormal-looking 2nd metatarsal head, usually flattened and perhaps more sclerotic.

frostbite. An injury produced by cold in which the affected tissues are frozen. The hands and feet, since they are farthest from the heart and have a more tenuous blood supply, and the face and ears, which are usually the most exposed portions of the body, are the areas most usually involved. The principal effect of cold is to impair the circulation of blood to the affected area. When the body is chilled, the blood vessels in the skin contract, particularly in the extremities, reducing the amount of heat loss by radiation into the surrounding atmosphere. Thus, body heat is conserved at the expense of lowering the skin temperature. Under such circumstances, in areas that are more severely chilled, blood vessel constriction may become so severe that circulation almost totally ceases. Cold also damages the capillaries in the affected areas, causing blood plasma to leak through the walls, thus adding to the tissue injury and further impairing circulation by allowing the blood to sludge inside the vessel. As the circulation becomes severely diminished, the nervous system shuts down and all sensation of cold or pain is lost. Unless the tissue is rewarmed promptly, the skin and superficial tissues actually begin to freeze. With continued chilling, the frozen area enlarges and extends to deeper levels. Ice crystals form between the cells and then grow by extracting water from within the cells. The tissues may be injured physically by the ice crystals and by dehydration and the resulting disruption of osmotic and chemical balance within the cells. Symptoms include progressive numbness, anesthesia, prickling sensation, and mild to severe pain. Signs are yellowish white area of hard skin; subsequently, according to degree, erythema; vivid cyanosis; blisters; pallor; or sloughing of skin. Complications may be gangrene and lowered local resistance to cold.

fungus infection. Athlete's foot is caused by an organism whose distribution is universal and whose growth on human skin is favored by warmth, moisture, and breaks in the skin surface. It is not highly contagious but tends to occur among members of a sports team when they are subject to similar conditions. Tinea cruris (jock itch) is a fairly common and disabling fungus infection involving the groin area, perineum, and on some occasions the scrotum.

G

galeazzi fracture (Piedmont fracture). A fall onto the outstretched hand. Symptoms are local pain and disability. Signs are deformity, swelling, tenderness, and/or crepitus on motion over distal radioulnar area. Complications are malunion or nonunion.

gallbladder disease, acute. The gallbladder is a saclike organ on the undersurface of the liver in which bile is stored until it is discharged into the small intestine. For reasons that are poorly understood, the bile salts may be precipitated, forming gallstones. Subsequent contractions of the gallbladder to expel bile into the intestine are painful. The condition known as chronic cholecystitis or chronic gallbladder disease is characterized by recurrent episodes of colic pain and tenderness in the right upper quadrant of the abdomen. Those attacks are rarely associated with jaundice. The ingestion of fried or fatty food is usually associated with belching, indigestion, and abdominal pain. An individual with acute gallbladder disease usually has a history of chronic cholecystitis. However, in an acute attack, he or she typically suffers the rather sudden onset of a much more severe, sharp pain, located immediately below the ribs on the right. The pain may be intermittent or continuous and may radiate through to the back or the shoulder blades. Vomiting is common; diarrhea is rare. The individual appears ill and is frequently jaundiced. The urine is often dark, and the stools may be light gray or clay-colored, particularly 2 to 3 days after the onset. Right upper-quadrant abdominal tenderness is present and may be very well localized. The points of maximum tenderness, rebound tenderness, and referred pain are all in the right upper quadrant. The attack usually subsides spontaneously within 1 to 2 days.

ganglion. The most frequent location of a ganglion is the dorsoradial aspect of the wrist. A ganglion arising usually from the wrist joint, but occasionally from the interphalangeal joints, metacarpo-phalangeal joints, or tendon sheaths, can cause a degree of disability out of proportion to its size. In a true sports injury, the athlete often has sustained a sprain of the wrist. The ganglion may have been present for some time but contained entirely within the wrist joint capsule. The minor injury may produce enough weakness of the joint capsule to allow herniation of the ganglion between the extensor tendons. As a rule the synovial hernia (ganglion) will appear as a small, discrete, sometimes extremely hard nodule lying directly over the tendon or the joint capsule. It is often impossible to tell whether the primary involvement is a tendon or joint. The consistency of the tumor may vary from that of bone to a soft, fluctuant, obviously liquid mass. That difference in consistency is more apparent than real and is due to the degree of tension within the sac, since it uniformly will be found to contain a clear, gelatinous, viscous fluid that is blood-tinged only following aspiration or recent trauma. The wrist has a particular predilection for synovial hernia.

genitourinary infections. Gonococcal urethritis is the most common genitourinary infection in athletes. Mycoplasma urethritis is being identified more frequently at present. The secretion is light and glairy, as opposed to the thick, white discharge of gonococcal infection. Both infections are transmitted by sexual contact. An occasional case of urethritis and prostatitis will be due to a staphylococcal or streptococcal infection. Cystitis is unusual as an isolated phenomenon in male athletes but is more common in females. Some anomaly or infection in the upper genitourinary tract should be suspected. If prostatitis involves the seminal vesicle on the right side, it may be mistaken for acute appendicitis. The organism is usually a staphylococcus or a streptococcus. It is best treated by system administration of antibiotics and prostatic massage. Pyelitis is more common in females generally. The basis is usually some congenital anomaly involving the ureter or kidneys. Although the infection responds to the administration of appropriate antibiotics, the rate of recurrence is high.

glenohumeral dislocation, anterior (subcoracoid dislocation). A leverage force on the abducted arm, as in making an arm tackle; less frequently, a fall or blow to the shoulder from the rear. Symptoms are pain and disability.

glenohumeral dislocation, downward (subglenoid dislocation). A leverage force on the abducted arm, as in making an arm tackle. Symptoms are pain and disability. Signs are deformity with deltoid flattened and head of humerus displaced downward, head of humerus palpated in axilla, arm fixed in about 45° abduction. Complications are associated fracture of humerus, scapula, and nerve and vascular injury.

glenohumeral subluxation, anterior, recurrent. A leverage force on the abducted arm, as in making an arm tackle; forced abduction and external rotation, as in throwing, swimming, (backstroke). Symptoms are pain, momentary disability, sensation of shoulder slipping out of place, usually spontaneous relief with change of position of arm. Signs are (before reduction) obvious deformity with humerus head prominent anteriorly, marked muscle spasm, or loss of function; (after reduction) sense of uneasiness on forced abduction and external rotation of arm and head of humerus palpable slipping against glenoid rim. Complications are dislocation and chronic instability.

glomerulonephritis, acute. A disease of the kidneys that usually follows a "strep throat" or some other streptococcal infection by a few days or a few weeks. The disorder appears to be caused by an allergy to streptococcal bacteria. In mild cases, which are more common, swelling or puffiness of the face, blood in the urine, and headache are the most common symptoms. More severe cases are also characterized by edema, visual disturbances, delirium, convulsions, and coma. A low fever, loss of appetite, nausea, and vomiting may be present in mild or severe cases. With antibiotics, the incidence of glomerulonephritis has been reduced through the treatment of the initial streptococcal infection with penicillin.

gluteal contusions and strains. Contusions, especially to the ischial tuberosity and the well-developed athletic buttocks, are frequently seen in clinics. Incidence is high in hockey and field sports. Just walking may be aggravating, but pain is usually not severe. Swelling and bleeding may be extensive but is reduced quickly if cold (ice pack) is applied immediately. Recurrent bleeding is always a problem, but its likelihood is reduced if cold application is continued for 3 or 4 days. Full healing without reinjury will usually take place within a month.

golf injuries. The amount of strain placed upon the body tissues when one is striking a golf ball varies considerably from that of an ungainly weekend player to that of a smooth-flowing professional. Almost every muscle in the body is involved at 1 time or another from the intrinsic muscle of the feet to the sternomastoids and the strains placed on the components of the locomotor system. The greatest strain in golf falls upon the back. Strains of the lumbar joints and less frequently those of the cervical and thoracic spine are the most common injuries encountered. Minor congenital abnormalities of the vertebrae may predispose to injury. Local muscle strains are far less common than joint disarrangements, which may vary from minor ligamentous strain to a full prolapse of an intervertebral disk with nerve root pressure. The presence of relatively stiff areas in the spine from old osteochondritis or the early wear-and-tear changes of spondylosis are frequent predisposing factors. Strains usually occur when a mobile joint adjoins a stiff one. There are also more subtle influences, such as the splinting action of the diaphragm, extending down to the 3rd lumbar vertebra, if the breath is held in an attempt to give added power to the shot. In the older spine degenerative changes of spondylosis cause narrowing of the neuro foramen and mushroom bulging of the disks, with increased liability to root pressure. Considerable lateral and rotational strain may be placed on the knee joints, especially when one is playing from an awkward position with the feet at different levels. Most of the tendon lesions, such as tennis elbow, medial ligament strain at the knee, lateral ligament strain at the ankle, and the occasional occurrence of painful heel in the middle-aged or elderly, are due to underlying degenerative changes in the fibrous tissue structure concerned with the superimposed trauma of the game acting as the trigger, which starts off inflammation. If a full golf swing hits the ground or a hard object other than the ball, an isolated fracture of the wrist may result. The mechanism appears to be one of violent contraction of the flexor carpi ulnaris insertion through the pisiform hamate ligament. Roentgenography may show a fracture of the hamate.

golfer's elbow. A condition that is the opposite of tennis elbow in that it affects the common flexor origin on the medial side of the elbow. It includes periostitis and subperiosteal hematoma, common flexor origin strains, and sprains of the medial ligament. Ectopic calcification is not unusual and is quite often seen in excellent tennis players. In golfers it seems to be most common on the right side and is thought to be due to taking too big a pivot in the chip shot.

golfer's hip. This condition, in addition to occurring in golfers, often is found in people who have never seen a golf course, including those who are not athletic. It is common among golfers, because the golf swing is probably the only athletic maneuver in which the hips go through so great a range of various motions in conjunction with the back. When the disorder occurs, it is usually caused by a faulty swing, which leads to abnormal stresses on the hip muscles created by the improper distribution of forces. Golfer's hip is usually nothing more than a preexisting bursitis of the hip that is aggravated when one happens to play golf. Bursitis of the hip usually occurs in 1 or both of the hip bursae. The 1st is the greater trochanteric bursa, which is situated at the "point" of the hip, the greater trochanter, and overlies the abductor muscle attachment. That bursa tends to become inflamed as a result of the repeated contraction of the abductor muscles when they are fatigued or weak. The basic stance in golf is the leg spread, or hips-abducted stance. The basic motion in the golf swing, aside from the rotation of the shoulders, is the swing and rotation of the hips. When that motion is performed, and especially when it is done improperly, while the hips are abducted, it tends to put an even greater strain on the abductor muscle than usual. Another way the bursa can become chronically inflamed is in sudden twisting and rotating motions of the lower back and hip while the legs are straight and the feet firmly planted on the ground. The force of the twist, instead of being dissipated into the ground through a swing of the legs, is concentrated in the iliopsoas muscles' tendinous terminus at the hip. The stress and overload pile up at the muscle site of attachment, and inflammation of the bursae, 1 on either hip, follows. Those inflammations, either singly or in combination, are what is known as golfer's hip. When they develop as a result of playing golf, they are caused by the constant recurring traumas produced by a faulty swing. When they already exist for other reasons, playing golf will merely aggravate them.

gracillis strain. Excessive forcible flexion of the hip, as in doing the splits. Symptoms are pain along the edge of the pubic ramus radiating along the inner aspect of the thigh and disability. Signs are, graded by degrees of severity, local tenderness and swelling, pain elicited on passive abduction of thigh, ecchymosis, possibly palpable defect. Complications are persistent disability, which is prone to recurrence.

groin pulls. The word *groin* describes nothing more than that area of the midline of the body where the thighs are joined to the torso. It might be called the pubic region, since the principal bones in the site are the pubic bones of the pelvis. By a "groin pull" is meant a tear in 1 of the hip adductor muscles, those muscles that flow down along the interior of the hips and attach to the thigh bone. Tears in those muscles usually come about because of sudden, intolerable adduction stresses, such as when one tries to close the thighs against a stronger opposite force or when the legs are forced suddenly apart and the muscles are overstretched. Groin pulls are deep tears in the fibers of 1 of the hip adductor muscles, either at the top of the inner thigh or on the lower pelvis itself. They can be worrisome and annoying but are hardly ever serious. Conditioning and strengthening of the groin muscles will normally prevent them.

gymnastic injuries. Fractures and dislocations occur in falls from gymnastic apparatus. The trampoline also can cause cervical spine fractures or dislocations. The majority of the injuries occur when the trampolinist lands improperly on the bed of the trampoline. The stunt most often associated with injury is a front drop. Other feats linked with injury include the back drop, back somersault, and front somersault. The majority of injuries in trampolining are minor. Studies have shown that those gymnasts who are completely immersed in a special event develop characteristic trauma as a result. Shoulder problems of the ring specialist were sited and the "wrist splints" of the gymnast on the pommel horse. The latter problem is apparently an overuse injury of the forearm and wrist that is analogous to the injury of the soft tissue attachments at the tibia in the runner. The gymnast with wrist or forearm splints may have pain in the midforearm or at the wrist. It is believed that most all-around gymnasts are eventually troubled with the problem. The pattern of injuries in men's gymnastics differs from that in women gymnastics largely because of the pursuit of different events. Although men perform free exercises of tumbling and vaulting, as do women gymnasts, men tend to dominate the activity on the rings, parallel bars, and pommel horse. A study of injuries and epidemiologic data related to girls and gymnastics revealed that the major activities in which the injuries occurred were tumbling, exercising on uneven bars, horse vaulting, using the balance beam, engaging in general activity involving more than 1 event, and performing free exercise other than tumbling. The ankle was the most injured body area; injuries included ankle sprains, fractures, and dislocation. Nearly all of the ankle sprains were inversion-type injuries during tumbling and free exercise. Backward tumbling is a dominant maneuver in tumbling and free exercise and was the major activity linked with the injuries. The lower back was the second-most-important injured body area. Other injury sites include the foot and the knee.

H

hamstring pulls. The hamstring muscles are the long, thick muscles along the rear of the thigh that are the primary knee flexors. They are highly prone to running injuries. They take the form of a tearing apart of muscle fibers, usually when sprinting, and can incapacitate the weekend athlete for weeks on end. When one runs at full speed, tremendous pressure is exerted on the hamstring muscles as the knee travels rapidly through the flexion-extension process. When the muscles are weak or unconditioned, they often cannot stretch as far as the legs do. Like all muscles, when the stresses are repeated, as in a 30- or 40-yard sprint in pursuit of a pop fly or long pass, the hamstrings can snap. The sensation of a hamstring pull is similar to that of a plantaris rupture. It feels as though the person has been whacked across the back of the thigh with a hot poker. The fibers in the muscle will tear apart suddenly, and the individual will pull up lame with an intensely searing pain. Further running will be impossible, and even walking will be difficult. A hamstring pull is not a serious ailment but can be discomforting for the 8 to 10 weeks it takes for a major tear to heal.

hamstring strain. Muscular discoordination, poor body mechanics, altering stride, inadequate warmup, fatigue cramps, sudden violent stretch or contraction. Symptoms are sudden acute pain and subsequent discomfort at the area of involvement and disability. Signs are graded by degree of severity: tenderness to tenseness at area of involvement, usually at ischial tuberosity, middle of posterior aspect of thigh, or popliteal region; gap or bunching possibly palpable; possible hematoma. Complications may be prolonged disability and recurrence.

hand fractures. Such injuries are common in most sports; for example, in hurling, hand fractures may account for a quarter of all fractures. Fractures in that area almost always unite, but finger stiffness is a handicap both in sports and in everyday living; malunion is less disabling than stiffness.

hand injuries. The bones of the hand and wrist are connected by joint capsules and ligaments. Each bone, except the carpals, is joined by tendons that flex or extend the joints on the dorsal and palmar surfaces. At the proximal levels, intrinsic muscles of the hand also produce motion on either side. The hand's location at the end of the extremity and its function expose it to a wide variety of traumatic episodes. The most common contusions of the hand in the athlete come as a result of direct impact, such as from a foot on the outstretched hand with the fingers extended or from a blow of the fist against an opposing blunt object with the fingers closed. Very often those will result in a combination of an abrasion and a contusion or a contusion and a laceration. The most common injuries to the fingertips are direct contusions, such as a blow from a hard missile like a baseball or a jamming of the fingertip against an object, and crush injuries. Subungual hematomas, a collection of blood beneath the nail, often form. The "mallet" or "baseball finger" is caused by a sudden flexion force on the distal interphalangeal joint while the finger is actively extended, such as when the player is poised to catch a ball. The extensor tendon ruptures at or near its insertion on the terminal phalanx and can no longer actively extend the terminal joint. The counterpart of the mallet finger, the "jersey finger," is caused by a sudden, forceful extension of the DIP joint while held in flexion, typically when a tightly held jersey is torn out of the grasp of a would-be tackler. An avulsion of the long flexor tendon can result. Injuries of the proximal finger joint can occur in the same manner as described for the fingertips. In addition, forceful twisting injuries may occur as a result of grabbing or being grabbed or catching fingers on an opponent's clothing or equipment. The thumb has only 2 phalanges and 1 interphalangeal joint. Generally, all of the injuries described for the fingers can also affect the thumb. Because the MCP joint of the thumb is more exposed than its counterparts in the fingers, it is subject to an injury peculiar to that joint, in which there is a rupture of the ulnar collateral ligament of the thumb. It is seen in many contact sports, such as football and wrestling, as well as in skiing. It is caused by forceful abduction of the thumb away from the hand, with the MCP joint in extension. On examination there is usually local tenderness on the ulnar side of the MCP joint. Contusions of the thenar and hypothenar eminence are seen, especially in baseball, hockey, and handball players. They follow trauma and appear as tender, painful swellings of the fleshy areas at the base of the thumb or the little

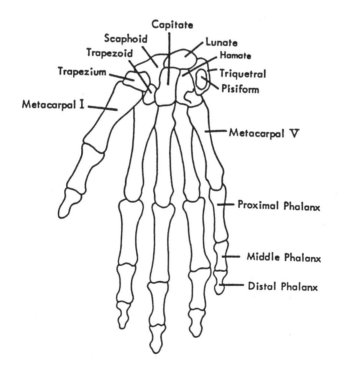

Bones of the Hand.

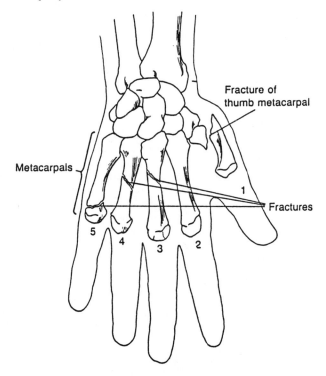

Metacarpals

Fracture of
thumb metacarpal

1

Fractures

5

4

3

2

Common Fractures of the Hand

finger. Metacarpal fractures, particularly of the neck of the 5th metacarpal, are relatively common. They are caused by a direct blow to the MCP joint with a clenched fist, as when striking a hard object. Ordinarily, the MCP joint is depressed, and there is tenderness, swelling, and angulation on the back of the hand.

handlebar palsy. An overuse injury experienced by bicyclists occasionally seen, which is a neuropathy secondary to injury of the deep palmar branches of the ulnar nerve (handlebar palsy). The trauma results from prolonged severe pressure on the handlebars during long races. The clinical picture is one of muscle weakness and wasting in the intrinsic muscles of the hands without sensory impairment.

hay fever and asthma. Sensitivity to plant pollens, to dust, to certain foods, and to other allergens may lead to hay fever or asthma or both. Hay fever is characterized by a watery discharge from the eyes and nose, and about half of all hay fever attacks end in asthma. In asthma the symptoms usually are due to a spasm of the involuntary musculature of the bronchial tube walls. It constricts the tubes so that the individual cannot exhale easily. He or she experiences a sense of suffocation and has labored breathing (dyspnea). Athletes may have to curtail physical activity during hay fever or asthmatic episodes.

head and neck trauma. Obstruction within the upper airway is the 2nd most common cause of death resulting from head and neck trauma. Thus, the priority concern in any anterior neck injury is impairment of the airway. In that regard, the cricoid and thyroid cartilages are quite vulnerable to direct trauma of the neck. Any injured person tends to hyperventilate. Thus, ventilation is not difficult to assess. A minor airway obstruction may soon become suddenly life threatening or be delayed for several hours after injury. The larynx may be crushed between a blunt object and the anterior cervical spine, leading to cartilaginous fracture, subluxation, and/or dislocation. The most common fracture of the thyroid cartilage is that of a vertical anterior split between the thyroid notch and the cricothyroid membrane, producing avulsion of the anterior vocal cord attachment and hematoma.

head injuries. Participation in many sports carries some risk of injury to the head and is more pronounced in body contact and vehicular sports. Boxing by its very nature causes indirect head injury in which the point of impact is the chin with concussive effects probably transmitted to the brain stem from the skull base. Punches to the side of the head may cause shearing damage because of the abrupt lateral or rotational movements with tearing of bridging vessels. Secondary injury may occur when the head strikes the floor of the ring as the boxer falls. In football trauma can result from hard contact between players, by striking the ground, and sometimes from an opponent's fist or shoe. In motor and motorcycle racing the vehicle or ground causes the damage. In swimming, the injury may be caused by diving with the head extended or striking the bottom of the pool, river, or seabed, particularly where there are rocks. In any head injury it is the brain damage that matters the most. It is well recognized that a fatal brain injury may occur without blemish to the scalp or a skull fracture. The simplest form of brain injury is concussion, the essential feature of which is its reversibility, with complete recovery occurring within a few seconds or minutes. Electroencephalogram studies have confirmed that changes in rhythm do not persist for more than 4 minutes. In more severe cases there may be brain laceration or contusion, particularly if the skull is fractured. Secondary complicating factors, such as hemorrhage, cerebral edema, and late infection, may ensue. In head injuries there is usually a loss of consciousness; confusion, irritability, headache, nausea, vomiting, photophobia, and double vision are often present. Serious signs are increasing confusion, dilated or irregular pupils, rapid and feeble pulse, rapid respiration, and weakness and sensory disturbances, including ataxia, in the limbs. Skull fractures are classified as simple or compound; linear or depressed. Classically a boggy swelling is found over the fracture. Blows to the nasal or frontal region may injure the delicate cribriform plate with resulting rhinorrhea. A black eye appearing some hours later with little or no damage to the skin around the eye and with a flame-shaped subconjunctival hemorrhage indicates a fractured anterior fossa. Blood in the ear that does not clot because of admixture with cerebrospinal fluid indicates a middle or posterior fossa fracture. The latter fracture may also produce a boggy swelling at the nape of the neck or behind the mastoid process. The simplest head injury in sports is a concussion. Its essential feature is sudden loss of consciousness at the moment of injury with full physiological recovery within a few minutes. The loss of consciousness is so transient that there may not be time for accurate observations, but there is often pallor, slowness, and feebleness of the heartbeat, shallow breathing, and abolition of reflex function. The changes occurring in concussion are reversible, and there are no visible structural abnormalities.

headache. A common ailment suffered by all but a very few individuals and usually attributed to tension, migraine, abnormal sinus, tumor, vascular disorders, or hysteria. Often-neglected causes are excessive eyestrain, overall postural strain, and/or trauma to the cervical spine. Headaches caused by viscerosomatic reflexes from the gallbladder, stomach, and duodenum are much more common than suspected. Nausea or vomiting with headaches is usually considered to have a neurologic basis of a vascular nature. However, a vagal disturbance owing to upper cervical function may be the offender. Rarely can any specific cause for a headache be identified. The disorder is frequently thought of as a disease in itself, although it is often only a symptom of another illness or disorder. The pain of a headache may be located in the back of the neck, behind the eyes, or in all areas in between. Little significance can be attached to the location of the pain except for those cases in which it is limited to 1 side of the head. Undilated headaches are frequently caused by a vascular disorder, such as migraine. A severe, persistent headache in an individual who usually does not suffer from headaches may be a sign of serious imbalances and/or disease. Headaches associated with confusion, forgetfulness, dizziness, nausea, and vomiting and occasionally convulsions or loss of consciousness may be the result of an acute increase in blood pressure (hypertensive encephalopathy). That disorder usually occurs in persons with preexisting hypertension but requires prompt treatment to avoid brain damage. Headaches associated with fever and a stiff neck are characteristic of meningitis. Following a head injury, headaches of increasing severity may be indicative of the development of a blood clot or a tumor within the skull. Aspirin, every 4 hours, relieves the pain of most headaches.

heart.   The bulk of the wall of the heart is made up of cardiac muscle, the myocardium. It is lined with a thin membrane, the endocardium, and is enclosed in a sac formed by a 2-layered serous membrane, the pericardium. A thin film of fluid in the pericardial sac prevents friction between the layers. The human heart is really a double pump, each half quite separate from the other. The right side serves as a pump for the pulmonary circulation. Its upper chamber, the right auricle, or atrium, receives venous blood, with its reduced load of oxygen, from the tissues, via the superior and inferior venae cavae. It passes the blood into the lower chamber to the right ventricle, which drives it into the lungs, where it gives up its increased quantities of carbon dioxide and takes on fresh supplies of oxygen. The left side serves as a pump for the systemic circulation. Its upper chamber, the left auricle, receives the freshly oxygenated blood, via 4 pulmonary veins, from the lungs, passes it into the lower chamber, the left ventricle, which then pumps it into the aorta, and on around the body to supply the tissues with oxygen and nutrients.

heart disease classification.   There are many ways of classifying heart disease. The 3 layers of the heart wall form the basis for 1 grouping of heart pathology, as follows: (1) Endocarditis, which means "inflammation of the lining of the heart cavities" but which usually refers to valvular disease. (2) Myocarditis, or inflammation of the heart muscle. (3) Pericarditis, referring to diseases of the serous membrane on the heart surface as well as that lining the pericardial sac. Another more generally used classification of heart disease is based on causative and age factors. On that basis, the more common kinds of heart disease are (1) Congenital heart disease, that is, present at birth. (2) Rheumatic heart disease, which begins with an attack of rheumatic fever in childhood or in youth. (3) Coronary heart disease, which involves the walls of the blood vessels that supply the muscles of the heart. (4) Degenerative heart disease, which is most common after the age of 45 and is due to deterioration of tissues, such as muscles, and the prolonged effects of various disease conditions.

heart function.   The function of the heart is to maintain an adequate supply of blood to all the tissues of the body. The supply of blood is maintained by rhythmical contractions of the heart. Those contractions occur at a rate of about 60/min or less in the average healthy adult. Atrial contraction occurs first, followed by ventricular contraction, and there is a short period of time when both chambers relax and fill with blood. That series of events is called the cardiac cycle. The following series of events occurs in the cardiac cycle: (1) The atria contract, filling the ventricles, called atrial systole, which lasts about 0.1 second. (2) As atrial contraction ceases, the ventricles contract. The mitral and tricuspid valves are then closed, and blood is pumped out into the aorta and pulmonary artery. That phase is called ventricular systole and lasts about 0.3

seconds. (3) The ventricles then relax, and the pulmonary and aortic valves close to prevent backflow of blood into the ventricles. At the same time the mitral and tricuspid valves open. Blood from the inferior and superior venae cavae then flows into the right atrium, and blood from the pulmonary veins flows into the left atrium. The tricuspid and mitral valves are open at this time, and the blood flows onward into the ventricles. That period, when both the atria and ventricles are relaxed and filling with blood, is called diastole and lasts about 0.4 seconds.

heart, myocardium contusion.   A direct blow to the chest, such as in baseball or boxing. Symptoms are local pain. Signs are tachycardia, fibrillation of auricles, ventricles, arrhythmia. Complications are cardiac failure, rupture of myocardium aneurysm, valvular incompetence, perforation of septum, traumatic pericarditis, and possible death.

heart problems (young athletes).   Many children who have had rheumatic heart disease have recovered with minimal valvular and myocardial damage and are able to participate safely and effectively in sports. However, each case must be evaluated individually. The great majority of young persons who have congenital heart disease, with or without surgical correction, will not present themselves for sports participation. The exceptions might be those who have small intra-auricular or intra-ventricular septal defects and no cyanosis or functional deficits and those who have had surgical ligation or a patent ductus arteriosus. They, too, should be evaluated individually. Young persons may suffer from coronary artery disease. Since the initial occlusion in a young individual (under 20) is frequently fatal, there may be no previous warning of the condition. The occurrence of precordial pain with any of the usual types of radiation should be carefully investigated before and during exercise. Positive identification of coronary disease should lead to a therapeutic exercise program rather than sports participation. Sinus arrhythmia is the chief cause of irregular heart activity in young persons and is normal up to age 35. Premature beats are the next most common and are often associated with air swallowing and other benign upper gastrointestinal conditions. Neither of those should prevent activity in sports. Paroxysmal atrial flutter and/or fibrillation is potentially more serious but is not an uncommon finding in competitive athletes.

heart rates.   A slow-resting heart rate, which is often slightly irregular, is very common in endurance athletes. It may be as slow as 30 beats/min. For a healthy athlete (without congenital disorders), the slower beats (30 to 50) are good evidence of an efficient cardiovascular system. If the heart rate is very slow, the effect of vigorous exercise should be to remove the vagal tone and increase the heart rate to well over 100 beats/min. However, the exercise target heart rate is age dependent. If the bradycardia is caused by congenital complete heart block, the heart rate may rise to 90 beats/min or even slightly more, but a normal pulse rate response to exercise will not be possible. Congenital complete heart blocks would have to be confirmed by a stress ECG recording but of itself may not preclude competitive sports, since maximum oxygen uptake levels in those people may fall within the range of normal for nonendurance athletes.

heart sounds.   During the cardiac cycle 2 heart sounds can be heard over the chest wall. The first is caused by the closing of the A-V valves (near the beginning of ventricular systole). The second is caused chiefly by the snapping shut of the semilunar valves at the beginning of ventricular diastole. When a doctor examines a heart with a stethoscope, he or she gains information about the state of the heart valves. Any disease that damages them tends to reduce their efficiency and may alter the quality of the heart sounds. Additional "murmurs" may be heard. Heart valves, for example, are frequently affected in rheumatic fever. The inflamed endothelial lining may heal with scarring. That may distort the valve flaps so that when they shut they do not meet properly and so fail to close off the cavity of the ventricle from that of the auricle. In those circumstances, blood can lead back through the A-V valve as the ventricular muscle continues to contract in ventricular systole. As blood leaks through the "incompetent" valve in ventricular systole, an additional "murmur" can be heard over the chest wall.

heat acclimatization for endurance training. Heat acclimatization may reduce the risk of heat stroke in those engaged in such sports as marathon runs. Physiologic studies of heat acclimatization have shown that training alone without acclimatization improves blood flow to the muscles. However, after acclimatization and training, there is an even greater improvement in muscle blood flow so that better performance can be expected at similar work loads after acclimatization. In normal individuals before endurance training, fairly high temperature loads are necessary to induce sweating. After training, however, lower temperatures reflexively activate sweat rate, and a further increase in sweat occurs with a rise in central temperatures. After acclimatization, however, sweat rates increase rapidly at considerably lower temperatures of skin and central core temperature so that cooling and sweat evaporation start much earlier than in nonacclimated athletes. Heat acclimatization can be achieved by exposure to hot and humid environments or by adjusting the microclimate through heavy sweats and windbreakers under cool environmental conditions. Once acclimatization has been achieved, which usually requires about 10 days of heat training, it will last for a period of 7 to 10 days after heat exposure has ceased.

heat balance. The body is a relatively inefficient machine. It performs best in such sports as distance running and cycling, but even during such activities 75 percent or more of the caloric content of the food consumed appears as heat rather than athletic endeavor. If the activity is brief, the heat can be stored within the body as a rise of temperature. A modest heating of the active muscles is valued by most athletes as a "warm-up" for competition, but an excessive rise of core temperature can be dangerous. For the body temperature to remain constant, heat production must balance heat loss. Heat production depends on the type and on the amount of food eaten and on the degree of activity of tissue cells, especially of the "active" tissues, such as the liver and skeletal muscles. Some 90 percent of the energy released by the oxidation of foodstuffs appears in the body as heat. It is dispersed to the tissue fluids that surround every living cell and is transported rapidly throughout the body by the bloodstream. The human body, like any other hot object in space, loses heat from its surface to its colder surroundings by: (1) radiation, the direct transfer of heat through the air in the same way as the sun heats the earth, and (2) convection, heat lost by warming the air in contact with the body. That air expands and rises away from the body. Cold air flows in to take its place. That in turn is warmed, expands, and rises away from the body. Convection currents are thus set up. (3) conduction, heat lost to a colder object with which any part of the body is in direct contact. The amount lost from the body in those ways depends on the caliber of the small blood vessels near the surface of the skin and on the amount of blood flowing through them. If the skin's blood vessels are dilated, more blood comes to the surface and more heat can be lost by radiation, convection, and conduction. In temperate zones, heat lost that way averages about 21,000 kilocalories per day. In addition, small amounts of heat are used in warming ingested food and fluid and inspired cold air; small amounts are lost in the feces and in urine, since they leave the body at around 27°C. If those were the only methods of heat loss available to the human body, however, it would be unable to lose heat when the environmental temperature was higher than its own. In such conditions the body would, in fact, gain heat from its surroundings by radiation, convection, and conduction. When the outside temperature rises or heat production activity of muscles increases, other mechanisms come into play.

heat cramps. Muscle cramps are severe, spasmodic contractions of 1 or more muscles that most frequently involve the legs or abdominal muscles. The cramps may last up to 15 minutes or, on rare occasions, even longer. The involved muscle is sometimes sore for several days afterward. Frequently cramps can be stopped almost instantly by stretching the involved muscle. For example, a cramp in the calf muscle can often be abolished by extending the leg and pointing or pulling the toe upward as far as possible. Fibrillating (gently rolling) the cramped muscles is often effective for relief. Kneading or pounding the muscle is less effective and may contribute to the residual soreness. No etiology can be identified for most muscle cramps, although salt deficiency may be a common cause. Under circumstances in which increased losses of salt could occur, muscle cramps, heat cramps, or salt cramps, as they would then be called, are indicative of salt depletion. Oral administration of salt and water should provide prompt relief from repeated episodes of cramps.

heat exhaustion. Can involve individuals in excellent physical condition and is caused by prolonged physical exertion in a hot environment. In such situations the blood vessels in the skin can become so dilated (enlarged) that the blood supply for the brain and other vital organs is reduced to inadequate levels. Dehydration may also cause a mild reduction in blood volume. The result is a physiological disorder that is similar to fainting and is rarely serious unless complicated by some coexisting disease. Lack of acclimatization to heat or even minor degrees of dehydration or salt deficiency make an individual more susceptible to heat exhaustion. At the time of onset the individual feels faint and is usually aware of rapid heart rate. Nausea, vomiting, headache, dizziness, restlessness, and even loss of consciousness are not uncommon. Most important from a diagnostic standpoint, the individual's temperature is not significantly elevated and may be below normal. The presence of sweating and the skin color are variable.

heat loss. More than 80 percent of heat loss occurs through the skin. The remaining 15 to 20 percent is dissipated via the respiratory system and through the urine and feces. Networks of blood vessels in the deeper part (corium or dermis) of the skin are capable of bringing considerable quantities of blood near the surface so that heat can be dissipated to the outside. That can occur in several ways. Heat can be transferred to the surrounding air (conduction). Heat also travels from its source in the form of heat waves or rays (radiation). If the air is moving so that the layer of heated air next to the body is constantly being carried away and replaced with cooler air (as by an electric fan) the process is known as convection. Finally, heat loss may be produced by evaporation. Any liquid loses heat during the process of changing to the vapor state. The rate of heat loss through evaporation depends upon the humidity of the surrounding air. When it exceeds 60 percent or so, perspiration will not evaporate so readily and one feels uncomfortable unless some other means (such as convection) can be resorted to. If the temperature of the surrounding air is lower than that of the body, excessive heat loss is prevented by both natural and artificial means. Clothing checks heat loss by trapping "dead air" both in its material and its layers. That noncirculating air is a good insulator. An effective natural insulation against cold is the layer of fat under the skin. Even though the skin temperature may be low, the fatty tissue prevents the deeper tissues from losing too much heat. That layer is on the average slightly thicker (about 5 percent or more) in the female than in the male. There are individual variations, but as a rule the degree of insulation depends on the thickness of the layer of subcutaneous fat. Other factors that play a part in heat loss include the volume of tissue compared with the amount of skin surfaces.

heat production. Heat is produced when oxygen combines with food products in the body cells. The amount of heat produced by a given organ varies with the kind of tissue and with its activity. While at rest, muscles may produce as little as 25 percent of the total body heat. When numbers of muscles contract, the heat production may be multiplied hundreds of times. Under basal conditions (rest) the abdominal organs, particularly the liver, produce about one-half of the body heat. But during vigorous muscular activity that ratio is greatly changed. While the body is at rest, the brain may produce 15 percent of the body heat, but an increase in activity in nerve tissue produces very little increase in heat production. The largest amount of heat, therefore, is produced in the muscles and glands. However, the circulating blood distributes heat fairly evenly throughout the entire body. The rate at which heat is produced is affected by a number of factors. When the body is at complete rest (basal condition), the glandular organs, such as the liver, continue to add some heat constantly with slight variation. But the amount of heat produced in muscles during activity is hundreds of times as great as during rest. In addition to those causes of variations, certain hormones, such as thyroxine from the thyroid gland and epinephrine (adrenaline) from the medulla of the adrenal gland, may increase the rate of heat production. The intake of food also is accompanied by increased heat production. The reasons are not entirely clear. Perhaps more fuel is poured into the blood, and there is therefore more energy readily available for cellular "combustion." The glandular structures and the muscles of the digestive system generate additional heat as they set to work. That does not account for all the increases, however, nor does it account for the much greater increase in metabolism following a meal containing large amounts of protein. Whatever the reasons, the intake of food definitely increases the chemical activities that go on in the body and thus adds heat production.

heat-related illnesses. Range in severity from heat cramps through mild heat syncope to fatal heat stroke. Heat cramps, heat syncope, heat exhaustion, and heat stroke can occur in climates that are not excessively hot. The accumulating metabolic heat and large sweat losses of the exercising individual can induce heat-related disorders even on mildly warm but humid days. There is an added risk when the environment is both hot and humid. Those illnesses are not always manifested as separate clinical entities; there are distinct areas of overlap among them. Heat exhaustion from salt depletion may accompany exhaustion from water depletion, which in turn can be accompanied by syncope. The all important differentiation between heat exhaustion and impending heat stroke is not always clear. There are considerable individual differences in thermoregulatory responses to exercise and heat tolerance. Some individuals respond with mild physiologic changes; others react with high body temperatures and excessive sweat loss. Cystic fibrosis is characterized by excessive sweating in warm environments and after exercise. Sweat in that disorder contains abnormally high amounts of sodium and chloride. Hypohydration and salt deficiency may precipitate heat exhaustion or heat stroke. Febrile states, irrespective of cause, can predispose to further hyperpyrexia when metabolic heat production is high. The hypothalmic thermal control may be malfunctioning and behaving in an unpredictable manner. Gastrointestinal infection or any other condition manifested by diarrhea or vomiting may contribute to hypohydration, heat exhaustion, and heat stroke during exercise in hot, humid weather. Insufficient acclimatization is probably the single most important cause of heat illness. Overweight or obese individuals may participate in school football, in wrestling or track, and on field teams. Obese individuals, when exercising in hot climates, respond with high body temperatures and more cardiovascular strain than do leaner individuals. Obese individuals also have a greater rise in core temperature at a given level of hypohydration and a lower tolerance to prolonged exercise in heat. Prior heat illness predisposes the exercising individual to a greater risk of subsequent heat illness.

heat storage. The average body can store heat to accommodate full effort for only a limited time. A continuous exchange of heat between the body and its ambient environment is necessary to maintain thermal homeostasis. The skin especially, along with the lungs and excreta, provides the means to accomplish that exchange. Hyperthermia results if maximum heat storage is not dissipated through a combination of losses from surface conduction, wind convection, and especially perspiration evaporation, along with antiradiation-gain factors, such as reflective clothing. During athletic activity general body temperature increases slightly for about 10 to 15 minutes, whereafter a plateau (dependent upon dissipation rate) is reached with continued exertion. The temperature within muscle tissue increases rapidly during the first 5 minutes of work. That tends to improve muscle physiology by dilating intramuscular blood vessels and reducing tissue viscosity.

heat stroke. Condition is due to excessive heat storage and can occur under any adverse condition that makes it difficult or impossible to dissipate heat by radiation, convection, and sweat evaporation. Neurologic abnormalities in heat stroke include loss of consciousness, which may appear suddenly, or there may be a sense of impending doom. Headache, dizziness, weakness and confusion, and sometimes euphoria may precede a coma. A number of circulatory abnormalities occur during heat stroke, including a high pulse rate with wide pulse pressures, and often supraventricular tachycardia. The cause of heart failure and impaired cardiac output during heat stroke is either a myocardial injury or the result of an increase in pulmonary vascular resistance. Severe dehydration and electrolyte imbalance are not common in acute heat stroke. Severe dehydration, however, is present if sweating has been prolonged before the heat stroke, such as is usual after prolonged exertion. Acute tubular *necrosis* occurs in some individuals and is related to thermal injury to the kidneys, circulating pigments and a reduction in renal blood flow. Hepatic abnormalities and jaundice with histologic evidence of liver damage have been found. Treatment must be instituted immediately. All untreated cases are generally fatal owing to brain damage; the degree of residual damage in nonfatal cases is directly related to the amount of elapsed time before treatment is begun. Heat stroke is one of the few true medical emergencies.

heat stroke relating to marathon running. The growth of interest in long-distance running has led to serious problems in many endurance events during climatic conditions favoring heat stroke when sufficient precautions are not taken. The well-trained, heat-acclimated athlete may compete under conditions that would ordinarily cause heat stroke in the poorly trained or those trained in cold environments. There are several climatic and situational factors that may lead to heat stroke, even in relatively cool ambient conditions, under continuous and high endogenous heat production, such as that seen in marathon or ultramarathon competition. These factors are as follows: (1) At the beginning of a race, running speed is usually fast, and large amounts of blood are shunted from the skin and other organs to active muscles. (2) Increased body temperature normally accompanies strenuous muscular activity and leads to sweating. (3) If the environment is hot or, particularly, humid and windless, decreased evaporative heat loss from sweating by convection and radiation from the skin occurs. The decreased blood flow through the skin at a time when cardiac output must be maintained to sustain continuous muscular activity contributes to decreased convection and radiation and, therefore, considerable reduction in heat transfer from the body core to the surface. (4) The normally high sweat rates contribute to dehydration. (5) Once dehydration appears, the high cardiac output cannot be maintained, and skin blood flow is further reduced because of decreased intravascular volume and the overriding need to supply adequate blood to active muscles. That becomes a vicious cycle, which leads to heat stroke.

heat syncope. Players who fail to adequately "warm down" after an event or spectators who stand for longer periods in the heat may lose consciousness from inadequate cerebral blood flow because of a reduced volume associated with a reduced cardiac stroke output, excessive sweating, relaxed superficial veins, and cutaneous vasodilation, which lowers systemic blood pressure. Added to that, players often have an accumulation of fluids within active muscles, and standing spectators frequently present extravascular edema in the lower extremities. Either athlete or spectator may have a superimposed vasovagal attack featuring general muscular vasodilation and a reduced cardiac rate. Syncope may also be associated with heat exhaustion or sunstroke. When one is in doubt, an unconscious or stupored subject with a temperature exceeding 104°F should be treated as a victim of heat stroke until a firm diagnosis can be made.

heat tolerance. Exercise in a hot environment causes a magnification of normal response to physical work, and increases in core and skin temperature, metabolic heat production, sweat rate, pulse rate, and systolic blood pressure. Those responses assist the body in shedding excess heat by convection, radiation, conduction, and evaporation. Women generally have a 10 percent to 12 percent greater surface area to mass ratio than do men. That greater ratio helps increase heat loss in moderate heat stress. But in cold or extreme heat, the larger area may provide too little protection from the ambient temperature. Women with large subcutaneous fat deposits have greater resistance to heat loss in air or water. In contrast, marathon runners who have lower than average fat deposits and a higher surface area to mass ratio lose heat more rapidly. In general, women and men respond similarly to heat at rest. Tolerance to exercise in heat appears to be related to the degree of acclimation and conditioning. With repeated exposure to work in heat, both men and women develop lower mean core and skin temperatures, a decreased heart rate, and an increase in the amount of time they can withstand the stress. Men usually have a higher sweat rate than do women.

heel bursitis. Bursae are small sacs of fluid located near prominent bones or around moving body parts. They function as shock absorbers. Occasionally after chronic trauma or overuse, these sacs become enlarged and inflamed. Bursitis often occurs with heel spur syndrome but is more frequently seen in the back of the heel between the Achilles tendon and the heel bone. That presentation, called retrocalcaneobursitis, is brought about by abnormal pressure from the shoe counter, which creates a shearing force within the bursal sac. Athletes with high-arched feet are particularly prone to retrocalcaneobursitis because their heel bone is prominent. That condition usually starts as an area or redness or blister formation at the back of the heel. The heel movement that causes bursitis is predominantly a side-to-side motion or inversion and eversion of the heel. Heel bursitis should be distinguished from Achilles tendonitis. If an athlete hops or jumps barefoot indoors and if there is no pain associated with that, bursitis should be suspected.

heel spur. A bony growth occurring on the underside of the heel bone. The growth appears in response to an abnormal pull from the planta fascia. Initially, only the bone covering or periosteum is involved, but later a bony spur gradually appears. The abnormal stress that causes plantar fascitis also causes the heel spur. Instead of afflicting the fascia in the arch of the foot, the stress is at the ligament's origin on the heel bone. In addition to bone and ligament involvement in a large number of cases, there is also bursitis and nerve entrapment. The pain is usually most severe during the initial stages, when only the periosteum is involved. Pain (from spurs) will be present on weight bearing and on firm application of pressure over the base of the heel.

heel stress fractures. Stress fractures are small breaks in bones that can occur in almost any bone subjected to continuous trauma. Stress fractures are characteristically seen during basic training for military duty and become known as march fractures. Stress or march fractures in athletes are usually seen in the metatarsals but also in the heel bone or leg bones. Metatarsal stress fractures usually are due to 1 metatarsal bearing a disproportionate amount of weight. The weight imbalance is seen with Morton's foot and also in a pronated foot. In Morton's foot the first metatarsal is abnormally short, leaving weight bearing predominantly to the 2nd, 3rd, and 4th metarsals. The 5th metarsal can elevate because it, unlike the 1st, has an independent joint movement. It therefore rarely sustains a stress fracture. Weight imbalance in a maximally pronated foot allows the 1st and 5th metatarsals to elevate, leaving the mid-region of the foot to bear most of the weight.

hematoma. The athlete is more prone to hematoma formation, since he or she is regularly exposed to the type of trauma likely to cause hematomata. Hematomata can be defined as a collection of pooled blood within a relatively restricted area. Pooled blood is not blood that has infiltrated through soft tissues, but rather blood that has collected in a localized area and maintained its identity as blood. Pooling will occur in many situations, in many locations, and from varying types of trauma, since the basic prognosis from the pathological standpoint is bleeding within the tissues. In hematoma formation bleeding takes place into the tissues, and by virtue of pressure from the hemorrhage, the blood makes a space for itself that it wholly fills by pushing other tissues away. That may be extremely extensive, as in hematoma formation up and down the fascial planes of the back following a serious vessel rupture in the vicinity of the spine; or it may be extremely localized, as in the collection that forms between the skin and the periosteum over the shin. After a hematoma develops, the body's reaction is to make an inflammatory response enabling it to cope with the blood pool. The response increases local tenderness and heat similar to that seen in cellulitis for 2 to 3 days until the stage of reaction inflammation subsides. A large hematoma is never absorbed; it undergoes organization, fibrosis, and scar.

hemoglobinuria. In a healthy person hemoglobinuria may be noted after prolonged walking or running. It is often associated with boxing, karate, and wrestling, and after hard trauma, and it is seen in players who assume a forced crouching position, such as football linemen and baseball catchers. In the latter group, minor renal dysfunction and nephroptosis are often related. Hemoglobinuria or hematuria is rarely seen in females. Severe injuries, severe infections, and other disorders cause the destruction of red blood cells. As those cells are broken down, the hemoglobin pigment they contain is released into the bloodstream and is excreted by the kidneys. Urine containing that pigment is faint pink to deep red in color and resembles bloody urine. Renal failure sometimes follows disorders producing hemoglobinuria. Occasionally strenuous exercise alone results in hemoglobinuria, and red blood cells may be evident in a routine urinalysis of a specimen obtained shortly after a vigorous sport. The condition is usually benign and disappears with rest.

hemorrhage. Acute hemorrhage consists of sudden or rapid loss of blood from the circulatory system within a few minutes or hours as a result of an opening or openings in the system. Life is generally threatened if blood loss reaches 25 percent to 50 percent of total volume. Concealed bleeding is difficult to estimate. The body in general and the cardiovascular system in particular react to stress of an injury to the circulatory system by shock, which is apparent after sudden loss of 15 percent or more of the circulating blood volume. The seriousness of hemorrhage lies in both the rate and the quantity of blood volume reduction, which are related to the number, type, and location of the vascular structures opened. Whenever an artery or vein is opened, the injured vessel constricts and, if severed, retracts into the tissue, thereby reducing the size of the opening and facilitating clot formation. In addition, other blood vessels temporarily constrict as a part of the general reaction to injury. That generalized vasoconstriction helps maintain blood pressure by reducing the capacity of the circulatory system. At the site of injury, blood tends to clot and plug the opened vessel. If vasoconstriction and blood clotting are unsuccessful, the resulting blood volume reduction causes a fall in blood pressure which, among its other effects, facilitates clot formation. If hemorrhage persists, the person dies from lack of oxygen and other nutrients.

hepatitis. A virus infection that selectively involves the liver. The virus is spread principally by fecal contamination of water, but contaminated food, personal contact, and contaminated injection needles, syringes, and similar instruments are also important routes of infection. The onset of hepatitis is usually rather insidious and follows an incubation period ranging from 3 weeks to 6 months. The earliest symptoms are loss of appetite, general malaise, and easy fatigability. Later a low fever and nausea and vomiting appear. Many individuals have a peculiar loss of taste for cigarettes. In those with more severe infections, the symptoms gradually increase in severity. Light-colored stools and dark urine may precede the appearance of jaundice by several days. Vague upper abdominal discomfort and tenderness may be present, particularly in the right upper quadrant, but severe pain is absent. After the appearance of jaundice, some individuals experience ill-defined joint or muscular pains. A highly variable skin rash may be present, and some people have generalized itching. The severity of the disease runs a full range from cases so mild that one does not realize he or she is ill, to the relatively rare fatalities. When jaundice does develop, it usually last 3 to 6 weeks. Malaise, easy fatigability, and loss of appetite may persist for several more months.

hernia, incarcerated. A hernia (or rupture) is a protusion of the intestine from its proper location within the abdominal cavity. The most common site for the protrusion is in the groin, where it may extend into the scrotum. Usually, such a hernia is easily reduced (pushed back into the abdomen) and has existed for months and even years. The hernia itself does not constitute an emergency, but the involved intestine may be trapped in the abdominal position, resulting in an intestinal obstruction. The surgical repair of a hernia is a relatively minor operation.

hernia, muscle. Excessive physical activity; congenital defect. Symptoms are mild pain on activity and muscle easily fatigued. Signs are fusiform bulges appearing in long axis of muscle on vigorous contraction, usually in lower extremity; defect variable in size and usually reducible. Complications are disability and secondary entrapment neuropathy.

herpes simplex (cold sores or fever blisters). A viral infection that produces small, painful blisters on the lips and skin of the face and occasionally inside the mouth. Herpes sores often accompany such diseases as pneumonia or meningitis and sometimes result from sunburn of the lips or face. Initially a small, painful swelling appears, which rapidly develops into 1 or more small blisters containing a clear fluid and surrounded by a thin margin of inflamed skin. The blisters may rupture, particularly if they are traumatized, resulting in bleeding and crusting. Fever or other symptoms are rarely experienced. The blisters usually heal in 5 to 10 days. Although uncomfortable and unsightly, they usually cause no significant disability. Athletes with herpes in exposed areas should not participate in contact sports until lesions have healed, because of the opportunity of transferring infection to abraded skin in close body contact (herpes gladiatorium).

high altitude pulmonary edema. Probably the most dangerous of the common types of altitude illness, resulting from filling of the air sacs (alveoli) of the lung with fluid that has oozed through the walls of the pulmonary capillaries. As more alveoli fill with fluid, oxygen transfer from the air to the pulmonary capillaries is blocked. A marked drop in the oxygen concentration in the blood results, producing cyanosis, interference with cerebral function, and ultimately death by suffocation. The causes of high altitude pulmonary edema are not clearly understood. Studies have established that individuals with the disorder develop a much greater increase in pulmonary artery pressure than usually occurs as part of altitude acclimatization. However, the increase in pulmonary artery pressure alone is not an adequate explanation for the fluid collection. It appears that some alteration of the small blood vessels that allows the fluid to leak into the air spaces must take place. High altitude pulmonary edema severe enough to cause physical incapacity is usually associated with rapid ascents by unacclimatized individuals who engage in heavy physical exertion after arrival at high altitudes. More rapid ascents and higher altitude are associated with a greater incidence of the disorder. However, high altitude pulmonary edema occurs as low as 8,000 feet, rarely ever lower.

high fiber diets. The most significant food sources of fiber are unprocessed wheat bran, unrefined breakfast cereals, and whole wheat and rye flours. Additional sources include some fresh and dried fruits, raw vegetables, and legumes. Dietary fiber adds bulk to the diet. It appears that of all the sources, wheat bran is the most effective in increasing fecal bulk. Because most sources are relatively low in calories, the increased bulk in the digestive tract greatly facilitates transit time. A high fiber diet also produces softer, more bulky, and more frequent stools and contains twice as much carbohydrate, fat, and protein. A high fiber diet has been found to lower blood cholesterol and especially low-density lipoprotein (LDL) and cholesterol levels. The intake of crude fiber in the diet has dropped significantly since the turn of the century. While the intake of fiber from vegetables has remained more constant, that from potatoes, fruit, cereals, and dry peas, and beans has declined over the years. Coincident with that reduction of dietary fiber has been an increase in a host of ailments including: coronary heart disease, cholesterol gallstones, diabetes, obesity, hiatal hernia, peptic ulcer, constipation, diverticulosis, hemorrhoids, varicose veins, and cancer of the colon. All have been linked to overconsumption of sucrose and highly milled starches and the underconsumption of fibrous materials in the diet. Although some of the assumptions still remain controversial, fiber, by adding bulk to the feces, will usually eliminate chronic constipation in many individuals. To the extent that the stool is soft and one does not have to strain, the problem of hemorrhoids is lessened. Obesity can be combatted by a high fiber diet, and its control affords a reduction in adult onset of diabetes and problems of varicosities. The antiobesity and cholesterol-lowering effect of fibers has contributed to a beneficial effect on heart disease. The cholesterol-lowering effects account for the alleviation of cholesterol gallstones. The transit time of feces may also be a factor in hiatus hernia, ulcers, and colon cancer.

hip dislocation—anterior. Forcible abduction and external rotation of hip as from fall onto feet or knees; crushing injury to back or pelvis with hip in abduction. Symptoms are severe pain and disability. Signs are thigh maintained in position of abduction and external rotation, perhaps slight flexion or extension, head of femur palpable in abnormal position, lateral surface of hip flattened, greater trochanter displaced inward. Complications may be conversion to posterior dislocation, associated fracture, rupture of femoral vessels, contusion of femoral or obturator nerve, aseptic necrosis of head of femur, traumatic arthritis.

hip dislocation, posterior. Violent force that approximates knee and pelvis, causing flexed thigh into internal rotation and adduction, or, with hip flexed, strong backward thrust on femur may snap head out of acetabulum posteriorly. Symptoms are severe pain, inability to bear weight or move limb, and disability. Signs are hip fixed in abnormal position of flexion, adduction, and internal rotation; apparent shortening of limb; trochanter unusually prominent; buttock on affected side unusually prominent; head of femur palpable in its abnormal position beneath gluteal; and/or tenderness of passive motion. Complications are shock; sciatic nerve palsy, traumatic arthritis, and aseptic necrosis of femoral head.

hip injuries. The articulation of the femur with the pelvis forms the hip joint, a ball and socket joint. The joint is encased in a tough fibrous capsule lined by synovial tissue that nourishes the joint. Three extremely strong ligaments, the iliofemoral, pubofemoral, and ischiofemoral, surround the joint anteriorly and posteriorly and reinforce the capsule. Of numerous bursae about the hip joint, the 2 most important are the trochanteric bursa, located just behind the greater trochanter and deep to the gluteus maximus and tensor fascia femoris muscle, and the iliopsoas bursa, located between the capsule and the iliopsoas muscle anteriorly. Motion of the hip joint includes flexion, extension, abduction, adduction, circumduction, and rotation. The primary flexors of the hip are the iliopsoas, rectus femoris, and adductor muscles. The primary extensors of the hip are the gluteus maximus and hamstrings. The trochanteric and iliopsoas bursae may become inflamed from overuse, such as in jogging. If the trochanteric bursa is involved, usually there is aching pain after running. If the iliopsoas muscle is involved, the pain is more medial and anterior in the groin. Falling on, or being hit upon, the greater trochanter of the femur may cause inflammation of the greater trochanteric bursa. Such an injury is followed by pain and occasionally by swelling. Examination occasionally reveals an antalgic gait, in which a short step is taken on the painful side. Contusion of the iliac crest, avulsion of the muscles attaching to the crest, or even a fracture of the pelvic rim produces pain along the crest of the ilium. The athlete complains that he cannot run without pain; in fact, he may not be able to run at all. Following contusion to the greater trochanteric area, the athlete may complain that his hip snaps or slips out when it is in certain positions. Often that is not painful but merely bothersome. On examination, with flexion of the hip, the click may be palpated over the greater trochanter. That probably represents the iliotibial band or the gluteus muscles moving back and forth over the bony prominence of

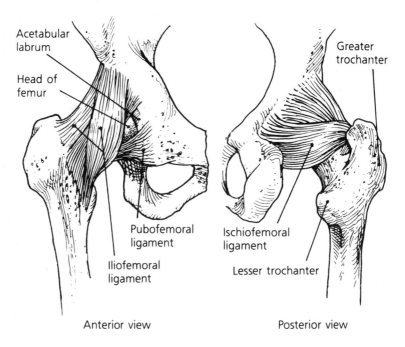

Anterior view   Posterior view

Hip joint.

the trochanter. With so many people becoming involved in long-distance running, stress fractures are often showing up in the lower extremities. If a runner complains of pain in the pubic area or in the hip area not associated with tenderness or swelling or any other physical findings, a stress fracture might be suspected.

hip pointer. A sports term for severe pain and inflammation over the greater trochanter of the femur, just lateral to and slightly forward of the hip joint itself. That can come about either through a direct blow (this is the "point" of the hip closest to the skin) or through a recurrent stress on the muscle site of attachment at the greater trochanter. Either way, inflammation and swelling of the bursa occurs, and the pain can be so intense and disabling that the ailment will also be mistaken for a fractured hip. When the pain and inflammation are the result of a blow, there is about a 2-to-3-week recuperation period. When the pain and inflammation seem to develop spontaneously, the probability is that there has been a tendency to overindulge each time one is engaged in a "leg" sport that calls for frequent, sudden, and extended hip abduction. That could come during any number of sports; i.e., tennis, skiing, horseback riding, and dozens of others. When a person is constantly abducting poorly conditioned muscles, they become fatigued. The tired and weakened muscles, unable to stand up under the punishment, transfer their overloads to the thigh bone. The bone has other things to worry about, however, so it hands the stresses back to the connecting tissue at the greater trochanter. The burden falls upon the tissue, and it becomes inflamed. It, in turn, causes the greater *trochanter* bursa to become inflamed and swell.

hip, snapping (clicking hip). Chronic trochanteric bursitis with bursal thickening may be contributory. Usually not painful but annoying and distressing, especially to hurdlers. With knee flexed, active internal rotation of hip causes the snapping noises.

hip sprain. Excessive forcible torsion of extremity. Symptoms are pain in groin and occasionally in buttocks or lateral aspect of hip, identified by motion or weight bearing. Signs are graded by degree of severity: flexion position assumed with body bent forward, decided limp, muscle spasm, decreased abduction or internal rotation of hip or both, tenderness and possibly swelling. Complications may include persistent disability.

hip strain. Excessive forcible repetitive use of hip external rotators. Symptoms are pain near posterior margin of greater trochanter radiating across buttocks to ischial tuberosity, especially on running or jumping, and disability. Signs are graded by degree of severity; local tenderness, pain elicited by active external rotation or passive internal rotation of hip.

hives. Often caused by a food allergy—chocolate, seafood, and fresh fruit being the most common offenders—but can also occur as an allergic reaction to many substances, including thorns, insect bites or stings, drugs, and occasionally even drugs as common as aspirin. The hives appear quickly following contact with the allergen, are usually widely scattered, and consist of red or white, raised wheals or "bumps." The appearance of the hives is accompanied by rather intense itching. Hives may rapidly appear and disappear several times from a single exposure. Repeated exposures to the same substance usually produce the attacks indefinitely. The condition is more miserable than serious. Treatment consists of administering an antihistamine.

hockey injuries. The potential causes of injury in ice hockey are numerous, including those produced by the opponents, puck, skates, ice, boards, and goal posts. The most common injury is lacerations; the most common fractures are those of the nose, cheek, and jaw. Loss of teeth happens in hockey. One study regarding the National Hockey League found that major injuries of all types occur once in every 2 games, a major injury being defined as one that keeps a player out of play at least 3 weeks. Three minor injuries occurred per game during a season of 70 games. An average of 1 facial laceration occurred per game. Sprains, strains, and avulsion injuries were the next most common category of injury. Knee, ankle, wrist, elbow, and hand injuries were also common. There were various types of fractures, including nasal fractures, rib fractures, and hand fractures, with spearing and jabbing with the upper end of the stick producing several rib fractures. Six concussions were recorded in players not wearing a helmet and 2 in those wearing a helmet. The rest were lacerations of the hand, acromioclavicular separations and torn menisci at the knee. Nasal fractures and facial laceration were caused by high sticking. Fighting within the game has accounted for many of the same injuries. The major cause of injury in professional hockey appears to be high sticking. Although eye injuries are not excessive, they produce a significant amount of handicapped players. One study showed that 15 players in the group of 11 to 15 years of age were most often injured. The hockey stick rather than the puck produced the most injuries.

humerus, epicondylitis, lateral. Repeated sudden jerky, vigorous pronating movement of extended forearm and wrist, as in tennis strokes. Symptoms are pain in elbow, first intermittent, later persistent, radiating to forearm, wrist, possibly fingers, and grip, which causes sharp pain. Signs are local tenderness over front of external epicondyle, pain with extension of hand against resistance, lack of pain wih flexion against resistance.

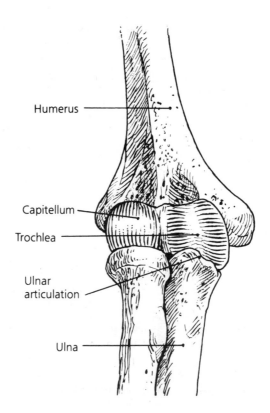

Humerus

Capitellum

Trochlea

Ulnar articulation

Ulna

The humerus.

humerus, epicondylitis, medial. Repeated sudden jerky, vigorous supinating movement of forearm and wrist, as in throwing. Symptoms are pain on medial side of elbow, radiating to forearm, wrist, and possibly fingers and weakness of hand and grip, which causes sharp pain. Signs are local tenderness and occasional swelling.

humerus, fracture, medial epicondylar epiphyseal avulsion (Little League elbow). Excessive repetitive vigorous stress on flexor-pronator muscles while one is throwing a baseball, usually between ages of 9 to 14. Symptoms are pain during flexing and pronating of forearm. Signs are swelling and tenderness. Complications may lead to permanent limitation of movement of the humerus.

humerus fracture, shaft. Direct violence, fall onto arm at side, forcible muscular action, as in throwing or hand wrestling. Symptoms are local pain and disability. Signs are shortening of humerus, swelling, abnormal mobility, crepitus. Complications could lead to radial nerve injury, vascular injuries, nonunion, nonangular or rotary deformity.

hyperhidrosis. Excessive feet sweating (usually associated with scales, fissure, maceration, and a strong odor) can often be managed with an antiperspirant powder. It is more often seen in overweight athletes. The fetid odor (bromhidrosis) is the result of perspiration and cellular debris being decomposed by yeasts and bacteria. The individual's perspiration often contains a high amount of urea. Sweat gland overactivity may also occur in the palms, axillae, groin, infra mammary region, or have a general distribution. The cause of localized excessive sweating is unknown. Hyperhidrosis of the palms and soles is often considered psychogenic. Generalized hyperhidrosis may have an endocrine, febrile, or central nervous system basis. A rash, which can be confused with ringworm, may be associated.

hyperthermia. The average body can store heat to accommodate full effort for only a limited time. A continuous exchange of heat between the body and its ambient environment is necessary to maintain thermal homeostasis. The skin especially, along with the lungs and excreta, provides the means to accomplish that exchange. Hyperthermia results if maximum heat storage is not dissipated through a combination of losses from surface conduction, wind convection, and especially perspiration evaporation, along with antiradiation-gain factors, such as reflective clothing. During athletic activity general body temperature increases slightly for about 10 to 15 minutes, whereafter a plateau (dependent upon dissipation rate) is reached with continued exertion. The temperature within muscle tissue increases rapidly during the first 5 minutes of work, which tends to improve muscle physiology by dilating intramuscular blood vessels and reducing tissue viscosity.

hyperventilation syndrome. Hyperventilation, overbreathing, is usually not due to a disease or injury. That may be confusing to the observer who watches an individual breathing very deeply and very rapidly. The "hyperventilation" syndrome is usually of traumatic emotional origin. As the individual breathes rapidly and deeply, an abnormally large amount of carbon dioxide is lost through the lungs, altering the acid-base balance and the pH of the blood and producing the typical symptoms. Individuals who develop the hyperventilation syndrome are usually nervous, tense, and apprehensive. However, the disorder can occur in apparently stable persons. The first signs are shortness of breath, rapid pulse, dizziness, faintness, sweating, apprehension, and sense of suffocation. The individual often complains that "the air doesn't go down far enough." He, or more frequently she, breathes in gasps or takes frequent deep sighs. As the blood becomes more alkaline, numbness or tingling around the mouth and in the fingers appears. Those symptoms may subsequently increase to painful cramps or spasms of the fingers and hands. Spasms of the muscles of the hands and forearms are particularly frightening to the individual, who believes he or she is paralyzed. The shortness of breath is puzzling, since the regulatory mechanisms of the body would be expected to correct the hyperventilation. However, in this condition, those mechanisms are usually overriden by the emotion. The syndrome can be produced in the anxiety-prone athletic competitor.

hypothermia. A decrease in core body temperature to a level at which normal muscular and cerebral functions are impaired. Normal body temperature is within 1 degree of 98.6°F. At body temperatures between 93°F and 95°F muscular incoordination appears; at lower temperatures cerebral function deteriorates. Death caused by cessation of effective heart function occurs between 70°F and 82°F. It is recognized that most deaths that would formerly have been attributed to exposure or exhaustion are due primarily to hypothermia. Heat loss from the body occurs by radiation, convection, evaporation, and conduction. Hypothermia occurs most rapidly in a cold, wet, windy environment. Studies of survival in cold-water immersion resulting from boating accidents have shown that the duration of survival is related to several factors, including: (1) water temperature, at a water temperature of 32°F, death occurs in 15 minutes, while at 70°F survival for as long as 48 hours has been observed; (2) persons wearing heavy clothing survive longer; (3) victims who relax and float in the water have a longer survival time than those who swim or struggle because of lower evaporative heat loss from the lungs and slower depletion of energy stores that maintain body heat. The same general principles apply to hypothermia on land. A wet, cold, windy environment removes body heat rapidly. Exposed skin is the most important source of heat loss by radiation, convection, evaporation, and conduction. Heat loss, especially from wet skin, is greatly increased by wind. Heavy physical exercise increases heat loss by increasing evaporation from the lungs and sweating, which also depletes body fluids. Exercise in a cold environment requires more energy stores and a higher water intake than does equivalent exercise in a warm environment. Fluid loss results in a decrease in blood volume and blood pressure and increases the tendency for weakness, apathy, and collapse to develop if hypothermia occurs. The caused hypoglycemia and reduced core temperature may interfere with hepatic detoxification of alcohol. Moreover, alcohol may inhibit hepatic gluconeogenesis independently. Thus, hypoglycemia, apart from occurring in those who exercise for prolonged periods, may be additionally aggravated by alcohol ingestion. In spite of the lower core temperature and decreased shivering, the individual drinking alcohol feels less cold and judges the environment warmer than do those who did not take alcohol. Thus, exposure to cold water (water immersion) plus alcohol ingestion may combine to seriously reduce central body temperature. Alcohol intake during or after sporting events in cold weather is dangerous and may accelerate the fall in central body temperature, causing serious complications. In addition, alcohol potentiates exercise-induced cutaneous vasodilation with increased heat loss from the extremities.

hypothermia in runners. The clinical manifestations of hypothermia need to be recognized because of deterioration in judgment and strength of the exposed person, which occurs with great rapidity. With rectal temperatures below 30.2°C, clouding of consciousness and sometimes a restless stupor occur. Slurring of speech, ataxia, and involuntary movements are common. Pallor, cyanosis and edema of the skin of the face, slow cerebration, and a croaky voice may suggest the presence of hypothyroidism. The body is characteristically cold. That coldness is not being confined to the extremities but is also found in covered portions and in the axillae groins. The pupils are abnormally dilated or may be pinpoint and react sluggishly to light. Muscle tone is increased, and the individual may show a generalized rigidity and neck stiffness. At that stage shivering is characteristically absent. When it occurs, in exposed runners, it must be recognized as attempts by the body to counteract rapid heat loss and as a warning of impending hypothermia. During hypothermia deep tendon reflexes are sluggish, and a delayed relaxation of the ankle jerk like that seen in myxedema has been observed. The plantar responses are often extensor and revert to normal with recovery. Clinically, hypothermia is thought to be present if the central body temperature is below 35°C, triggering normal thermoregulatory activity, and, provided consciousness is not impaired or another physical disability supervenes, that does not interfere with appropriate exercise and behavioral efforts at temperature conservation that are usually successful in restoring body temperature to normal. In a warm environment such a subject recovers rapidly without aftereffect. If the central temperature is between 32.2 and 24°C, there is depression of tissue metabolism, with progressive clouding of consciousness. Below 24°C, death usually occurs from ventricular fibrillation, and the mechanisms to prevent temperature drops, such as vasoconstriction and shivering, usually fail. The body continues to lose heat in those circumstances like an inanimate object without the modulating influence of the autonomic nervous system.

I

iliopectineal bursitis. Excessive repetitive running. Symptoms are pain over anterior aspect of hip about middle of inguinal ligament, possibly radiating down front of leg. Signs are hip usually held in flexion, abduction, and external rotation, and tenderness. Complications could lead to infection and persistent disability.

iliopsoas strain (groin strain or pull). Excessive forcible contraction of iliopsoas with thigh fixed or forced into extension. Symptoms are pain in groin, especially in hip extension or rotation, and disability in running or jumping. Signs are graded by degree of severity: thigh held in flexed adducted position, tenderness over anterior aspect of hip or near region of lesser trochanter along upper anteromedial aspect of the thigh. Complications could lead to recurrence and persistent disability.

ilium fracture, spine avulsion. Anterosuperior spine pulled off by tensor fascia femoris and sartorius during forcible running or jumping activity. Symptoms are local pain, especially on flexion or abduction of thigh, with disability. Signs are local swelling and a tenderness; fragment may be palpated. Complications may lead to recurrent and prolonged disability.

impetigo. Characterized by distinct, superficial vesiculopustules, especially around the mouth, which crust and rupture. The 3 types of impetigo seen in athletics are ecthyma, impetigo contagiosa, and Bockart's impetigo. Ecthyma invades the deeper skin, often producing ulcers, which result in scars. The common site is on or near the legs as a complication of scabies. Impetigo contagiosa arises as a small, red spot, which evolves into a nonitchy flat, raised sac filled with fluid having a straw color. When the sacs break, the oozing fluid carries the infection to adjoining areas and new lesions appear. Rather than breaking, the sacs usually dry into a yellow crust. Large blisterlike lesions about the size of a quarter are called bullous impetigo. Bockart's impetigo is characterized by small pustules at the base of hairs, no larger than a pinhead and thus often missed. If the pustules are left untreated, secondary infection may occur, leading to a severe septicemia. The first signs of any form of impetigo demand immediate medical attention.

influenza. A viral infection that is an acute, self-limiting disease of 5 to 6 days' duration. Although the infection is limited to the respiratory tract, the symptoms may suggest a generalized disease. Many different viruses produce the disorder (Influenza A is most common), but the disease produced by each type is identical. Spreading occurs by sneezing, coughing, or close contact with an infected person. Epidemics are common. The incubation period is short, only 1 to 2 days. The onset is heralded by chilliness, fever, weakness, lassitude, headache, loss of appetite, and aching muscular pains. Respiratory tract symptoms (such as a dry, hacking cough, sneezing, sore throat, nasal irritation, and hoarseness) are often present but are usually not severe. Fever is oscillating, usually lasting 2 to 3 days, and occasionally reaches 104°F. The pulse rate may be quite rapid. The throat is sometimes inflamed, and the nasal mucosa is often red and swollen, causing noisy breathing as a result of obstruction. The signs and symptoms of upper respiratory tract involvement usually differentiate influenza from other systemic infections. No specific treatment is available. Rest, inactivity, and ingestion of fluids work for many.

inguinal hernia. The development of a hernia is a common condition. The indirect type is a result of a congenital weakness in the region of the internal abdominal ring and can happen at any age. It consists of a sac of peritoneum protruding through the internal abdominal ring into which intestinal contents protrude. In that situation, the neck is always narrow and therefore is a potential site for intestinal gut strangulation. The presence of a hernia in an athlete, especially one competing in strenuous events, is a potentially dangerous situation. Strangulation and serious complications can occur at any time, such as in scuba diving, where an increase in intra-abdominal pressure from underwater pressure changes results in an especially dangerous situation. Any such hernia should be repaired surgically before the athlete competes again.

inner ear disorders. Characterized by vertigo, tinnitus, and hearing loss. Acute viral labyrinthitis is usually secondary from a cold or gastrointestinal infection. Hearing loss is rarely associated, but vertigo is usually severe. It is usually self-limiting in 1 to 2 weeks. A common cause of earache is often not within the ear itself, but from the adjacent temporomandibular joint, especially in gum chewers and brace wearers who have a subclinical arthralgia of the joint. Chronic tonsil, pharynx, or larynx inflammations are also common causes of referred pain to the ear. Other causes include cervical subluxation, sternomastoid and masseter trigger points, dental problems. In inner-ear barotrauma, injury to the inner ear is usually of an intrinsic nature, as it is well protected by surrounding bone. Impairment is usually the result of abnormal pressure changes or fistulae. Menier's syndrome features endolymphatic hydrops from pressure change in inner-ear fluids. Symptoms include paroxysmal dizziness, tinnitus, and a degree of deafness. The latter 2 may originate unilaterally and progress to both ears. It is often secondary to a number of metabolic disorders, but a common cause often overlooked is a cervical or upper thoracic subluxation.

intertrigo (chafing). Mechanical friction producing abrasion where skin surfaces are in contact, such as the groin, axillae, with sweat a contributing factor, obesity predisposing. Signs are erythema and mild maceration, which may progress to marked hyperemia, denudation, or erosion. Symptoms are pain and disability. Complications could lead to infection and cellulitis.

intestinal disorders. Indigestion may be due to a gastritis (inflammation of the stomach lining) or to an enteritis (intestinal infection). More often, the stomach and the small intestine are both involved so that the illness is known as gastroenteritis. The symptoms include nausea, vomiting, and diarrhea as well as acute abdominal pain or colic. Diarrhea, meaning "to flow through," is a symptom in which there is an abnormally frequent water bowel movement. Dysentery means "difficulty of the intestine" and usually refers to an inflammation of the mucosal lining, although deeper tissues also may be affected. The 2 main types of dysentery are bacillary dysentery, which is caused by rod-shaped bacteria that are transferred to food and water primarily by human carriers, and amebic dysentery, which is due to an infestation by a 1-celled animal called *Entamoeba histolytica*.

intestinal grippe. A condition characterized by acute onset of fever, nausea, vomiting, abdominal cramps, and diarrhea. Not all of the symptoms are invariably present or occur in that order. High fever may be present in the first 6 to 12 hours and then disappear spontaneously. Fever usually comes with the onset of diarrhea. Weakness and generalized aching pains, particularly during the period of fever, are common. A feeling of unusual fatigue may last for some days after other symptoms have disappeared. The feeling of weakness and fatigue appears to be due to involvement of the liver, since liver function studies frequently show significant changes. The infection appears to be mildly contagious and may spread through a whole team in short order. The incubation period is unknown.

intracranial hematomas. A few athletes develop intracranial hematomas after head injuries. Acute epidural hematomas usually occur if a hard, localized blow to the temple fractures the temporal bone and tears the underlying middle meningeal artery. Epidural hematomas occur most often in golfers or baseball players and rarely in helmeted football players. Athletes with those injuries typically have a lucid interval of minutes to hours before they deteriorate. The enlarging extradural hematoma increases intracranial pressure and causes headache, nausea, and vomiting. The hematoma may compress the adjacent frontal lobe cortex, causing weakness of the opposite arm and side of the face. Ultimately, the brain may be shifted enough toward the opposite side to compress the midbrain against the tentorium. That causes midbrain hemorrhages, which in turn may cause severe disability or death. However, the brain adjacent to the hematoma is usually not bruised or swollen, and removal of the clot will relieve the problem. Acute subdural hematomas are the common intracranial hematomas football players develop. The injury results from severe blows to the head that cause angular acceleration to the brain and tear vessels spanning the cortical-dural gap. Athletes, with acute subdural hematomas, may be unconscious from the moment of impact or may have a lucid interval. If they are conscious after the injury, they usually experience headache, nausea, vomiting, and perhaps focal seizures within a few hours. They then have decreasing levels of consciousness and increasing neurologic deficit as time passes. Intracerebral hematomas usually occur in boxers who do not recover consciousness after the blow. Intracerebral hematomas result from blows severe enough to shear intracerebral vessels. They are associated with cerebral contusion and edema and are best diagnosed by CAT scans.

intrapatellar bursitis. Direct blow over patellar ligament; excessive repetitive running or climbing. Symptoms are sharp pain with pendulum extension of knee and usually mild disability. Signs are tenderness over patellar ligament, fluctuant swelling on either side of patellar ligament, normal depression on either side of patellar ligament absent or limited motion of knee.

ischiogluteal bursitis. Prolonged sitting on hard surface, as in a rowing crew. Symptoms are pain over ischial tuberosity and radiating down back of thigh along hamstring. Signs are local tenderness, pain elicited by active extension of hip or active flexion of knee, or passive flexion of hip or passive extension of knee (straight leg raising). Complications are suppuration and calcification of bursa.

ischiopubic fracture, rami. Crushing violence, either in lateral or anteroposterior direction. Symptoms are pain in pubic and perineal regions, inability to bear weight, possible symptoms of shock. Signs are local swelling and evidence of trauma, such as abrasions, contusions, lacerations; inability to lift leg on affected side; acute tenderness on palpation; possible deformity. Complications may include rupture of urethra and urinary bladder or retroperitoneal hemorrhage.

ischium fracture, tuberosity avulsion. Excessive forcible action of long head of biceps femoris; forcible flexion of hip with knee extended, as in leading leg of hurdler. Symptoms are pain over ischial tuberosity and disability. Signs are local tenderness, crepitus, swelling; loose fragments that may be palpable; pain elicited by contraction of biceps femoris or on straight leg raising. Complications could lead to painful non-union, recurrence, or extensive heterotopic ossification.

J

jaundice. Produced by diseases of the liver. One of the numerous functions of that organ is to remove from the blood those pigments resulting from the normal destruction of the old red blood cells. That (waste product) pigment is excreted into the intestine through the bile ducts and, following further changes in the intestinal tract, imparts the normal brown color to the stool. In diseases that severely damage the liver, the pigment (waste product) is not removed from the blood. As a result, it accumulates in the body and imparts a yellow or bronze color to the whites of the eyes and later the skin. Since the pigment is excreted into the intestine in smaller amounts or not at all, the stool becomes pale or "clay-colored." The pigment is partially excreted by the kidneys, imparting a yellow to brown color to the urine. It also causes the foam produced by shaking when there is a yellow color instead of the normal clear appearance.

jaws and earache (swimming and diving). A common cause of earache in adults is pain in the ears from disorders of the temporomandibular joint, which also results in ears that are "blocked," itchy, and painful. The prime cause, in underwater swimmers, is forceful clenching of the teeth on the mouthpiece of the snorkel or regulator. The onset of symptoms is probably due to the presence of several factors working together, including a tendency in affected subjects to grind or clench their teeth. If there is faulty dentition owing to lack of teeth or their malposition or if dentures are unsatisfactory, the condition may cause subconscious irritation leading to faulty habits of moving the jaws and grinding the teeth. Rarely is the joint physically affected, but the many muscles that move the joint tend to develop contraction to protect it even to the point of spasm, causing aches and pains similar to backache and pain. Pain can arise at the site where the muscles are attached to the bone of the skull, in the jaw, or in the muscle itself and is referred to the face, forehead, or the temples.

joints. Joints are the central focus of bones, muscles, tendons, and ligaments that make up the musculo-skeletal system, thereby giving the body mobility and flexibility. They are also the most frequent site of sports injuries. The 3 most common types of joints in the body are the ball-and-socket (hip, shoulder), the hinge (knee, elbow), and the modified hinge, often called a "saddle joint" (ankle, thumb). The ball-and-socket joints are the largest and anatomically the least complicated. They allow for the greatest range of motion, and except for dislocations (which usually occur from sudden injuries) and inflammation of the bursa, little goes wrong with them under ordinary athletic conditions. However, inflammation of the bursae—flat, membranous sacs that protect the movements of the joints from interference by other tissues—can be very painful ailments. They go under the name of bursitis and occur most frequently in the ball-and-socket joints, the hip, and the shoulder. The hinge joints are smaller structures but somewhat more complicated than the ball-and-socket joints and are subject to a greater variety of ailments. The range of motion they permit is limited. For instance, the knee and elbow joints are limited to forward-backward articulation only, with the backward articulation (flexion) capable of full range and the forward articulation (extension) capable of half the range. The third type of joint in the body is the modified hinge or saddle joint, of which the ankle is the most readily visible example. The ankle connects the foot to the leg. It is called a "saddle" joint because the major bone of the joint, the talus or ankle bone, is shaped like an inverted saddle. The movement of that joint, where the lower end of the leg bone, or tibia, meets the top of the ankle bone, is limited, as in the movement of the elbow or the knee, to flexion and extension. The ankle joint is held together by an assortment of tendons, ligaments, and muscles and just as subject to injuries and ailments involving the components as are other joints. A joint is classified by its structure and may be described as fibrous, where fibrous tissue unites the bone ends. Where some slight movement occurs, it is called a syndesmosis; where no movement occurs, a suture. Where cartilage unites the bones, either temporarily or permanently, the joint is termed cartilaginous. Synovial joints are those surrounded by a fibrous capsule, where the bones can move easily upon each other because they are plated with smooth articular cartilage and lubricated and nourished by synovial fluid. The fibrous capsule of a joint may be thickened in areas of stress to form a ligament. Sometimes accessory ligaments are found within the joint to give added strength. A joint performs 2 functions; to transmit stress to fixed parts of the limb while other joints are moving, and itself to permit movement. Joints transmit stress while they are stabilized by muscular activity, and the least muscular activity is required when the stress is transmitted through the center of the joint.

joint disorders. Joints are subject to certain disorders of a mechanical nature, examples of which are dislocation and sprains. A dislocation is a derangement of the parts of the joint. A sprain is the "name" for the wrenching of a joint with rupture or tearing of the ligaments. The most common type of infection is arthritis, meaning "inflammation of the joints." There are many different kinds, a familiar form being rheumatoid arthritis. The condition is crippling, characterized by swelling of the joints of the hands, the feet, and other parts of the body as a result of inflammation and overgrowth of the synovial membrane and other joint tissues. The articular cartilage is gradually destroyed, and the joint cavity develops adhesions; that is, the surfaces tend to stick together, so that the joints stiffen and are ultimately rendered useless. The cause of rheumatoid arthritis is still unknown, though some types of streptococci are suspected. Arthritis also can be brought on by such infections as rheumatic fever and gonorrhea. The joints, as well as the bones proper, are subject to attack by the tuberculosis organism, and the result may be a gradual destruction of parts of the bones near the joints. The organism is carried by the bloodstream, usually from a focus in the lungs or lymph nodes, and may cause considerable damage before it is discovered. Degenerative joint diseases usually occur in older people. They occur mostly in joints involving weight bearing. Various degenerative changes in the joints include the formation of spurs at the edges of the articular surfaces, thickening of the synovial membrane, atrophy of the cartilages, or calcification of the ligaments. Gout is a kind of arthritis basically caused by a disturbance of metabolism. One of the products of metabolism is uric acid, which normally is excreted in the urine. If there happens to be an overproduction of uric acid or for some reason not enough is excreted, the accumulated uric acid forms crystals, which are deposited as masses about the joints and other parts of the body. The joint becomes inflamed and extremely painful. Any

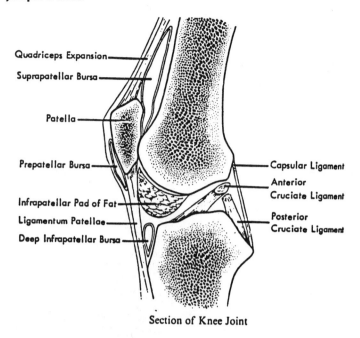

Quadriceps Expansion

Suprapatellar Bursa

Patella

Prepatellar Bursa

Infrapatellar Pad of Fat

Ligamentum Patellae

Deep Infrapatellar Bursa

Capsular Ligament

Anterior Cruciate Ligament

Posterior Cruciate Ligament

Section of Knee Joint

joint can be involved, but the one normally affected by gout is the great toe. A joint may be injured in a number of ways, including a direct blow leading to contusion of the capsule or injury to cartilage or bone. An unexpected or excessive force to which the protective mechanism of the joint does not have time to react—or which it cannot develop the tension to withstand—may cause damage, as may overuse of an unconditioned joint or faulty or abnormal technique leading to low-grade repetitive stresses on the joint. External penetration of the joint may occur as well as damage to supporting structures.

jumper's knee. An amalgamation of several conditions. The athlete with the condition is almost always involved in some type of repetitive activity, such as jumping, climbing, kicking, or running. The common sports with this complication are basketball, volleyball, high jumping, long and triple jumping, football, figure skating, tennis, racketball, climbing, and long-distance running. Over the infrapatellar or suprapatellar regions, there is often pain of insidious onset, which disappears with rest. A sensation of weakness occurs, giving way to fullness around the knee. When the symptoms are marked and the athlete persists with sports, an acute episode, namely, a "giving away" of the knee, is experienced. Occasionally there may be a complete rupture of the tendinous attachment to the involved pole. The poles of the patella or the patellar tendon may be tender. Effusion is rare, but sometimes there may be a snapping sensation of the patella on full knee flexion. The athlete is usually tall, and there may be abnormalities of the extensor mechanism such as patellar hypermobility and subluxation, patella alta, Osgood-Schlatter's disease, chondromalacia patellae, genu recurvatum, genu valgum, and external tibial torsion.

K

karate lump. It is not unusual for karate enthusiasts to scarify their hands and feet by striking a staw-covered pliable post (makiwara) in the course of several years of practice. The results can be scar tissue development over the injured part, mostly seen at the dorsal aspect of the 3rd and 4th metacarpophalangeal joints. Severe pain on flexion of the 3rd finger is typical. An entrapment syndrome may be produced as infiltrative scar tissue clamps the extensor tendon. In minor injuries transient swelling and painful metacarpophalangeal joints occur. Occasionally hand and wrist fractures are present. Remarkably, a large number of hands severely abused by such a severe form of hand conditioning show no visible soft-tissue calcification or damage to the metacarpal heads.

kidneys. There are 2 kidneys, which are covered by a fibrous tissue capsule. Deep in the capsule is an outer cortex, where the "filtering" units lie, and an inner medulla, which contains "reabsorbing" tubules and collecting ducts, which convey formed urine to the pelvis of the kidney for passage to the ureter and the urinary bladder. Each time the heart beats, about a quarter of the left ventricle's output of blood is distributed (via the renal arteries) to the kidney's for filtering. The renal artery divides into a number of interlobar arteries, each of which distributes blood to 1 "lobe" of the kidney tissue. Those vessels in turn branch out into arching or arciform arteries, which lie at the junction of the cortex and medulla. At intervals, the arciform artery gives rise to straight arteries. They lie parallel to each other and run from the cortico-medullary junction up into the cortex. From both sides of the straight arteries, afferent arterioles take origin. Each divides into approximately 50 capillaries, which stay looped together to form a glomerulus, where filtration takes place.

kidney disease. Nephritis means inflammation of the kidney tissue. The term includes not only the results of infection but also the results of certain degenerative changes in the kidney that may occur. Sometimes the category or disorder is given the general name of Bright's disease. Bacteria or their toxins may involve the kidneys following such infections as "strep" sore throat, scarlet fever, or many of the other contagious diseases. Whatever the cause of the nephritis, the effects upon the kidney are similar. The tiny clusters of capillaries in the nephrons become inflamed and sometimes blocked, as in the case of an infection. They may collapse for the lack of blood, as in arteriosclerosis. One characteristic symptom of nephritis is edema, an abnormal accumulation of fluid in the body tissues or cavities, showing up as a puffy, swollen condition of the area involved. In nephritis 1 cause of edema is the destruction of the nephrons, causing a great deal of albumin (blood protein) to escape into the urine. Because of the deficiency of albumin in the blood, the fluid part of the blood can now escape through the walls of capillaries and into the tissues. Chronic nephritis can lead to a sometimes fatal condition known as uremia, which means an accumulation of urinary constituents in the blood. The cause of the disorder is the inability of the kidneys to remove the poisonous substances from the blood. A prolonged destruction of nephrons can ultimately render a kidney completely useless. Kidney stones, or calculi, are made of certain substances, such as uric acid and calcium salts, that precipitate out of the urine instead of remaining in solution. They usually form in the renal pelvis, although the bladder may be another site of formation. The causes of the precipitation of stone-building materials include infections of the urinary tract and stagnation of the urine. The stones may vary in size from tiny grains (resembling bits of gravel) to large masses that fill the kidney pelvis and extend into the calyces. The stones may be swept into the bladder by the urinary stream, causing excruciating pain as they pass through the duct (ureter) that connects the kidney with the bladder. The symptoms produced by a kidney stone usually appear suddenly and are characterized by sharp, stabbing pain, which may come and go in waves of increasing intensity. The ache usually begins in the back at the level of the lower ribs but frequently radiates around the side to the lower abdomen and into the groin or scrotum. The individual typically writhes in agony and is unable to lie still. Bright, red blood is often found in the urine but may be present in only small amounts. Discomfort on urination and increased frequency of urination are common. Nausea, vomiting, and cold sweats normally occur; chills and fever may be present but are not typical. A kidney stone rarely requires emergency surgical care and is not associated with any danger of severe blood loss. The pain may last for 24 hours or more but usually subsides spontaneously in a shorter period of time as the stone is passed into the bladder.

kidney function. The kidneys have 3 main functions. The first is excretion. The use of proteins by the body cells (in the form of amino acids) produces, among other waste materials, those containing the chemical element nitrogen; the chief waste product of that category is urea. The urinary system is the specialized mechanism of excretion for the nitrogenous waste material. Certain salts from the blood plasma also are excreted. The 2nd function of the kidneys is as an aid in the maintenance of water balance. The 3rd function of the kidneys is to help regulate the acid-base balance of the body. Acids are a category of chemical substances, which in the body are produced by cell metabolism. They may take the form of solids, liquids, or gases. Bases, also called alkalies, are another category of chemicals. They have the effect of neutralizing acids (the product of an acid-base reaction is salt). Certain foods can cause acids or alkalies to form in the body. In order that all the normal body processes may take place, a certain critical proportion of acids and bases must be maintained at all times, and this despite the fact that the person may take varying quantities of acid-forming and alkaline-producing substances as food. Acid substances are constantly being removed from the body in various ways, including the exhalation of carbon dioxide, which serves to remove carbonic acid. The kidneys are constantly removing both acid and alkaline substances, which may be present in excess, and they are able to manufacture ammonia at certain times. Ammonia neutralizes acids, and that is another example of the kidney's ability to help maintain the acid-base balance.

kidney injuries. Kidney contusion comes from a direct blow or fall. Symptoms are acute pain in the lumbar area, which may be progressive, or red urine or both. Signs are obvious distress, shock, tenderness in the flank, and pains sometimes associated with rib fractures. Kidney laceration is caused by a direct blow, fall, sudden violent muscular action, diseased kidney, congenital anomaly vulnerable to slight trauma. Symptoms are acute pain in lumbar area and upper abdomen, increasing with activity;

nausea and vomiting; red urine. Signs are obvious distress, shock, tenderness, muscle spasm, ileus with abdominal distension, bulge in flank or tachycardia. Complications could lead to severe shock and hypertension resulting from renal scarring.

Kienbock's disease. The condition is variously called osteitis, osteochondritis, or malacia of the lunate and is most common in the adolescent. In this condition there is definite involvement of the lunate with bony changes, the bone going through various stages, i.e., atrophy followed by sclerosis and later decalcification, often with fragmentation resulting in marked change in shape of the bone. The athlete gives a history of pain in the wrist that may or may not be associated with an injury. Despite adequate treatment, the pain does not resolve. Examination reveals tenderness in the wrist, most marked over the lunate area. Wrist motion is limited. The pain is worse with active motion. X rays show increased density of the lunate bone in the early stages. In the later stages collapse and loss of normal architecture occur.

knee bones. Skeletally, the knee is formed by the vertical joining of the thigh bone, the femur, to the 2 bones of the lower leg, the tibia and the fibula. In the design of the leg, the femur can be considered the equivalent of the humerus, the long upper bone of the arm. In the knee the thigh bone, or femur, does not connect directly with both lower leg bones; it connects only with the large one, the tibia. At the lower end, the thigh bone broadens out and forms into knuckles, 2 outer knobs and a center notch. At the upper end the larger of the 2 lower leg bones, the tibia, widens and flattens into a corresponding configuration. At the very end of the tibia, there are 2 condyles, inner and outer, with a projecting ridge separating them. That ridge fits into the center notch of the lower end of the thigh bone, and the flat surfaces of the 2 condyles fit against the rounded surfaces of the 2 projecting knobs, also called condyles, of the thigh bone's lower end. That conjunction of surface constitutes the skeletal design of the knee joint. The articulating surfaces at the lower end of the femur and the upper ends of the tibia, where the 2 bones meet to form the knee joint, are covered by a glistening, rubbery, cartilage-type lining that secretes a lubricating fluid that reduces friction between the 2 opposed bodies when they move against each another.

knee injuries. The knee joint movement is helicoid or spiral in character, consisting of large, rounded condyles of the femur and the much-flattened condyles of the tibia. The fibula does not take part in the joint. The patella articulates with the patellar surface of the femur, and thus the knee joint consists of 3 joints in 1: a joint between the patella and the femur and between each tibial condyle and femoral condyle. The vicinity of the knee is quite susceptible to injuries of the muscle-tendon unit since violent muscular activity is involved in the normal function of that vulnerable joint. The athlete with an unstable knee complains of its giving way. There is a lack of thrust when the knee bears weight, particularly on stairs or uneven ground. The unstable knee is caused by an injury to the ligaments or joint capsule or both, a tear of the anterior or posterior cruciate, or a partial rip of a collateral ligament associated with a capsular laceration. The knee is a highly vulnerable joint and is particularly liable to contusion either by a fall directly on the front of the knee or by a blow from the side. Contusion is usually followed by local tenderness, ecchymosis, and overlying abrasion.

Chondromalacia of the patella is not well understood. There are several theories of its cause. One is that it is precipitated by a single episode of trauma, such as falling on the flexed knee. Or it may be caused by multiple episodes of small trauma. In some instances it is caused by an abnormally lateral attachment of the patellar tendon, creating a displaced patella with flexion. That places the patella more in contact with the femoral condyle. There also may be a genetic predisposition, with some individuals having a less resilient cartilage covering on all joints. Whatever the cause, the athlete complains of vague pain within the knee, perhaps localized behind the patella. There may be some swelling and increased discomfort when he or she goes up and down stairs. Running on hills will increase the pain. With increased interest in distance running, more knee problems are being seen. As an athlete increases his distance, his posterior muscles, particularly the Achilles tendon muscles, become overdeveloped and shortened, which may cause abnormal stresses about the knee, exacerbating chondromalacia.

Inflammation of the patellar tendon at its attachment to the inferior pole of the patella will create problems in the athlete who runs or jumps. The individual will complain of pain as he or she pushes off, as in jumping. The runner will complain of pain for a long period of time. There is usually no swelling. Examination usually reveals tenderness only at the inferior pole of the patella. In long-distance runners there is usually tightness of the Achilles tendon group and the hamstring group. There are many bursae around the knee, all of which are prone to inflammation, either following direct trauma or through overuse. The bursae become swollen to protect contiguous moving parts. The athlete complains of pain in one of the areas of the bursa. Examination reveals localized tenderness and localized swelling.

Swelling in the popliteal area, either nondescript or well delineated, may indicate a Baker's cyst, the diagnosis applied to a mass in that region whether it be caused by bursitis of the semimembranous or the medial gastrocnemius. The athlete complains of a full feeling in the popliteal area, particularly on extension of the knee. The mass may be palpable, and it may vary in size on any given day. Recurrent dislocation of the patella is more common in girls than in boys. Several factors may predispose to recurrent dislocation. Patella alta, or high-riding patella, is thought to be one. The patella is not well seated in the intertrabecular groove and has a greater likelihood of displacing laterally. Underdevelopment of the lateral femoral condyle allows the patella to dislocate laterally. Genu valgum, in which the quadriceps tendon is more lateral, predis-

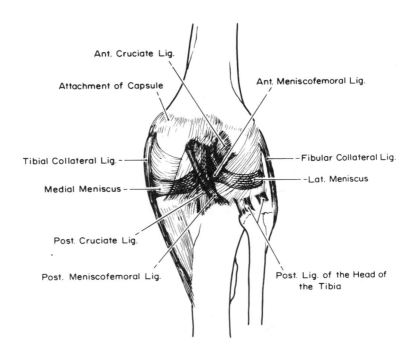

Knee anatomy, posterior view.

poses to dislocations. That is particularly true in women, with the wide pelvis causing the femur to be internally angulated and placing the knee in a relative valgus position. Examination reveals 1 or more of these conditions. Usually there is some subpatellar crepitus, indicating roughness of the patellar cartilage. The patella usually dislocates when the knee is flexed. The athlete may resist attempts to dislocate the patella because it is uncomfortable.

Injury to the medial collateral ligament (Pellegrini Stieda Disease), producing either a partial tear or a hematoma, may lead to calcification within that area. It is most frequently found in the proximal portion of the medial collateral ligament attachment on the femur. The athlete complains of soreness and discomfort in that area with strenuous activity. There may be some swelling. With the advent of interest in long-distance running, many athletes have complaints of knee pain. The runner usually experiences onset of pain after several miles. The knee becomes progressively more painful so that running is no longer possible. A short time of walking will usually relieve the symptoms. Common areas of pain are the medial joint line and the lateral joint line. Examination reveals no knee abnormalities. However, examination of the foot and ankle usually reveals loss of flexibility of the Achilles tendon. The runner will not be able to dorsiflex the foot beyond neutral with the knee extended. In runners who complain of medial knee pain, the configuration of a normal or cavus arch combined with slight valgus is often seen. In runners with lateral knee pain, just the opposite, or a planus foot with genu varum, is common.

knee ligaments and tendon injuries. The triad of chondromalacia, tendinitis, and ligament strain can all occur in the runner's knee syndrome. Ligamentous strains, however, are more prevalent in sports requiring quick movements in a side-to-side fashion. That motion puts a greater twisting force on the knee joint. The 3 reasons athletes develop soft tissue strains around the knees are (1) lack of proper condition for the activity, (2) unnatural activities leading to unusual stresses, and (3) inherent musculoskeletal weakness. When vigorous activity is attempted without preparation, the muscles are often too weak to effectively stabilize and coordinate knee motion. That state puts excessive stress on muscle tendons and ligaments that are responsible for maintaining joint stability. The stress results in fatigue and damage to soft tissue structures. Participation in a sport that requires unnatural body movements may cause knee injury. Little can be done to change the activities required, but a thorough conditioning program before serious participation will allow the supporting elements of the knee more time to adapt to the increased load. Musculoskeletal weaknesses in the feet and legs are major contributors to overuse knee injuries. When faulty foot mechanics throw the leg and thigh bones out of alignment with every step, the supporting tissues cannot maintain stability without some signs of fatigue. Anatomically, the leg is divided into 4 muscular compartments. The front, or anterior compartment, houses muscles responsible for raising the foot on the leg. The lateral compartment lies on the outside of the leg and contains muscles that pull the foot away from the midline of the body (foot abduction). They also function in supporting the ankle. The posterior compartment has the large calf muscles causing foot plantar flexion, the movement of the foot allowing one to stand on his toes. The posterior group also includes muscles for flexing the toes and the posterior tibial muscle, which helps maintain the arches of the foot. The leg unit consists then of large muscles originating from either of the 2 leg bones to exert their force on the foot below.

knockdown shoulder. A ligamentous injury that grades from minor subluxation to full dislocation. It is due to injury of the acromio-clavicular joint. It can result from a fall on the point of the shoulder or onto an outstretched hand or to a downward blow on the shoulder. It is seen in contact sports, such as soccer and rugby and in horse-riding sports after a fall.

L

laceration. A separation of the skin with relatively sharp edges. Ordinarily in athletics this is not a cleanly incised wound, as with a knife or razor blade. Instead, it is a combination of a contusion and a lacerated wound in which the lacerated edge is jagged and irregular. The wounds may be of any degree, from an extensive tearing of the skin with considerable separation of the skin edges to a fissurelike injury with little external evidence of damage.

Lacrosse, field hockey, hurling, shinty injuries. All these games have in common the following—they are team games involving teams of between 10 to 15 players. They are all running games and are played using a "stick" or "club" with which a hard ball is struck, caught, or thrown. The last 2 are Gallic games played respectively in Ireland and in Scotland. Impact injuries are produced by the ball, the stick, or the club and by accidental collision and falls. Indirect injury is caused by running and cutting, the knee and ankle being the commonly involved areas. For protection in lacrosse, wear head and face guards. For protection in field hockey, goal keepers should wear protective gloves, pads, and special heavy boots. Players may wear shin pads. In hurling a head helmet may be worn. Contusions and lacerations are fairly common. Fractures are rare and are commonly associated with twisting injuries to the ankle. Falls may produce fractures about the wrist and elbow and shoulder—commonly the clavicle.

lactic acid system. When stored adenosine triphosphate (ATP) and phosphocreatine (PC) are substantially reduced, additional short-term energy is available from anaerobic metabolism of glycogen. Glycogen is broken down to lactic acid in this 2nd anaerobic system. ATP (for high-density activities lasting as long as 3 minutes) can be supplied by the lactic acid (LA) system. Training procedures increase production of ATP from this anaerobic system and thus enhance the performance potential for strenuous activities lasting 1 to 3 minutes. However, in the process lactic acid accumulates in the muscles and blood which may contribute to symptoms of fatigue and muscle soreness. During heavy exercise lactic acid accumulates within muscle tissue as a result of oxygen demands exceeding oxygen supply. Choking of performance, because of excessive competition or poor pacing, may lead to early anaerobic demands on metabolism, resulting in lactate accumulation. It is witnessed as a premature distressing hyperventilation. Local muscle weakness may also induce premature breathlessness. The hyperventilation from premature lactate accumulation can cause an athlete to exceed normal ventilation adjustments where oxygen delivered to the circulation is less than the corresponding demand for oxygen consumption. It is thus important for an athlete to avoid lactate accumulation until late in the activity. Marathon runners usually operate just under their lactate threshold until their final sprint.

larynx injuries. The larynx, or voice box, is located between the pharynx and the windpipe. It has a framework of cartilage that protrudes in the front of the neck and sometimes is referred to as the Adam's apple. The larynx is considerably larger in the male than in the female. At the upper end are the vocal folds. Those cordlike structures serve in the production of speech. The nasal cavities, the sinuses, and the pharynx all serve as resonating chambers for speech. The larynx may be crushed between a blunt object and the anterior cervical spine, leading to cartilaginous fracture, subluxation, and dislocation. The most common fracture of the thyroid cartilage is that of a vertical anterior split between the thyroid notch and the cricothyroid membrane, producing avulsion of the anterior vocal cord attachments and hematoma. Laryngeal injury usually produces a louder stridor than does tracheal injury, but stridor may be absent if the obstruction is severe enough to completely obstruct the airway. Besides stridor, other signs and symptoms of laryngeal fracture may be loss of cartilaginous landmarks from edema, *dyspnea*, *dysphonia* from paresis or hematoma, pain increased by neck motion, dysphagia, subcutaneous emphysema, and local tenderness.

leg. Anatomically, the leg is divided into 4 muscular compartments. The front or anterior compartment houses muscles responsible for raising the foot on the leg. The lateral compartment lies on the outside of the leg and contains muscles responsible for pulling the foot away from the midline of the body (foot abduction). Those muscles also function in supporting the ankle. The posterior compartment contains the large calf muscles causing foot plantar flexion, the movement of the foot allowing an individual to stand on his or her toes. The posterior group also has muscles for flexing the toes and the posterior tibial muscle, which helps maintain the arch of the foot. The leg unit consists of large muscles originating from either of the 2 leg bones to exert their force on the foot below.

leg injuries. Contusion is very common in the lower leg since in most sports it is exposed to direct blows. The nature and severity of the injury depend upon the site of the direct trauma. Much of the tibia is superficial and therefore has very little protective coating. Direct blows to the posterior aspect of the leg may cause hemorrhage of varying degree but seldom result in myositis ossificans traumatica. Contusions over the proximal fibula may injure the peroneal nerve. The symptoms will vary according to the extent of injury to the nerve. Strains of the muscles and tendons of the leg are frequent in runners and jumpers. The diagnosis of a sprain to a muscle or tendon is based upon the history of the mechanism, at the point of tenderness, and the degree of disability. In shin splints the injury expresses itself in the form of painful swelling of the leg muscles, especially the anterior and posterior tibial ones, which may be acute or chronic. It arises from a variety of causes, chiefly from the prolonged hard running of the untrained or poorly conditioned athlete. Repeated running on very hard surfaces may also induce a chronic state. Following vigorous exercise, especially in an unconditioned athlete, rapid swelling may occur within the anterior compartment, which may lead to early interference with the blood supply and muscle necrosis. Pain, cramping, muscle spasms, paresthesias, and numbness are signs of anterior compartment syndrome. Dislocation of the head of the fibula results when a twisting force is applied to the knee, rotating it internally, and at the same time direct force is applied to the head of the fibula, levering it out of the shallow socket in which it lies. Isolated fractures of the tibia and fibula occur but are not unusual. Fractures may also be due to direct violence, as in football, or indirect violence (particularly rotational strains), as in skiing. Shin splints or shin soreness is fairly common among athletes who complain of pain in the front of the leg on exercise. The problem may be due to stress fracture, to tibia and anterior syndrome, or to tendoperiostosis or tibialis posterior syndrome. Differentiation may be made at the site of the pain and the fact that the mode of onset varies. Tendoperiostosis usually occurs on the medial side of the leg at the medial tibial border. Pain occurs during exercise and may be quite severe although normally well localized. There is no hint of direct trauma. The condition is due to microtraumatic elevation of the periosteum by the jerk of the attached muscle fascia during exercise.

leg overuse compartment syndrome. The overuse compartment syndrome is frequently manifested by a dull generalized ache in the anterior or lateral leg compartments. There is pain on pressure, without significant increase on moving the foot. That is because the pain is within the compartment, not in the muscle. The pain is a result, not of lactic acid accumulation, which gives a constant soreness with motion of the foot, but of muscle inflammation and excessive pressure in an unyielding space. The swelling is a result of overexertion and, if severe enough, can impede blood supply to the muscle-causing cramping. The pain varies from mild soreness to intolerable cramps made worse by weight bearing. The complaint is normally seen in the poorly trained athlete. Proper conditioning will usually strengthen muscles sufficiently to withstand increased demand. Muscle spasms attributable to foot or ankle trauma may also be present as generalized compartment pains in the leg.

ligament injuries. Like tendons, ligaments are dense, stiff, very strong bands of fibrous tissue. The major difference between the 2 is in their functions. Whereas tendons attach muscle to bone, ligaments attach one to another. Ligaments go from 1 bone to the next and hold them together in their proper relationships. They are more flexible than tendons, so that a certain amount of motion can occur at their connecting joints, but at the same time they have (like tendons) a low amount of elasticity. Thus they can be stretched only to a limited degree before they rupture or "tear." Once ligaments have been torn, they do not generally repair themselves. When ligaments are either partially or completely torn, they release the normal tension holding a joint's parts in their proper relationship and the joint loosens. Such looseness can provoke all sorts of further complications, such as: instability, trick knee, arthritis, and so forth. It can also have a deleterious effect on nearby areas of the body. A ligament can be repaired only surgically, that is, through a procedure of removing the section of ligament that is torn or ruptured and inserting other tissue to replace it. Ligaments are numerous throughout the body. Not only do they join every bone to every other bone; they also are an integral part of every articulating joint. The principal function of ligaments in joints is to provide a checkrein effect so that joints cannot overextend in an unnatural direction and tear or pull apart all the muscles and other structures surrounding them. Probably the most frequently noticed ligaments are those in the knee, but ligaments have equally vital functions throughout the body. The ligaments of the spine, for instance, hold the spinal column in its proper alignment. Each of the 24 vertebrae in the back and corresponding discs represents a joint; thus there are 24 small articulating joints in the spine. The various spinal ligaments keep them connected and in line and prevent the spine from overextending under normal conditions.

Injuries involving the knee are very frequent in basketball. The medial semilunar cartilage is most often damaged with the torsion and lateral stress applied to the knee. In violent, twisting movements, either collateral ligaments may be torn. When the force is continued, the semilunar cartilage of the cruciate ligament may be involved. At times the medial collateral ligament, medial semilunar cartilage, and anterior cruciate ligament are damaged. In skiing, the knee joint is 2nd only to the ankle in its susceptibility to injury, with the injuring force being abduction, with some rotation; 56 percent of all torsion injuries to the lower limb result in a knee injury, and 29 percent

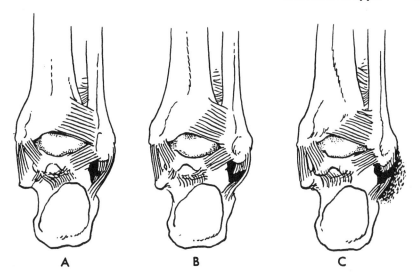

A   B   C

Drawings showing (1) partial tear of ligament, mild (1st-degree) sprain; (2) moderate (2nd-degree) sprain, with more complete tear but still integrity of ligament; (3) severe sprain with (3rd-degree) tear and loss of integrity.

are associated with an ankle sprain and with injury to the opposite knee. The medial collateral ligament is damaged along with the lateral in the cruciate ligaments. The common injury of the knee is a partial tear of the deep fibers of the medial collateral ligament between their attachments to the femur and the meniscus. In football the sprain of the medial ligament is usually a combination of direct and indirect violence, resulting from a blow on the outside of the knee as the player's leg is stretched out, the blow being caused either by a tackle or a falling opponent. The torn meniscus is usually the semilunar, the one on the inside of the joint; it is torn by rotation of the femur on a bent knee, as when a fullback tackles and pivots at the same time. The ankle is particularly vulnerable in football players. Fractures to the joint, or just above the joint, are often caused by sliding tackles; sprains are caused by forced abduction or adduction, movements that may result in ligament sprain, joint sprain, or cracked or chipped malleoli. In tennis most of the tendon lesions, such as tennis elbow, medial ligament strain at the knee, lateral ligament strain at the ankle, and the occasional occurence of painful heel in the middle-aged or elderly, are due to underlying degenerative changes in the fibrous tissue structure concerned, with the superimposed trauma of the game acting as the trigger that starts off inflammation.

limb bones, lower. The lower limb is attached to the trunk by the pelvic girdle, which is formed by the 2 hip bones, which articulate with each other in the midline anteriorly and with the sacrum posteriorly. The lower limb is composed of 3 segments: the thigh, which has 1 bone, the femur; the leg, which has 2 bones, the tibia and the fibula; and the foot, which is composed of the tarsal bones (7), the metatarsal bones (5), and the phalanges (14).

limb bones, upper. The upper limb is attached to the trunk by the shoulder girdle, which is made up of 2 bones, the clavicle anteriorly and the scapula posteriorly. The shoulder girdle is attached to the trunk by 1 joint, the sternoclavicular joint, and the muscles. The shoulder girdle is able to move in several directions, and its movements are important in the range of movements that are possible with the upper limb. The upper limb consists of 3 segments: the upper arm, which has 1 bone, the humerus; the forearm, which has 2 bones, the radius and the ulna; and the wrist and hand, which is made up of the carpal bones (8), the metacarpal bones (5), and the phalanges (14).

Little League shoulder.   The technical name for this ailment is osteochondrosis of the proximal humeral epiphysis, but it is more commonly known as "Little League shoulder." Up until the adolescent stage of development, the growth of the musculo-skeletal system is incomplete. The bones, especially at the joints, must have the ability to expand with the rest of one's growth. As a result, the ends of the bones have sectors called "growth plates." They are usually immune from damage in normal childhood and preadolescent activities. But in certain sports the growth plates of youngsters can be damaged by excessive and recurrent stresses on those areas. That is especially true of the shoulder and elbow growth plates of the humerus in the throwing sports, such as baseball. The growth plates represent the weakest links in the young musculo-skeletal chain. In the adult those areas are no longer present, and stress is absorbed instead on the ligaments, tendons, and the bones themselves. But in the shoulders of baseball-playing youngsters up to the age of 15, it is the growth plate at the top of the humerus that is required to bear much of the stress in repeated hard throwing or pitching. With repeated stress on the growth plate at the top of the humerus, the bone loses its blood supply and becomes devitalized. The symptoms are acute pain in the shoulder upon any attempt to throw a ball, followed by an insistent full ache that becomes more severe with subsequent efforts. Similar ailments can develop in and around the growth plates of the elbow in preadolescent tennis players as well. Fortunately, damaged or debilitated bone regenerates and heals. However, if youngsters are allowed to continue competing when that situation develops, their shoulders or elbows can develop serious complications and weaknesses that will affect their joint function later in life.

liver damage.   Direct trauma to the upper aspect of the right side of the abdomen in sporting injuries can lead to hepatic damage. In most cases the injury is minor, a hematoma or a small laceration, but damage to the liver may be more serious, the symptoms being similar to those of ruptured spleen, except that the initial pain and tenderness are referred to the right side of the abdomen and the right shoulder tip. Subsequently, the extent of the peritoneal hemorrhage again determines the general state of the injured person.

long, continual-stress injuries.   Long-maintained stresses are by nature subtle in their effects. The only tissue in the body that can sustain stresses indefinitely without being harmed is bone. Articular cartilage and the intervertebral discs also have to sustain such stresses and are highly modified for that purpose, although they often suffer ill effects from so doing. All the other soft tissues of the body, muscle, tendons, ligaments, etc., are harmed if they are subjected to mechanical forces for too long. Such forces are usually those of traction and may be comparatively small. If applied for a short time, they do not harm, but if continued indefinitely, they set up (in the affected tissue) a cycle of changes, which leads to pain and disability. The conditions so produced are usually called strains and are basically traumatic in origin, the results of excessive mechanical force applied to the body tissue.

long-distance running temperature regulation.   Thermoregulatory responses during long-distance running events have been measured. The health and performance of marathon runners do depend to a great extent on their thermoregulatory capacity. The circulatory system transfers metabolically produced heat from active muscle tissue predominantly to the surface for dissipation through convection, radiation, and sweating. The factors that overload the cardiovascular system or reduce sweat evaporation will markedly decrease the performance of the heat-losing mechanisms and increase the risk of overheating. Marathon racers should, therefore, not be running when the ambient temperature or the humidity is high. Core temperature in finishing marathon competitors of 40°C or greater has been observed even under cool conditions. During such long-distance runs, the body temperature is directly dependent on the metabolic rate or body weight or both, so heavier competitors will have higher rectal temperatures than lighter athletes when running at the same pace. Since dissipation of heat depends also on sweat evaporation, large losses in body water occur during long-distance races. Those who are not suitably hydrated before a long-distance race may have an inordinate rise in body temperature and be unable to complete the distance.

lunate dislocation. Forcible hyperextension and compression of the wrist, as in a fall onto a hand. Symptoms may include local pain and disability. Signs may be swelling on the volar surface of the wrist, the hand held in slight flexion, tender depression palpable on the dorsal surface, and a palpable mass deep in the volar surface beneath the flexor tendon. A lunate injury may be seen in any athlete from a fall on the outstretched hand, but it is most common in boxers whose hands are carelessly wrapped. Damage to the median nerve is a complication. The clinical picture is one of anterior wrist swelling, with stiff and semiflexed fingers. The lunate usually dislocates posteriorly or anteriorly, disrupting its relationship with the neighboring carpals and the distal radius. Complications with a lunate injury may include: median nerve injury, traumatic arthritis and aseptic necrosis.

lungs. The organs in which external respiration takes place, that is, where blood and air meet through the medium of the extremely thin and delicate lung tissues. There are 2 lungs, set side by side in the thoracic cavity. As soon as each bronchus enters the lung at the hilum, it immediately subdivides. Those branches or subdivisions of the bronchi resemble the branches of a tree. Each individual bronchial tube subdivides again and again, forming progressively smaller divisions. The smallest are called bronchioles. Those tubes are assorted sizes containing small bits of cartilage, which give firmness to the walls and serve to hold the tube open so that air can pass in and out easily. As the tubes become smaller, the cartilage also decreases in amount until finally, in the most minute subdivisions, there is no cartilage at all. At the end of each of the smallest subdivisions of the bronchi tree (called terminal bronchioles) there is a whole cluster of air sacs, resembling a bunch of grapes (alveoli). Each air sac is made of 1 cell layer of squamous (flat) epithelium. That very thin wall provides an easy passage for the gases entering and leaving the blood, which is contained in the millions of tiny capillaries of the alveoli.

lung disease, chronic. Can be the result of chronic infection (such as tuberculosis), slow-growing tumors, small airway infection (bronchiectasis), or chronic obstructive disease. Emphysema (dilation of the alveoli and formation of small or large cysts owing to destruction of the alveolar walls) is the result of long-standing chronic lung disease, most often obstructive diseases. Both obstructive diseases and emphysema usually result from long exposure to air pollution, particularly cigarette smoking or heavy smog. Most individuals with chronic lung disease are aware of their problem and are not likely to venture into such endeavors as mountain climbing or peak performing sports. However, in the early stages, these diseases may not be detectable except with severe exertions or at high altitude. The first signs of chronic obstructive lung disease or of emphysema may be a decrease in the respiratory reserve (pulmonary vital capacity). That reserve is the extra breathing capacity that is called on during exertion. Respiratory reserve is also called upon during activity in high altitude or whenever infection in part of the lung, shock, or loss of blood decrease the availability of oxygen to the body.

lung injuries. The lung may suffer contusion, and a small hemoptysis results. With proper treatment sports can be resumed in 2 weeks in most cases. In a more serious accident, the opposite lung may be affected as well with a mixture of edema, interstitial hemorrhage, atelectasis, and alveolar hemorrhage. Such serious injuries may need intermittent positive-pressure respiration. Subcutaneous emphysema follows an escape of air from a damaged lung or air passage, which then finds its way into the chest wall, mediastinum, and subcutaneous tissues by way of a rupture in the parietal pleura. It is occasionally associated with an open chest wound, and when there is a rapid accumulation, a torn bronchus may be suspected. Lung lacerations do not bleed freely, because of the low pulmonary arterial pressure.

lymphadenitis and lymphangitis. Inflammation of the lymph nodes and lymphatic vessels frequently accompanies infection and it is particularly prevalent following abrasions of the hand and infection around the feet, such as ingrown toenail or severe athlete's foot. The involvement of the lymph system is due to the drainage from the infection. The symptoms may be increasing pain in the local lesion followed by appearance of red streaks extending toward the neighboring glands (lymphangitis). The red streaks have local heat and tenderness but are not particularly painful. Soreness will develop in the regional lymph glands, which may become swollen and inflamed (lymphadenitis). Only occasionally will they go on to suppuration.

lymphatic system. Composed of (1) a plexus of minute vessels, called lymphatic capillaries, which start minutely in the tissues and contain a fluid called lymph; (2) lymphatic vessels, which are formed by the union of the lymphatic capillaries and which ultimately empty their contents into the bloodstream; (3) lymph nodes, which are composed of lymphatic tissue and through which all the lymph is filtered before it is returned to the bloodstream; and (4) collections of lymphatic tissue, which are found at various sites in the body. The lymphatic capillaries form a network in the tissues. The walls of the lymphatic capillaries are more permeable to larger molecules than are the blood capillaries. They are important for returning tissue fluid and molecules of larger size to the bloodstream. If the lymphatic drainage from a region is obstructed, then fluid accumulates in the tissue spaces. The lymphatic capillaries can drain particulate, waste, and pathogenic matter from the tissues. When an infection occurs in the tissues, white cells with ingested bacteria may also pass into the lymphatic capillaries.

M

mallet finger. A more serious version of baseball finger, with more potentially disabling consequences. It occurs when the tip of the finger is impacted by a moving object, such as a ball, and the distal or farthest interphalangeal joint is hyperflexed (bent) at the same time as its extensor tendon is contracting. As one is opening or extending a finger, it is struck on the tip, and its distal joint is forcibly bent downward. What happens is basically the collision of 2 opposing forces within the finger, the flexing force versus the extending force. Something has to give, and since the flexing force of the impacting object is greater than the extending force of the joint's extensor tendon, the tendon gives. The tendons in the fingers are extremely tough and resistant to tearing, and the distal extensor tendons are no exception. It is not the tendon itself that gives; rather, it struggles to combat the overload brought about by the impact. The result is that the tendon pulls a piece of bone off the spot at which it attaches to the distal phalanx. The extensor tendon is no longer attached or is only partially attached to the bone beyond the joint. It is therefore no longer, or only marginally able, to extend the joint; therefore, the joint remains in a flexed position, and the finger takes on a mallet-head configuration. The deformity may become permanent unless it is treated immediately and properly.

mandible fracture (fractured jaw). Symptoms may be local pain, especially on movement, and inability to occlude teeth forcibly. Signs may include: swelling, local tenderness, crepitus, deviation to fracture side, restricted movement. Complications may lead to osteomyelitis and malocclusion. Fracture of the mandible is a possible injury in most all sports.

meniscus, lateral tear (torn cartilage). Forcible hyperflexion of the knee, with foot fixed firmly upon the ground, femur rotated outward upon tibia, while knee is adducted and flexed, as in squatting with heel against buttocks for long duration in duck-waddle-type exercise; discoid may be predisposing. Symptoms may be recurrent effusion, instability, weakness, pain, snapping sensation upon full flexing or extending. Signs may include effusion, tenderness along joint line, anterolaterally or posterolaterally; pain elicited at lateral side of knee by rotary stress; positive McMurray test with tibia internally rotated and adducted; audible and palpable click coming out of deep flexion. Complications could be traumatic arthritis, meniscus cyst, concomitant ligamentous instability.

metacarpal fractures. Boxers frequently damage the first metacarpal bone especially when they are training with heavy punching bags and poorly taped hands. Generally, the fracture is transverse, a quarter of an inch distal to the carpometacarpal joint, and reduction is performed by pulling on the abducted thumb and levering the metacarpal outward against the operator's thumb, thus correcting the bowing. Spiral fractures and transverse fractures of the other metacarpal shafts with only slight displacement do not require reduction. Another common boxing fracture is of the 5th metacarpal neck. As in any metacarpal neck fracture, slight displacement may not be a problem, but an ugly lump in the palm needs accurate reduction, which is produced by direct thumb pressure in the palm. Fractures and dislocations of the phalanges are common, the typical goalkeeper's injury. The dislocation or fracture is usually easily reduced and maintained by a malleable splint or plaster.

metacarpophalangeal dislocation. Extreme or abnormal extension of the metacarpal bones of the palm of the hand, which can create a deformity. Signs are obvious deformity, proximal phalanx displaced dorsally, slight flexion of the proximal interphalangeal joint, head of metacarpal prominent in palm. Symptoms may be pain and limitation of motion.

metacarpophalangeal strain. Extreme or abnormal extension of the metacarpal bones of the palms of the hand causing a severe strain. Symptoms may be pain and varying degrees of instability. Signs are graded by the degree of severity. There is local tenderness, with pain being felt on motion.

metatarsal fracture, base. Excessive or forcible movement of the foot so as to bend the part toward the dorsum or posterior aspect of the body; the movement of the foot backward at the ankle. Symptoms are pain, disability in running and jumping. Signs may include sharply localized tenderness, swelling, ecchymosis. Complications may cause persistent disability.

metatarsal fracture, head. Fracture caused by stubbing toe under foot, weight falling on the foot. Symptoms may be pain localized to the metatarsophalangeal joint. Signs may include localized swelling, tenderness, stiffness, or deformity. Complication may be traumatic arthritis.

metatarsal fracture, neck. Fracture caused by stubbing toe under foot, weight falling on foot. Symptoms may be local pain and disability in walking and running. Signs may include local swelling and tenderness just proximal to joint, involved metatarsal head prominent in sole of foot, limited motion. Complications are metatarsalgia, malunion, or nonunion.

metatarsal fracture, shaft. Crushing injury, as in weight falling on the foot. Symptoms may be generalized pain of foot and some disability. Signs may include extensive swelling, pain elicited by axial pressure in line of shaft, crepitus demonstrated on gentle flexion and extension. Complications are prolonged disability, metatarsalgia, callosity, malunion.

metatarsal stress fracture. Stress fractures are small breaks in bones that can occur in almost any bone subjected to continuous trauma. Stress fractures in athletes are usually seen in the metatarsals but also frequently in the heel bone or leg bones. Metatarsal stress fractures are usually due to 1 metatarsal bearing a disproportionate amount of weight. The weight imbalance is seen with a Morton's foot and also in a pronated foot. In Morton's foot the first metatarsal is abnormally short, leaving weight bearing predominantly to the 2nd, 3rd, and 4th metatarsals. The 5th metatarsal can elevate because it, unlike the 1st, has an independent joint movement. It therefore rarely sustains a stress fracture. Weight imbalance in a maximally pronated foot allows the 1st and 5th metatarsals to elevate, leaving the midregion of the foot to bear most of the weight. Therapy includes fracture, healing with time, and the balancing of the forefoot with orthoses. Stress fractures in the heel and leg bones are due to body impact at heel contact and does not respond to orthotics.

metatarsalgia. Morton's syndrome (metatarsalgia) exhibits a pain at a small spot near the proximal end of 1 of the 3 outer toes. It is especially debilitating in track and almost always associated with compression of the foot by tight shoes, resulting in pinching of the external plantar nerves between the metatarsal bones. The syndrome triad consists of (1) a 1st metatarsal bone that is shorter than the 2nd, (2) hypermobility at the naviculocuneiform and medial- and inter-cuneiform articulations, and (3) posteriorly displaced sesamoids. Differentiation must be made from postural strains, neuroma, arch fractures, subluxations, exostoses, and tendon avulsions. There are toe pains, foot fatigue, and pronation complaints that are often associated with plantar callous patterns, bunion, corns, and intermetatarsal neuroma. The sesamoids are displaced posteriorly, there is hypertrophy of the 2nd metatarsal joint, the foot is pronated, and the arch flattened with abnormal weight balance and distribution.

middle ear barotrauma. In rapid pressure changes, such as in diving or in an airplane descent, the drum herniates inwardly if the Eustachian tube does not afford pressure equalization. The negative pressure within the middle ear causes slight hemorrhages and extracts fluids from adjacent tissues. A weakened drum may rupture in a deep descent, resulting in severe vertigo as water enters the middle chamber. Prevention is made by avoiding clogged ears or nasal congestion before descent.

miliaria. "Prickly heat" or "heat rash" manifests as a series of pink, pruritic, papulovesicular lesions under protective gear, such as shoulder pads and rib pads, worn during warm-weather activities. It is not unusual in football linemen. No protective uniform can be considered "cool" for the overweight athlete, and the disorder is brought on by excessive sweating and a distinct lack of perspiration or a partial obstruction, such as congenital, to the ducts of the sweat glands, forcing sweat to escape into the epidermis.

mineral needs. Sweat contains less sodium chloride (0.1–0.4 percent) than blood (0.9 percent). Thus, unless fluid intake is large, the sodium content of the plasma tends to rise during competition. Potassium ions "leak" from the active muscles, partly as a consequence of glycogen depletion, and there is thus some tendency to hyperkalemia. Mineral deficiencies are incurred in the hours following competition when muscle potassium is restored and the body is dehydrated. A single incident in a hot environment is rarely sufficient to cause any problem, but a cumulative mineral deficit can arise from an extended exposure in training or a succession of heats. The normal salt loss in a temperate climate is 12 g/day, but a man who sweats profusely can lose up to 8 g/hr from a total body pool of 175 g. A loss of 0.5 g/kg causes lassitude, weakness, giddiness, fainting, and muscle cramps, while a deficit of 0.75 g/kg leads to apathy, stupor, and a marked fall of blood pressure. In the absence of supervision, more acute salt deficiency may occasionally develop, with marked weight loss, constipation, scant urine, and other signs of dehydration, such as nausea, vomiting, sunken eyes, inelastic skin, and circulatory failure. Once vomiting has begun, it leads to a vicious circle of further salt loss and dehydration.

molluscum contagiosum. A mildly contagious disease, affecting the skin and conjunctivae, most likely to be seen in mature athletes. It features round, firm, smooth, waxy, translucent, skin-colored, crateriform papules (2 mm to 10 mm in diameter) containing caseous matter and peculiar capsulated bodies. The condition resembles large "whiteheads" often appearing on athlete's genitals, pubic area, eyelids, or buttocks, as a small asymptomatic patch containing about a dozen lesions. Sometimes a large single molluscum may grow to 30 mm in diameter. An area of dermatitis may surround the lesion patch. The incubation period appears to be from 2 to 7 weeks. The disease is contagious as long as active lesions are present. Contact sports, especially wrestling, should be avoided. Participation in other sports is discretionary if the lesions can be adequately covered.

Morton's foot. Described as the "Grecian foot" with the short big toe and the long 2nd toe. It is a hereditary deformity, common but not disabling among sedentary individuals. However, in athletes, especially middle- and long-distance runners, it can lead to problems associated with overuse. Anatomically, Morton's foot consists of an abnormally short 1st metatarsal bone, which is extremely hypermobile at its base. There is posterior and lateral displacement of the sesamoid bones and a thickening of the 2nd metatarsal cortical areas. The 2nd metatarsal is usually abnormally long as compared with the rest of the metatarsal bones. This foot is a problem because of the shortness of the 1st metatarsal bone, the lateral aspect of the foot, especially when the 2nd metatarsal bears more than its share of weight. That allows the foot to become hypermobile and to flatten or pronate. The architecture is disturbed, and the foot does not function properly during the last part of the gait cycle. That, together with hypermobility at the base of the 2nd metatarsal, produces an injury-prone foot. If there is also a secondary deformity, such as rear foot varus or forefoot varus, the runner can expect more than his or her share of lower extremity injuries. The foot strikes the ground more than 5,000 times during a 1-hour jogging period, and that exerts strain on a foot that is already weak. A survey (over several years) showed that more than 30 percent of those with lower leg injuries also have Morton's foot.

Morton's neuroma. Neuritis, inflammation, or irritation of a nerve can be a troublesome problem for athletes. Morton's neuroma, a common neuritis, is characterized by localized pain between the 3rd and 4th metatarsal heads, often radiating into the 3rd and 4th toes, although other interspaces may be involved. The pain is increased by tight shoe wear and is relieved by going barefoot. The medial and lateral plantar nerves converge between the 3rd and 4th toes, where the junction becomes enlarged. Tight shoes compress the metatarsal heads against the nerve, producing a painful neuroma. Once the pain starts, it is often difficult to control. It is a common problem in women, but it may occur in men. The pain usually develops after activity has been going on for a time.

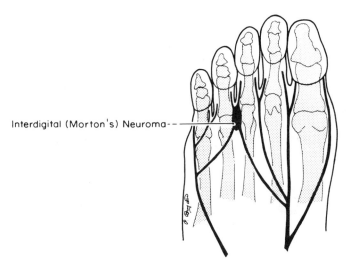

Interdigital (Morton's) Neuroma

motor unit (muscles). The basic functional unit that initiates movement in muscle tissue is called the motor unit. It consists of a single alpha motor neuron, its axon, and all the muscle fibers innervated through the axonal branches. The number of muscle fibers in 1 motor unit varies widely. There is a general agreement that muscles controlling fine movement and adjustments have the smallest number of muscle fibers per motor unit, whereas large coarse acting muscles have large units. Thus, it has been estimated, for example, that motor units of human extraocular muscles contain 5 to 6 muscle fibers, human laryngeal muscles 2 to 3 fibers, and the medial head of the human gastrocnemius, 2,000 muscle fibers per motor unit. The individual fibers of a motor unit may be widely scattered and intermingled with fibers of other motor units.

mountain sickness, acute. A term applied to a group of rather widely varying symptoms caused by altitude. The primary cause is undoubtedly the decreased oxygen in the blood, which is related directly to the altitude attained. However, the mechanism by which the reduced oxygen produces the varied features of acute mountain sickness is uncertain. Evidence suggests some alteration of the cells lining small blood vessels is present that allows water to leave the vessels and accumulate in the tissues in an abnormal manner. That change apparently is associated with a reduction in water excretion by the kidneys. The symptoms of acute mountain sickness depend on the height attained and the rate of ascent, usually begin within a few hours of ascent, and begin to decrease in severity on about the 3rd day. Common symptoms may include: headache, dizziness, fatigue, shortness of breath, loss of appetite, nausea, and vomiting, disturbed sleep, and a general feeling of being unwell (malaise). Drowsiness and frequent yawning are common. Anxiety attacks and hyperventilation may occur. Cheyne-Stokes breathing may be present during the day and is common at night, when it may interfere with sleep. A cerebral form of mountain sickness, caused by the effect of oxygen lack or possibly abnormal fluid collection on the brain, may have as the principal symptoms headache, dizziness, memory loss, confusion, and a decrease in mental acuity. In severe cases disturbances in gait, nerve paralysis, psychotic behavior, hallucinations, or coma may be seen. High altitude pulmonary edema may be present in this type of acute mountain sickness and may not be suspected. The cerebral form of acute mountain sickness is more commonly observed at altitudes in excess of 14,000 feet. Acute mountain sickness occurs with increasing frequency at higher altitudes. Between 8,000 and 10,000 feet occasional individuals have symptoms; above 14,000 feet most have symptoms.

muscles. Skeletal muscles are primarily voluntary muscles, containing their own nerves and their own blood supplies. The muscles are attached to bone by tendon in 2 areas. The area of attachment that is the least mobile is called the origin; the opposite mobile end is called the insertion. The origin and insertion of some muscles may vary, depending on which joint is fixed at a certain time in a period of motion. Usually the origin is the proximal end, and the insertion is the distal end. Anatomically, the insertion is always tendinous, whereas the origin may in some cases be muscular or fibrous. Tendons are stronger structures than muscles. They are composed of nonliving fibers and are more capable of sustaining trauma than muscles are. To protect muscles from underlying bony prominences, connective tissue pads are present. To protect the tendons from those same projections there are bursae and tendon sheaths. Fluid in the bursa provides a cushion to protect the tendon. Within the tendon sheath, a synovial-like fluid is produced to lubricate and allow the tendon to glide effortlessly. Trauma to the muscle or tendon increases the fluid in either of those spaces, causing pain and limitation of motion.

The strength of the muscle and the amount of movement the muscle can produce depends on several different factors: the actual number of muscle fibers being stimulated by the nerve, the position of the insertion at the time of activation, and the type of muscle. Muscles contract in 3 ways. An isotonic or equal tension contracture is the shortening of a muscle fiber without great variation in the strength of the contraction; an isometric contraction is one in which opposing muscles work with equal strength but there is no movement of the part and thus no shortening of the muscle; an eccentric contraction occurs in a movement that can be carried out only by gravity. The muscles that oppose this movement must first contract and then gradually lengthen. Of the 3 types, eccentric contraction exercises are the most efficient in increasing strength. Muscles may be damaged by direct blows, which may cause bruising and some disruption of fibers, or self-induced tears. Muscle tears may be complete or incomplete. Complete tears may be seen dramatically in the upper-arm biceps muscles when the long head of the biceps is torn and bending the elbow up causes the unattached end of the muscle to appear as a lump halfway down the forearm. A similar appearance is seen at the front end of the thigh, where the rectus femoris muscle may be damaged in a direct blow or torn in a kick, or at the back of the thigh in the hamstring muscles, which are often torn in sprinters. Partial muscle tears involve

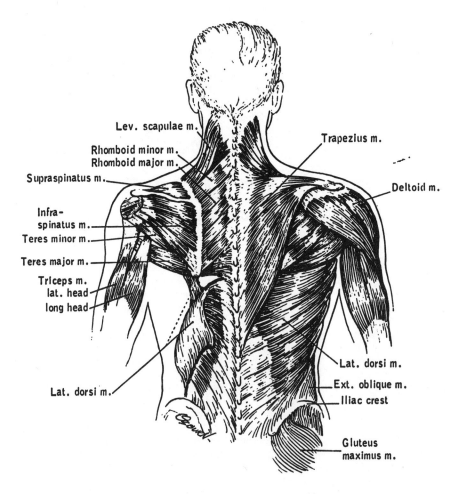

Muscle attachments about the shoulder.

only part of the muscle (central) or toward the edge of a muscle bundle (peripheral). It is not immediately possible to differentiate between a peripheral and a central tear. At this time a central tear is usually more painful, loss of function is more evident, and bruising is unlikely unless there is associated superficial contact injury. A peripheral tear allows drainage by gravity of the hematoma, or bruise, along tissue planes, and often spectacular bruising appears close by, while the original site of the injury is much less tender.

muscle cramps. Cramps are characterized by spontaneous, prolonged painful muscle contraction, usually occurring in the voluntary weight-bearing muscles. They often develop during sleep or soon after violent exertion and may vary from slight contraction to violent spasms. Cramps frequently follow drinking ice water or other cold drinks too quickly or in too large a quantity after exercise, but in the cramp phenomenon, all motor units fire and cause the spasm. Most muscle cramps (including heat type) are often caused by excessive potassium and calcium salt loss. However, other factors may be involved, such as muscle anoxia, cold, a blow or strain, or some undetermined reason. Swimming too soon after a meal increases the danger of active extremity cramps, because much of the general circulation is diverted to the abdomen for adsorption purposes. Hormonal factors and PMS may be involved in the female athlete, especially before or during the menstrual period.

muscle disorders. Myalgia means "muscular pain," whereas myositis is a term that indicates actual inflammation of muscle tissue. Fibrosis means "inflammation of connective tissues," particularly those connected with muscles and joints. Usually a combination disorder called fibromyositis is present. Such a condition is usually referred to as rheumatism, lumbago, or charley horse. The disorder may be acute with severe pain on motion, or it may be chronic. Bursitis is inflammation of a bursa, a cavity or sac filled with synovial fluid. The purpose of a bursa is to minimize friction. Some bursae connect with joints, others are closely related to muscles. Sometimes bursae develop spontaneously in response to prolonged friction. Some examples of bursitis are (1) student's elbow, in which the bursa over the point of the elbow (olecranon) is inflamed because of long hours of leaning on the elbow while studying; (2) housemaid's knee, in which the bursa in front of the patella is inflamed; (3) bursitis, which is common in those who must sit a great deal, such as taxicab and bus drivers and truckers. Housemaid's knee is a form of bursitis found in those who must be on their knees a great deal. Bunions are enlargements normally found at the base and medial side of the great toe. Usually prolonged pressure has caused the development of a bursa, which then has become inflamed.

muscle fatigue. The diminution of activity of a specific muscle or muscle group; that is, the mechanical output of the muscle decreases after a sufficiently prolonged and intense period of exercise. In isolated muscles that is seen as a decreasing contraction or tension production in spite of constant stimulation. As the muscle fibers become fatigued, their output per twitch decreases, but new units are then mobilized to compensate for the lost power. Although fatigue is localized in the neuromuscular system, the major cause of fatigue is chemical. It can be due either to accumulation of intermediate or final end products of energy metabolism (carbon dioxide, lactic acid, pyruvic acid, acid phosphates, etc.) or to the deficiency of energy-furnishing materials. The adequacy or inadequacy of oxygen supply to the muscles during exercise determines the extent of accumulation of the intermediate or end products of metabolism and influences the resynthesis of the energy-furnishing substances. Recovery from fatigue caused by lactic acid accumulation can occur within 1 hour; but if the depletion occurs in the glycogen stores, which are important in rebuilding the energy-rich phosphates, then the replenishing of those stores may take several days. Electrical changes occurring in muscle tissues during sustained contractions have been studied extensively, with researchers agreeing that with sustained contractions occurring in a state of fatigue, there is a reduction in the amplitude and a lengthening in the duration of the muscle action potential. Considerable modifications also occur in the organization of the electrical activity recorded from the whole muscle.

muscle function. Muscle is composed of contractible fibers that are responsive to impulses from the nerves. All the skeletal muscles (those muscles that are attached to the bones and are responsible for the motions of the skeleton) are controlled by the individual's conscious thought processes. All muscles are nourished on oxygen from the body's circulating blood system and are controlled by nerves that originate in the brain, descend through the spinal cord, and branch out into the muscles. One nerve may supply branches to many muscles, or 1 muscle may have several branches from different nerves. Therefore, the contraction of a particular muscle may be partial or complete depending upon the activity of the nerves that supply it. It is this blood-and-nerve supply system that accounts for such things as muscle strength, muscle tone, muscle function, and muscle ache. Muscles do not operate independently of one another. Muscles exist singularly and in groups. Within each group, muscles interact, and within specific areas of the body, various muscle groups interact with one another. The body is composed of large, medium, small, and miniscule muscles. Some lie near the surface of the skin; others are buried deep within the skeleton; but all function in an identical way. When a brain cell is activated, it sends impulses along specific nerves that feed the muscles. Those impulses instantaneously stimulate a muscle or group of muscles and cause them to contract. Contraction is the primary function of muscles and is what moves the skeleton. Muscles also serve to support the skeleton and hold it together in proper alignment. Many athletic ailments, such as trick knee, are directly responsible or traceable to weak muscle support around the affected joint area. Another group of ailments often brought about by poor muscle support is back problems. The muscles of the back and abdominal areas are designed not only to provide movement and mobility but also to support the spine. When those muscles become too weak to properly do the job, the spine loses much of its support and disk and vertebrae problems result.

muscle glycogen in endurance. Few athletic events place greater demands on the body's energy producing system than do endurance sports, such as distance running and cycling. The athlete must be content with high energy expenditure, both in daily training and maximal competitive efforts. One significant factor that limits the endurance athlete's capacity for work is nutrition. With extremely strenuous training, the performer may be chronically exhausted, which is probably related to muscle glycogen depletion. Intense training (daily) drastically reduces glycogen content in the exercised muscles. After 2 or 3 days of distance running, muscle glycogen is reduced to near zero. A diet containing 60 percent carbohydrate is inadequate to restore muscle glycogen to its pretraining level, and some individuals do not restore muscle glycogen despite 5 days of rest and carbohydrate ingestion. After prolonged exhaustive exercise, young men require approximately 46 hours to restore muscle glycogen to the preexercise level, in spite of consuming a diet composed of 90 percent carbohydrates. Muscle glycogen can be increased to well above normal by first depleting glycogen stores through strenuous exercise and then ingesting a high carbohydrate diet for 3 days. The resulting glycogen replacement is localized to muscles that have been exercised and is referred to as "muscle glycogen super compensation." A fat/protein diet following exercise, on the other hand, produces low incomplete replacement of the glycogen in the exhausted muscles. If carbohydrates are given without previous exercise, only mild increases occur. Since glycogen is essential for continued muscular work, large muscle glycogen stores (in the tissues to be exercised) reduce the chance of premature exhaustion during races lasting an hour or more. The exercise time to exhaustion can be increased by more than 100 percent by this means.

muscle injury. Damage to a muscle, whether intrinsic or extrinsic in origin, will result in tearing and disruption of the muscle fibers, connective tissue, and vessels and may occur in the belly of the muscle or at the origin or insertion of the fibers into tendon, aponeurosis, or periosteum. Normally, injury is restricted to only a few muscle fibers and their supporting connective tissues, in which case it may be called a "pull," "tear," or "strain." When a tear or strain occurs, both contractile and noncontractile elements are damaged, but such is the comparative strength of the muscle fibers that the major damage is probably incurred by the connective tissues, particularly the blood vessels. As a result of the injury, blood escapes into the extracellular and interstitial spaces of the muscle already somewhat engorged as a result of the hyperemia or exercise, thus producing the hematoma. In the more severe cases where the muscle sheath has also been damaged, the hematoma may expand into the potential space between the muscles. The degree of hemorrhage and hematoma formation is directly proportional to the degree of general muscle tone. When extrinsic violence is applied to a muscle, the subcutaneous and deep connective tissues are damaged as well and also become the site of hematoma formation. Bruising is normally the cause of muscle hernia. Hemorrhage from the site of injury will cease as intramuscular tension builds up, thus compressing the bleeding points. A muscle action that is not balanced by reciprocal inhibition of the antagonistic muscle (such as a blow or unexpected force) may result in rupture by sudden contraction or a less common injury to its antagonist by overstretching. Muscles previously weakened by fatigue or disease are more apt to rupture. Rupture is characterized by knifelike pain, followed by a sensation of extreme local weakness. If a complete tear occurs, the lesion is usually at the tendinous attachment to the muscle belly. Normal continuity is broken and quite obvious on palpation until obliterated by hemorrhage and swelling. Function is lost in proportion to the degree of tear. Muscle ruptures associated with nonpenetrating wounds are seen in both young and old. In youth they occur when a muscle is suddenly stressed beyond its tensile strength and the muscle fails at the musculotendinous junction. Such rupture is characterized by painful voluntary contraction, ecchymosis at an area of local tenderness, swelling, edema, and hemorrhage. Palpation will often reveal the defect. After the acute stage persistent weakness remains, and there is an increase in muscle bulk proximal to the rupture site upon contraction. In the elderly, muscle rupture occurs under minimal loads as a result of degeneration within the muscle's tendon. The ruptures are accompanied by considerably less pain, swelling, tenderness, and ecchymosis. However, they do present the later persistent weakness and increased bulk upon contraction.

muscle strength. The tension produced by a muscle is called muscular strength. However, in voluntary movements, various degrees of muscle tension may be developed in accordance with the purpose of the movement. The maximum level of tension is recorded isometrically and is termed muscular strength. The strength of a muscle is roughly proportional to its cross-sectional dimension. The girth of the arm includes, in addition to the muscles, the bone as well as subcutaneous adipose tissue. The size of the arm girth, therefore, is not necessarily in proportion to its strength. For athletes whose variance in subcutaneous fat is known to be much smaller, higher correlations are expected between muscular strength and arm girth. Muscular strength increases through training. In addition to their originally favorable physique of mesomorphic dominance, athletes go through intensified muscular training. Athletes specialized in certain sports events, however, demonstrated muscular strength not appreciably superior to that of the untrained. Among those sporting events, long-distance running actually does not require any exceptional muscular strength. However, such events as throwing, weight lifting, rowing, and judo require extra strength, and the athletes in those particular events need further intensified training to improve their performance. Muscular strength usually is measured in a static condition when muscles develop tension against a resistance, such as a spring, weights, or the equivalent. There is a close correlation between height and strength. Strength may be developed disproportionately, however, even in persons of relatively small stature by intensive training. Overloading muscles by isometric, isotonic, or isokinetic exercise may bring about enormous increases in strength over a period of time. With any type of training that increases strength, muscle size (added mass) will also increase in the exercised muscles. Strength in any one muscle is found proportional to its cross-sectional areas. Limiting factors in increasing muscle mass are the ability of the circulation to supply the muscle and the strength of the skeletal structure with its ligaments to be able to resist the force exerted without breaking or tearing.

muscle tendon strains. Soft-tissue damage is usually more painful and can be more serious than bone injury. Bone heals with calcification, whereas soft tissue heals with fibrous or scar tissue growths. The latter is different from the original soft tissue and lacks the elasticity or viability of the original tissue. Soft tissue also takes longer to heal than bone tissue. Bone tissue may actually be stronger after the healing process has taken effect, whereas soft tissue is usually weaker after repair. The most common muscle injury is strain of a few muscle fibers and associated connective tissue. Players refer to it as a muscle pull or tear. In strain both intrinsic or extrinsic muscle stress can produce torn muscle fibers, connective tissues, and vessels within a muscle belly or at its point of origin or insertion. A strain cannot affect a muscle and not the tendon or vice versa; thus the musculotendinous unit must be considered as a whole in case of a strain. Chronic strain is the result of prolonged overuse, which produces an inflammation at the tendinous attachment, musculotendinous junction, or within the tendon itself. As the activity continues, the inflammatory reaction progresses to calcification at the muscle origin or tendon insertion with possible spur development. Tendons with sheaths are more likely to become inflamed, with the inflammation spreading between the tendon proper and the sheath.

muscle tissue. Designed to produce power by a forcible contraction. The cells of muscle tissue are long and threadlike and are called muscle fibers. Skeletal muscles, which combine with connective tissue, form the body muscles proper. They provide for the movement of the body. That type of tissue is also known as voluntary muscle, since it can be made to contract by those nerve impulses from the brain that originate to form an act of will. The next 2 groups of muscle tissue are known as involuntary muscle, since they typically contract independently of the will. They are the cardiac muscle, which forms the bulk of the heart wall and is known also as the myocardium, the muscles that produce the regular contractions known as heartbeats. The visceral muscles (also known as the smooth muscles) form the walls of the viscera. Some examples of visceral muscles are those that move the food and waste materials along the digestive tract. Visceral muscles are found in other kinds of structures, such as tubular forms, as the blood vessels and tubes that carry urine from the kidneys. Even certain structures at the base of the body hairs have such muscle. When they contract, a skin condition results called "gooseflesh." There is a general disorder of muscles called spasm, a sudden violent and involuntary contraction of a muscle. A spasm of the visceral muscle is called colic, an example of which is the spasm of the intestinal muscle usually referred to as "bellyache." Spasms may also occur in skeletal muscles; if the spasms happen in a series, the condition may be called a convulsion. Muscle tissue, like nerve tissue, repairs itself (only with difficulty or not at all) once an injury has been sustained. Those tissues, when injured, become replaced frequently with scar tissue. A muscle contusion is a disturbance of muscle tissue in the nature of a bruise, resulting from a direct force over the muscle. There usually is little or no accompanying disturbance to the skin or subcutaneous tissue. However, muscles may be lacerated by sharp or pointed objects. A compound wound has the added problem of infection. After contusion, there is local swelling, tenderness, pain on motion, and mild function impairment. Muscle fibers have no break in their surrounding sheath. Following repeated intermittent trauma to a muscle, the normal resolution is interrupted, fibrous scarring occurring in the hemorrhagic areas and frequently followed by calcification (myositis ossificans).

myalgia (fibrositis). Or muscular rheumatism, is a generalized term referring to aching muscles associated with stiffness, tenderness, and varying degrees of disability increased by active motion. Everyone, sometime or another, has suffered from some form of stiff neck, pleurodynia, scapulodynia, lumbago, or sore leg muscles after unusual exertion or chilling. It appears to be the most common form of persistently recurring pain other than headache. Fibrositis is a better term than myalgia, since the changes occur chiefly in the white fibrous connective tissue of tendons, muscles, nerve sheaths, fascia, periosteum, joint capsule, and ligaments. Those changes are a hypothermic edema and proliferation of white fibrous connective tissues as a result of chilling, toxic influences, acute trauma, chronic strain, or physical fatigue. Thermal and barometric changes, calcium and vitamin B and E deficiencies, chemical intoxication, metabolic imbalances, and dampness and respiratory infections are important precipitating factors. Local infection is often an important factor, as is a malfunctioning colon. The early state is one of effusion, with a localized inflammatory serofibrinous exudate, causing puffy swelling. The exudate may be absorbed or organized by fibroblast invasion and proliferation of fibrous tissue. In the latter stages of fibrous thickening, fibrous bands and nodules sometimes form in the muscles and fascia as adhesions and press on arterioles and nerve filaments, producing contracture and atrophy.

myocardial infarction. A serious, acute medical emergency that may lead to sudden death. Chest pain is the most common initial symptom and may appear when one is at rest or active. The pain resembles agina pectoris but is usually more severe. The condition may last for 1 to 6 hours and is not usually relieved by nitroglycerin. Frequently, other symptoms and signs may be present, including: nausea, vomiting, difficulty in breathing, weakness, sweating, pallor, cyanosis, and cold extremities. The blood pressure may be low; the heart rate may be slow and occasionally irregular. Myocardial infarction is due to an insufficiency or complete obstruction of a coronary artery caused by the death (necrosis) of that part of the heart muscle that had been supplied by that artery or branch.

myositis ossificans. A frequent complication of the combination of contusion and hematoma involving the muscle near its origin on bone. The term is often used to include several conditions that may differ considerably. The name would imply inflammation of a muscle followed by ossification, but more often there is ossification of infiltrated blood along the muscle origin on the bone. The condition may appear as a simple exostosis having a broad base with a sharp extension into the muscle and may seem to be an involvement of the periosteum rather than the muscle. The muscle is merely displaced by the ossifying mass. In another type of so-called myositis ossificans, there is actually a plaque of bone lying within the muscle and separated from the bone by a layer of muscle. A third condition also called myositis ossificans is the ossification about a traumatized joint or a fracture site. A hematoma in those locations will ossify as a result of the repeated insult to healing tissue. In those instances there is no involvement of muscle whatever. Trauma is almost always the initiating cause of myositis ossificans. In the case of the long muscles, the cause may be repeated trauma such as that occurring to the upper arm as a result of the constant blows of the blocker in football.

N

neck and back fractures. Vertebral body fractures are relatively rare in sports. The mechanism is usually one of hyperflexion and the compression producing an anterior wedging of the vertical body. That may occur anywhere in the spine but is most common at the thoracolumbar junction. Since the spinal cord ends at the level of the second lumbar vertebra, cord damage is seen only in fractures above that level. In the lower spine the diagnosis is usually made on the type of injury and the degree of pain and disability and is confirmed by X ray. The well-known situations causing broken necks include diving into shallow water, faulty jumping on a trampoline, skiing, and horseback riding. However, fracture dislocation can follow apparently trivial injuries. Paraplegia or death may follow. The survival and future well-being of the athlete with such an injury may depend on proper first aid management.

neck and back, muscles and ligament injuries. Direct injuries (following a kick or blow) occur usually in contact sports and form an important group of sports injuries. They range from trivial trauma to hematoma formation. In the lower region injuries may at times result in a localized subcutaneous collection of serosanguineous fluid that may require drainage. Indirect injuries to muscles or ligaments are common. Muscle injuries particularly involve the erector spine group in the lumbar region. The typical story is one of a sudden or poorly coordinated movement followed by pain and tenderness (usually well localized in 1 area). Moving that affected part (either by stretching or resisting extension) will reproduce pain. Muscle injuries are particularly common in some types of athletes, including weight lifters, field event athletes who have to hurl missiles, and fast bowlers. Although back ligaments are quite strong, they may nevertheless be acutely overstretched and thus may become sprained. That occurs in a few typical sites, such as the lumbrosacral joint and in the interspinous ligament (sprung back). Ligaments are particularly likely to be sprained in injuries involving a fall in which there is a rotational strain to the lower spine or in bending and lifting. Ligamentous pain may also occur in sports that involve long periods of standing or crouching in a flexed position. The "whiplash" type of injury is not normally seen in sporting injuries, though hyperextension strains do occur, as, for example, in diving.

neck and spinal cord injuries. The range of force applied to the neck produces a variety of neck injuries, from cervical sprain to quadriplegia and death. Ten percent of spinal cord injuries occur during sports activities, the majority during diving, surfing, and football. Athletes with neck injuries usually have either immediate pain without neurologic deficit or immediate deficit with little pain, and there may be an unstable spinal fracture in either case. The most common neck injury is a cervical sprain, which usually occurs in football players, as they acutely angulate their necks in making a tackle. They may develop localized neck pain that is increased with movements in certain directions. Persistent deep pain may indicate a small cervical fracture of subluxation. Subluxations with fracture are ligamentous injuries. The onset of neurologic symptoms after cervical cord trauma may be delayed. Seventy-five percent of cervical cord injuries in athletes occur in water sports, with diving accidents accounting for three-fourths of those injuries; falls from surfboards or water skiis account for the remainder. Most diving accidents occur in water 5 feet deep or less. Vertebral body-burst fractures are usually present because the mechanism in those injuries, as in football injuries, is axial loading to the skull vertex. About half the injuries cause complete quadriplegia, and half cause incomplete quadriplegia. In football players pinched cervical nerves are the most common injury. Cervical nerve root injuries occur at some time in 50 percent of players, especially those with long, thin necks. Immediately after impact symptoms occur, sharply angulating the neck laterally and briefly compressing an upper brachial plexus root against the rim of a cervical foramen, an osteophyte, or a transverse process. Sudden pain and dysesthesia, and occasionally weakness, occur in the arm and hand, but symptoms subside in minutes. Symptoms persisting more than a couple of hours warrant spinal X rays. If the lateral force to the neck is severe, several roots or the upper trunk of the brachial plexus may be injured and the athlete briefly may be unable to use his or her entire arm. Arm weakness occasionally recurs 1 to 7 days after the injuries. That indicates a more serious injury and perhaps a permanent neurologic deficit.

nerve and vascular damage. Nerve concussion (neuropraxia) is common after kicks and blows to the limbs especially as a form of "dead leg" following a posterior thigh blow. The numb feeling usually subsides in a few hours. Intrathecal rupture of the nerve fibers, axonotmesis, occurs with a severe stretching injury or even a dislocation (e.g., axillary nerve damage with a shoulder dislocation) and may take several weeks to recover. Normally, recovery is complete. Nerve severance (neurotmesis) is normally found with a laceration or fracture, especially when there is gross displacement of jagged bone ends. Absent pulses, reduced warmth, pallor, and numbness may indicate vascular injury that might be due to direct rupture or pressure from increasing swelling or both or to a dislocated bone, intimal tears, bruised vessel wall, and arterial spasm.

nerve contusion. Nerve compression or pinched nerve. There is direct trauma, perhaps recurrent trauma, causing the swelling of a nerve under a ligament, and the condition may be in association with a fracture of an extremity. The symptoms may be dermatomal numbness and parethesia and weakness in the muscles involved. Signs may include: tenderness over site of contusion; hyperalgesia is created by weakness or paralysis of muscles supplied by the nerve. Complications are possible permanent loss of sensation and motor function of muscles supplied by the nerve.

nerves. Every voluntary muscle is innervated by at least 1 nerve with several branches. The components of the 1 or several nerves are not always derived from the spinal nerve. There may be 2 or more segmental levels of spinal localization involved in any 1 muscle. Destruction of any 1 peripheral nerve, or 1 spinal nerve, will not necessarily totally paralyze a whole muscle. The typical nerve has both motor and sensory functions. The sensory portion of the nerve is concerned with many modalities other than pain. Most of the sensory impulses involving the muscles do not reach the level of consciousness. The nerve fibers coming from the muscles and those coming from the joint must coordinate in order to produce orderly motion. They are predominantly proprioceptive fibers, which are very important in learning skilled movement. The motor nerve fibers to the muscle terminate on a motor end plate, which stimulates a certain muscle fiber. With that stimulation, an all-or-none contraction takes place within that fiber. That principle does not apply to the total muscle, or such things as fine movements and gentle grasp would not be possible. Thus, voluntary movements can be modulated in strength and in speed. Training teaches one how to control those movements to provide skilled movement. The main areas where nerves are damaged in sporting injuries are supraorbital in lacerations, infraorbital in zygomatic fractures, dental nerves in maxilla and mandibular fractures, brachial plexus in clavicular and traction injuries, axillary nerve in shoulder dislocations, radial nerve in humeral fractures, median nerve in elbow injuries, ulnar nerve in elbow dislocations, posterior interosseous with upper radial fractures or dislocations; digital nerves with finger injuries; median nerve with carpal dislocations, lateral popliteal nerve with fibular fracture, anterior or posterior tibial nerve injury with tibial fractures, digital nerves with foot injuries. Nerve concussion (neuropraxia) is common after kicks and blows to the limbs especially as a form of "dead leg" following a posterior thigh blow. Intrathecal rupture of the nerve fibers (axonotmesis) occurs with a severe stretching injury or even a dislocation, and it may take several weeks to recover. Nerve severance (neurotmesis) is commonly found with a laceration or fracture, especially when there is gross displacement of jagged bone ends.

nerve pinch. Especially common in sports, often seen in football "spearing" with the neck, in flexion, but those syndromes appear throughout the cranium, spine, pelvis, and extremities in many sports. Hardly any peripheral nerve is exempt. Terms used synonymously include: nerve compression, nerve contusion, nerve lesions, nerve pinch syndrome, nerve root syndrome, and nerve stretch syndrome. A nerve stretch syndrome is normally associated with sprains, lateral cervical flexion with shoulder depression, such as in football, blocking, and tackling, or dislocation. Nerve fibers may be stretched, partially torn, or ruptured almost anywhere in the nervous system from the cord to the peripheral nerve terminals. A nerve pinch syndrome may be due to direct trauma (contusion and swelling), subluxation, a protruding disc that results in nerve compression, or fracture (callus formation and associated posttraumatic adhesions). Any telescoping, hyperflexion, hyperextension, or hyperrotational blow or force to the spine may result in a nerve "pinch" syndrome, where pain may be local or extending distally. In sports, nerve pinch syndromes are less common than nerve stretch syndromes but are generally more serious.

nerve tissue. The human body is made up of countless structures, both great and small, each of which contributes something to the action of the whole. The aggregation of structures might be considered as an army, all of whose members must work together. In order to do that, there must be a central coordinating system and an order-giving "agency" somewhere. In the body, the central agency is the brain. Each structure of the body is in direct communication with the brain by means of its own set of telephone wires called nerves. The nerves (from even the most remote parts of the body) all come together and form a great trunk cable called the spinal cord, which in turn leads directly into the central switchboard of the brain. The entire communication system, brain and all, is made of nerve tissue. The basic structural unit of nerve tissue is called a neuron, consisting of a nerve cell body plus small branches like those of a tree, called fibers. One group of the fibers carries nerve impulses to the nerve cell body; another group carries impulses away from the nerve cell body. Neurons can be very long, such as the ones that reach from the big toes to the brain and involve but 1 cell. Nerve tissue is supported by ordinary connective tissue everywhere except in the brain. Here, the supporting tissues are of a special kind, the particular purpose of which nobody knows exactly. All the nerves outside the brain and spinal cord, called the peripheral nerves, have a thin coating known as neurilemma, which is part of the mechanism by which the peripheral nerves repair themselves when damaged. The brain and spinal cord have no neurilemma, so that if they are injured, repair is slow and an uncertain process. The insulating material of nerve fibers is called myelin, and groups of the fibers form "white matter," so called because of the color of the covering, looking very much like fat. Not all nerves have myelin. Some of the nerves of the system which controls the action of the gland, the smooth muscles, and the heart do not have myelin. The cell bodies of all nerve cells are also uncovered (without myelin). Since all nerve cells are gray to begin with and large collections of cell bodies are found in the brain, the great mass of brain tissue is termed "gray matter."

nervous system. Nerves are not isolated points but a complex network running throughout the body and reaching into its every area. A nerve is a cordlike or filamentous band of tissue composed essentially of fibers capable of conducting the electric impulses produced by the brain. Thousands of those bands or cords, large and small, are to be found in the body. The larger of them emanate from centers in the brain and travel through the spinal cord and, by means of hundreds of branches and subbranches (of all lengths and thicknesses), reach into every part of the body. Through its branches and subbranches, the nervous system coordinates and regulates the excitation of muscles, organs, and glands and directly conditions all behavior and activity. The nervous system has 2 major components: the somatic system and autonomic system. The somatic system is the combination of brain and spinal cord nerves that governs the voluntary actions, motions, and sensory feelings. The autonomic system is part of the peripheral system that governs the involuntary actions, motions, and feelings, such as those pertaining to circulation, digestion, and the like. Both systems are interrelated and are part of the central nervous system. In athletics the somatic system is more important, since it is directly involved in athletic activities and the ailments and injuries that derive therefrom.

neuromuscular system conditioning. Active physical conditioning has its effects on the functional state of the neuromuscular system. In this system, training will affect both the neural (input) component and the muscle function (output). Because the movement of the muscle is directed by several neural commands and feedback systems, it is often difficult to assess in which of the 2 components the changes caused by training have been most affected. Furthermore, it is often impossible to differentiate the pure effects of training from those of learning. Training causes a motor act to be learned. Thus, learning involves training either physical, mental, or both. The neuromuscular system has been developed to produce coordinated movements. For example, in a simple flexion-extension movement of the elbow joint, the agonist-antagonist activity should be fairly well coordinated. The effect of training on the coordination of the muscle in a complex movement, such as the knee circle mount on the horizontal bar, has been clearly demonstrated. Coordination of activity can also take place "inside" the muscle, that is, among several hundred motor units responsible for the muscular activity. A trained person possesses the ability to produce a greater force output than an untrained person, giving the same amount of neural energy. Conditioning and training should then lead to a reduction of the neural (EMG) energy activity needed by a muscle to reach a certain level of muscular tension or movement.

nitrogen narcosis and the bends. During assisted diving, a nitrogen narcosis may result from the effect of nitrogen on the central nervous system. The state is self-limited with adequate oxygen. The symptoms are a mild-to-moderate intoxication encouraging the diver to take abnormal risks or ascent at a higher than optimal rate. Rapid ascent may also produce rupture of the alveoli and tympanic membrane, middle ear problems, and bends. Bends result from nitrogen bubbles forming (and replacing oxygen) within the blood and tissues that block capillary blood flow. That leads to severe cramps, organic dysfunction, and neurologic systems. Symptoms may include ear pain, sinus pain, headache, confusion, aching muscles, and joints. Signs may include shortness of breath, cough, hemoptysis, and air in the subcutaneous tissues. Management of the bends and barotrauma requires immediate hyperbaric oxygen in a decompression chamber.

no panic syndrome. This is an underwater diving problem in which loss of consciousness can occur without warning or struggle. There are a variety of causes: (1) holding breath after hyperventilation to extend to breath-holding time; (2) distractional blackout when the diver delays surfacing because of interest in his underwater environment; (3) diffusional blackout in deep breath-hold dives because of increased pressure on lung gases; (4) dilutional blackout; the diver is hypoxic because of mechanical failure of a diving system using a carbon dioxide absorber; (5) valsalvic blackout when the diver skips breaths to conserve air supply; (6) tank blackout, owing to depletion of the oxygen content of tank air by rust formation when water has entered an iron tank; (7) cardiogenic blackout, caused by cardiac arrhythmias or infarction; (8) caroticogenic blackout by neck compression, owing to too tight a hood or diving suit neck; (9) carbon monoxide blackout, caused by contamination from the petrol exhaust of diver compressors used to fill diving tanks; (10) narcotic blackout caused by the effect of nitrogen under great pressure in deep dives; (11) hypothermic blackout, caused by a drop in core temperature; especially prone to occur in deep dives in low-temperature water or under ice; (12) concussive blackout, owing to accidental head blows from collisions or falling equipment; and (13) drug blackout, resulting from some not widely recognised effects of high barometric pressure on drugs that may be quite innocuous at normal atmosphere.

nose and sinuses (diving and swimming). As far as safe and pleasant swimming and diving is concerned, the state of the nose plays an important part. Any defect of the nose is liable to affect the Eustachian tube and make clearing the ears by inflating the middle era less easy or even impossible. Accordingly, the most common medical aid used by swimmers and divers is some form of nasal decongestant, and the most common cause of trouble is the common cold. Any of the usual conditions causing nasal obstruction (such as a deviated nasal septum, allergic rhinitis, vasomotor rhinitis (sinus), or true sinusitis) will need attention. One of the causes of nosebleeds in scuba divers is poor pressure equalization in the sinuses, causing the "sinus squeeze." Facial pain occurs and nonfrothy blood issuing from the nose or mouth may be coming from the sinuses. Prevention of many disorders arising from water activity is based on having a healthy nose or, when there is nasal congestion, the use of nasal decongestants.

nosebleed. The most common cause of nosebleed, also called epistaxis, is an injury or a blow to the nose. Other causes may include inflammation and ulceration, such as may occur following a persistent discharge from a sinusitis. Growths including polyps also can be a cause of epistaxis. Sometimes an abnormally high blood pressure or overheating of the body or both may cause the vessels in the nasal lining to break, resulting in varying degrees of hemorrhage. To stop nosebleeds, the individual should remain quiet with the head slightly elevated.

nummular eczema. A disorder often induced by trauma of winter temperatures, sometimes seen in sports played outdoors in cold weather, such as football, and most common in linemen who play without gloves or warm socks. It usually begins as a mild itchy skin infection of the hand, characterized by coin-shaped patches of vesicles and papules, which progress to a widespread secondary dermatitis characterized by oozing and crust formation, especially during cold weather. Lesions may normally be sited on the extensor aspects of the extremities and on the buttocks.

nutrition, dietary principles. For optimum support of athletic performance, appropriate timing of food intake is essential. Large, infrequent meals may cause discomfort during athletic performance and provide excessive calories. Meals before training or competition should be generally varied. The training diet should be the standard one for a particular sport. Ideally, 4 to 6 hours should elapse between the last meal and the beginning of competition. A time lapse of several days exists between carbohydrate ingestion and muscle glycogen storage. The food mix is important. Free carbohydrates should be avoided before prolonged competition, since insulin release often leads to reactive hypoglycemia, if physical activity is continued during the metabolism of sugar. The value of vitamin supplements is not definitely established. Many endurance athletes use megavitamin supplementation, but the effect upon their performance has not been validated. Endurance events require high caloric intake in the form of carbohydrates and fats and relatively little protein in proportion to the total calories consumed. The quantity of fiber in the diet is important when one is preparing for competition. For events lasting more than a few minutes, dietary fiber should not be taken, if possible, for a day or 2 to avoid gastrointestinal motility problems and the urge to defecate at inappropriate times.

nutrition, megavitamins. Megavitamin therapy is the use of 1 or several vitamins in amounts that are 10 or more times greater than those recommended by the Committee on Dietary Allowances of Food Nutrition or the National Research Council of the United States. In general, vitamins function as coenzymes or hormones or, when combined with body protein, form holoenzymes, which are usually referred to as enzymes. A vitamin is useful only when combined with its apoenzyme, and the apoenzyme that is manufactured per unit of time is limited. Saturation of apoenzyme occurs at vitamin levels that are roughly those recommended in the dietary allowances, and excess vitamins may become pharmacologic agents. A vitamin is an organic compound that the body cannot make in adequate amounts, that is, it is not a protein, fat, or carbohydrate. But it is necessary for normal human metabolism. Of the 13 vitamins needed, 4 of them are fat soluble and 9 are water soluble. Several growth factors, para-aminobenzoic acid, bioflavonoids, choline, insitol, lipoic acid, and ubiquinone, are necessary for other organisms, such as beneficial bacteria and possibly phagocytes or lymphocytes. Some of them are also used by humans but can be produced in the body as needed. There is no medically acceptable published data that indicate that healthy, usually active individuals need vitamin supplementation, provided they eat a diet that includes natural grains, fruits, vegetables, meat, and milk products.

nutritional homeostasis. The fuel required varies with the intensity and duration of activity, but in the vigorous effort typical of the athlete, a high proportion of energy is initially derived from carbohydrates. The proximate source is glycogen, stored within the muscle cell. That normally amounts to 1 to 5 g/100 g of wet muscle, or some 1,200 kcal (5.2 MJ) of energy in all. When carbohydrates are providing 75 percent of the needed energy, then fuel is available for about 80 minutes of activity at an expenditure of 20 kcal (0–08 MJ)/min. Blood sugar totaling 6 g = 24 kcal (0–10 MJ) is a negligible energy resource for strenuous physical work. However, there is a further labile reserve of glycogen in the liver (total 100 g = 400 kcal (1–69 MJ). That can be mobilized at a rate of about 1 g/min. The total reserves of energy stored as fat are, from the athletic viewpoint, almost infinite. A normally nourished male contestant may have 10 percent to 15 percent of his body weight, 10 kg or more, in the form of adipose tissue. That is equivalent to some 70,000 kcal (294 MJ) of energy, or (assuming expenditure at a rate of 10 kcal [0–04 kcal MJ]/min) 7,000 hours supply. Unfortunately, most of that fat is at some distance from the active muscles. Intramuscular lipids are soon exhausted, and subsequent usage is set by the rate of mobilization from depot fat and transport across to the active muscle cell membranes.

nutrition principles. No single food can guarantee adequate nutrition. To be well nourished, one must eat a variety of foods. That should include proteins which supply the essential amino acids (meat, poultry, fish, eggs, or nuts and vegetables), milk or milk products (cheese, ice cream, or yogurt), and fruits and cereals, some of which should be light milled or whole grain. Caloric intake must be balanced with output. The amount of physical activity is important in determining proper caloric intake. Alcohol has a high caloric content, and it may predispose to some forms of cancer, but in moderate amounts it may retard atherosclerosis. Calories are the same, regardless of their source. It is important to ingest only as many as are expended, to maintain proper weight. Consumption of 1 big meal a day rather than several tends to increase the number of intake over expended calories in a 24-hour period. It is better to have several small meals rather than 1 large one. Natural fluorides are essential for maintaining strong bones, and they may retard or prevent tooth decay. Other nutritional supplements are not generally necessary for most people who consume a balanced diet. Increased blood cholesterol may be a risk factor for cardiovascular disease. Cholesterol levels are influenced not only by cholesterol intake or by the type of fat ingested, but also by total caloric intake and expenditure. Cholesterol is also made by the body in the absence of exogenous sources, but that is not appreciably influenced by dietary cholesterol. Minimizing dietary (sodium) salt may be helpful in reducing hypertension in those afflicted. The salt used should be sea salt or iodized.

nutritional requirements, vitamins. Vitamin supplementation is a common practice among athletes seeking to improve performance. Selected vitamin deficiencies generally impair physical performance. There is only a little validated evidence to suggest that excessive vitamin intake may enhance performance. Nevertheless, a number of investigators recommend that athletes in heavy training increase their intake of vitamin B, C, and E. The B-complex vitamins, principally thiamine, play an important role in fat and carbohydrate metabolism. During muscular exercise thiamine requirements increase by 15-fold more than during rest, so daily vitamin B requirements increase in proportion to daily energy expenditure. Since the caloric intake of training athletes generally matches energy expenditure, it is likely that the need for additional B-complex vitamins is adequately met by diet. Protein foods and whole grains are excellent sources of those vitamins. The recommendations for vitamin C (ascorbic acid) supplementation has some theoretic justification. Like the B-complex vitamins, vitamin C has a role in oxidative energy metabolism. Some in vitro studies showed that increased ascorbic acid in blood results in a shift in the blood oxygen-carrying capacity, which could make more oxygen available to the muscles. Vitamin C is necessary to make the "cementing" substances like collagen, which helps to hold body cells together. It aids also in forming stronger scar tissues, which is important for healing muscles and tendons. Some studies have indicated that endurance performance of trained middle-aged men is greater when wheat germ oil, high in vitamin E, is added to their diet. Other studies indicate that some injuries may heal faster (and with reduced scar tissue) when supplemental E is taken internally or applied to a wound externally or both. However, there has been no validated evidence of beneficial effects of supplemental vitamin E alone. The normal diet provides about 20 to 25 units of vitamin E per day, well above that needed by the body. The richest sources are vegetable oils, whole grains, and eggs.

O

olecranon bursitis. A painful inflammation of a soft-tissue sac, which underlies the olecranon at the back of the elbow but does not connect with the joint. Its usual cause is either a direct blow or sustained pressure resting on the elbow. The bursa overlying the tip of the olecranon is frequently injured by direct trauma. The acute injury is often overlooked. Sometimes later the athlete realizes that there is a painless swelling over the tip of the elbow. There is no loss of motion. X rays are usually normal except for the soft tissue swelling. Occasionally in an acute case there may be a chip of the olecranon. In a chronic case there may be some calcification within the bursal area.

orbit blowout fracture. Trauma producing sudden increase in intraorbital pressure. It is caused by a blow to the soft tissues in the orbital area from a fist or other objects. Symptoms may be the diplopia, anesthesia, or hypesthesia of the cheek along distribution of infraorbital nerve; enophthlamos; or eye muscle imbalance. Signs may include ecchymosis, swelling, subconjunctival hemorrhage, hyphemia, or inability of the eye to rotate upward in a normal range. Complications are permanent visual disturbance, diplopia if untreated, glaucoma, or cataract formation.

Osgood-Schlatter disease. Apophysitis of the tibial tubercle is commonly called Osgood-Schlatter disease but is not a disease. There are actually 3 manifestations relating to Osgood-Schlatter disease. One is bursitis of the infrapatellar tendon bursa. The tenderness in that condition is elicited at a point slightly higher than the tubercle and is treated as a bursitis. The 2nd type is an aseptic necrosis of the tip of the epiphysis for the patellar tubercle of the tibia. The necrosis occurs in the patellar tendon attachment and is probably traumatic in origin and is initiated by a fracture or by an avulsion of the tip of the patellar tubercle. The 3rd type is a true epiphysitis involving the whole epiphysis. That type is not particularly frequent but generally is more severe than the others when it occurs. The symptoms of the latter 2 conditions are pain on direct pressure and pain on active use of the quadriceps, with rather sharp limitations resulting. It usually occurs between the ages of 10 to 15, with the child athlete, usually male, complaining of swelling at the tibial tubercle. Often a direct blow causes the initial problem. The pain is made worse by falling or running. Examination reveals a prominent area over the proximal tibia with localized tenderness. There may be tenderness at the proximal end of the patellar tendon, a symptom of a different entity called "jumper's knee." Swelling of the soft tissue is frequently seen.

osteoarthrosis. A disease of attrition affecting primarily the articular cartilage and later the bone around the edges of the articular cartilage. It is most commonly involved in the weight-bearing joints and is markedly precipitated by irregularity of the articular surface and damage of the articular cartilage caused by trauma or infection or where deformity of the bones leads to excessive stress being exerted on a part of the joint. Genu varum leads to osteoarthrosis of the lateral compartment of the knee. It is believed that joints that have been subjected to repeated trauma or have experienced recurrent sprains or fractures or have been the objects of repeated surgical interference will generally have a higher incidence of the disease than will joints spared injury. However, whether a normal joint subjected to normal or even heavy exercise wears out less rapidly is difficult to prove.

osteochondritis dissecans. An articular cartilage involvement occurring most frequently in the knee. The pathologic condition consists of the separation of a fragment of cartilage from the underlying matrix. This line of separation fills with granulation tissue. The separated fragment necroses because of poor circulation and, in effect, becomes a sequestrum. The articular cartilage does not increase at this stage but remains intact. The whole cycle of separation, necrosis, and regeneration may occur without any defect in the articular cartilage and may terminate in spontaneous healing of the condition. If enough of the fragment is absorbed to permit it to depress into the crater in the epiphyseal bone, fissuring of the cartilage and ultimate separation may occur. The age incidence coincides with the age of active athletes, namely adolescence and early adulthood. Thus, the condition is frequently seen in young athletes. There is no preventive measure of any value. The condition may be completely asymptomatic and be discovered only by incidental X rays. Normally there is a discomfort in the joint, sometimes accompanied by effusion, with symptoms of internal derangement. That may go on until there is actually locking of the joint if the fragment becomes free or if a flap of cartilage turns up and interposes between the articular surfaces.

osteomyelitis. An infection of the bone, often also involving the marrow, caused by pus-producing bacteria. The pathogens may reach the bone through the bloodstream or by way of an injury in which the skin has been broken. Further, an injury without a break in the skin may make the bone more susceptible to blood-borne infection. Because of antibiotic drugs, there are fewer reported cases today, as many of the bloodstream infections are prevented or treated early enough so that bone infection is less common. If those that do appear are treated promptly, the chance of a cure is usually excellent.

osteophyte, or a transverse process. Immediate pain and dysesthesia and occasionally weakness occur in the arm and hand, but symptoms subside in minutes. Symptoms persisting more than a couple of hours generally warrant cervical spine X rays. If the lateral force to the neck is severe, several roots of the upper trunk of the brachial plexus may be injured and the athlete (briefly) may be unable to use his entire arm. Arm weakness occasionally recurs 1 to 7 days after the injuries. That indicates a more serious injury and perhaps a permanent neurologic deficit.

osteoporosis, post-traumatic (Sudeck's atrophy). Following extremity trauma, bone (being reactive tissue, as are other tissues) undergoes rapid and extensive physiochemical changes under the influence of the circulatory and trophic disturbances that frequently follow injury. It is common for immobilized bones to lose considerable mineral salts and show osteoporotic areas on X ray examination. That type of disease atrophy has little clinical importance, as normal bone density and strength return quickly when function is resumed. It is essentially asymptomatic. Clinical osteoporosis can be differentiated from such disuse atrophy in that true osteoporosis is characterized by a patch decalcification of extremity bones in which there are coexisting signs of pain, vosomotor changes, and trophic disturbances. A neurogenic type of bone atrophy may become apparent long after the effects of the original trauma have subsided and after fractured bones have united in good position. Not infrequently, it manifests from 3 to 6 weeks after some apparently trivial injury to a polyarticular joint. It may be confused with "malingering" when insurance or compensation cases are involved. In the early states it is characterized by constant aching pain, hyperesthesia, local swelling, and hypervascularization, local heat, redness, marked joint stiffness, and abnormal submotor responses of the previously injured part. In late stages the skin may become atrophic, thin, and shiny, and there may be attrition of the nails, excessive hair growth on the part, and diffuse osteoporosis, as demonstrated on X ray films.

otitic barotrauma. As a result of rapid descent, as in an airplane or in underwater swimming, there is a change in the external pressure on the ear from low to high. If the Eustachian tube does not allow air in the middle ear, then the outside raised pressure usually pushes the eardrum inward, as the gas in the middle ear is compressed or squeezed. Pain in the ear normally occurs in the inexperienced diver after a change of pressure of 5 feet of water. But in the more experienced diver, the sensations are not so great, partly because the eardrum has been stretched on many occasions, and partly because one is naturally disinclined to take any notice of early warnings. As the eardrum does not stretch far enough to allow the pressure equalization, negative middle ear pressure extracts fluid from the blood vessels into the cavity of the middle ear (traumatic secretory otitis media). Bleeding into the middle ear then occurs. The small hemorrhages that occur into the substances of the drum are common in scuba divers and can be recognized up to 2 or 3 weeks later. They indicate poor technique of cleaning the ears or diving with nasal congestion. If the pressure changes are great, or if there is any weakness in the drum, it may rupture. That occurs in water pressure changes ranging from 9 feet to 90 feet (2.7 m–27 m) depending on the strength of the eardrum, which may be atrophic from childhood secretory otitis media. If water enters the middle ear through the perforation, dizziness or vertigo occurs. Such ruptures occur mostly in depths more than 60 feet (18 m) deep and can be dangerous to life.

otitis externa. An ear infection. The predisposing causes of otitis externa are prolonged immersion in the water with the removal of the normal earwax, probing of the ear with matchsticks or hairpins, or rubbing in or around the ear with a finger. It is known to be more common in tropical climates because the warmer water washes out the wax coating quicker, the humidity is greater, and airborne infections are more common. Wax in the ear is a normal protective secretion but, where present in lumps, prevents water from draining out freely, leading to maceration of the skin and making it susceptible to otitis externa. Infections from waterborn organisms are an unusual cause of otitis externa. It is not so in the case of chlorinated pools, and it is highly unlikely in the open sea because of the dilution factor. Waterborne infections may be a factor in untreated or overloaded pools or where sea pollution is high. The main symptom is itch, but there also may be ache or discharge from the ear. The latter may be thin and run out easily, or it may be thick and look like wet blotting paper. The skin itself is reddened and sometimes swollen and tender.

otitis media. The result of the normally air-filled middle ear chamber with an intact drum becoming filled with fluid because of impaired Eustachian tube function. That is usually the result of an inflammation spreading from a sore throat via the Eustachian tube. A feeling of fullness in the ear may progress to pain or a degree of deafness. As pressure builds within the chamber, the drum appears thick and red (blood) or yellow (pus) before possible rupture. The common cause in swimmers is usually poor technique, such as not expelling air when the nose is under water. The water may irritate the nasal mucosa, resulting in nasal congestion and infection.

outer ear barotrauma. The outer ear squeeze or "reverse ear" is not a serious condition, but it can make a person unfit for scuba diving, so it has a considerable nuisance value. Within the outer opening of the ear canal obstructed by the hood or ear plugs, on descent into water, a negative pressure develops, maintained by the elasticity of the neoprene hood, which prevents fluid from entering the outer ear canal. To get sufficient pressure differential to cause trouble, the diver needs to be at a depth of 30 feet to 50 feet (9 m to 15 m) as compared with 6 feet to 10 feet (1.8 m to 3 m) for middle ear trouble. The eardrum will bulge outward though seldom sufficiently to cause pain or rupture, and the skin capillaries rupture, forming blood blisters in the skin of the ear canal. The blisters can break spontaneously, giving a tattered look to the ear canal and eardrum.

outside agency injuries. The simplest and most usual cause of injury, taking many forms. Essentially, the damage is due to the influence of somebody or something unconnected with the person injured and ordinarily not in any way under his or her control. The outside cause may be the principle factor, but body activity, body momentum, or both may also be involved. The injuries produced by an outside agency can be classified in many ways. They may be direct, when the damage is done at the point of impact, or indirect, when the damage occurs some distance away from the point of impact, force being transmitted through the tissues themselves. The injuries may be "high velocity" or "low-velocity" depending on the speed at which the outside agency and the body come into contact. That factor determines to some extent the nature and depth of the tissue damage. The danger of injury from an outside agency varies in different games and sports, and quite often the injuries are produced accidentally in contact with another player.

oxygen. The total usable store of anaerobic energy is set at an oxygen equivalent of 75 ml/kg to 80 ml/kg. Aerobic metabolism thus yields about half of the energy used in an event of 1 minute duration, but the proportion rises to 88 percent with 5 minutes of activity, and 98 percent with 1 hour of activity. Aerobic power is normally measured as the maximum oxygen intake, the plateau of oxygen consumption reached during several minutes of progressively increasing activity on a large muscle task, such as uphill treadmill running. In theory, that provides the unequivocal expression of the ability of the cardiorespiratory system to transport oxygen from the atmosphere to the working tissue. In practice, results vary somewhat with the test modality (treadmill, bicycle ergometer, step test, arm and shoulder ergometers), and an athlete such as a kayak paddler may be limited by local systems (leg pain or weakness) rather than by true central exhaustion. Results are normally expressed in ml/kg min STPD, since the cost of many activities varies almost directly with body weight. Oxygen transport may be conceived as proceeding through a chain of resistance, including ventilation, the interaction between the diffusing capacity of the lungs and blood transport, blood transport itself, and the interaction between blood and the diffusing capacity of the tissues. For the ordinary sedentary individual, exercising under normal ambient conditions is by far the smallest conductance (20 l/min to 30 l/min) and thus the largest resistance is presented by the blood transport term. Alveolar ventilation (60 l/min to 80 l/min) also imposes some restriction upon oxygen transport, but the remaining terms are unimportant.

oxygen breathing. Increases maximal exercise ability owing both to an increase flow to the muscles of oxygen that is in solution in the blood and to a reduction in exercise ventilation. The additional oxygen amounts to only about 1.7 ml per 100 ml of blood, an increase of 8 percent, but sufficient to reduce the anaerobic metabolism and to lower the blood lactic acid level during strenuous exercise. Oxygen breathing also increases the efficiency of cardiac contraction and reduces the pulse frequency, so that the cardiac output tends to rise. By reducing acidemia, both those effects decrease ventilation on exercise. Oxygen breathing also causes an immediate reduction in ventilation within a few seconds before there has been any change in the level of circulation lactic acid. That reduction is believed to be a direct consequence of the rise in blood oxygen tension; it is an additional factor increasing exercise performance. The effect of oxygen illuminates the mechanisms that normally limit exercise. Its use increases maximum exercise ability and therefore maximum oxygen intake. At the same time, the ventilation minute volume during maximum exercise is not greater on oxygen than it is on air, which again suggests that sensations associated with breathlessness may be a limiting activity.

oxygen transport system. One of the major determinants of optimal health and fitness is the efficient operation of the mechanism necessary for bringing oxygen to the exercising muscles and burning it properly once it arrives there. Collectively this has been called the oxygen transport system. The first component of the system is the lungs. Each time oxygen is inhaled, the air is transported deep into the lungs and is brought into contact, across a microscopically thin membrane, with the blood in the lungs. The red blood cells bind oxygen. At the same time carbon dioxide, one of the body's main waste products, is blown out in the air exhaled. As fitness is increased, the lungs function more efficiently. There is greater oxygen uptake and carbon dioxide removal. Deeper breaths are taken, and breathing can be done more efficiently. Cigarette smoking is the major cause of poor lung function in most adults. Smoking severely injures lung tissues, interfering with oxygen uptake and carbon dioxide removal. Aging also reduces lung function efficiency. There is good evidence that a good fitness program may slow that deterioration. The next component of the oxygen transport system is the heart, which is basically a pump. The oxygen-rich blood from the lungs returns to the heart, which then pumps it to the rest of the body. In the average adult at rest, the heart may pump 4 to 5 quarts each minute at a pulse rate of 60 to 80. During intense exercise the pulse may rise to 200 or more. At peak activity the amount of blood the heart pumps each minute, called the cardiac output, may increase to 5 or 6 times above the resting level. With training, each heartbeat or contraction is more vigorous, pumping more blood in the body. The arteries, veins, red blood cells, and the exercising muscles are the other components of the oxygen transport system. The role of the arteries is to transport blood from the heart to the exercising muscle. But arteries are not merely passive conduits for the movement of blood. Fitness produces changes in arteries, improving their ability to expand and contract. Fitness may stimulate the growth of tiny new arteries in the exercising muscles to help improve the efficiency of the oxygen transport system. Another important adaptation occurs during training; a greater percentage of the blood pumped by the heart is directed to the exercising muscles and away from the other parts of the body, such as the kidneys and stomach. If blood flow to the kidneys is reduced, urine formation stops, which is a useful adaptation for the runner. There is usually no need to stop to urinate during a run; and if it is hot, the body fluids can be used to produce sweat rather than urine. But because blood flow to the stomach and intestine is reduced during the run, recently ingested food may ferment and not be digested adequately. Pain, cramps, and heartburn may result.

P

pain sense. A most important "protective sense." The receptors for pain are the most widely distributed sensory end organs. They are found in the skin, the muscles, and the joints and (to a lesser extent) in most internal organs (including the blood vessels and viscera). Pain receptors are not oval bodies as are many of the other sensory end organs, but apparently are merely branching of the nerve fibers, called free nerve endings. "Referred pain" is a term used in cases in which pain that seems to be in an outer part of the body, particularly the skin, actually originates in an internal organ located near that particular area of the skin. Those areas of referred pain have been mapped out on the basis of much experience. It has been found, for example, that liver and gallbladder diseases often cause referred pain in the skin over the right shoulder. Spasm of the coronary arteries that supply the heart may cause pain in the left shoulder and the left arm. One reason is that some neurons have the twofold duty of conducting impulses both from visceral pain receptors and from pain receptors in neighboring areas of the skin. The brain cannot differentiate between those 2 possible sources, but since pain sensations originate in the skin, the brain automatically assigns the pain to that more likely place of origin. Pain sense differs from other senses in that continued stimulation does not result in adaptation or remission. This is nature's way of being certain that the warnings of the pain sense are heeded. Sometimes the cause cannot be remedied quickly and occasionally not at all. Then it may be necessary to relieve the pain.

palpitations. Consciousness of the heart beat. It may become evident during training following illness, when the heart rate response to exertion may be temporarily greater than normal. Pounding of the heart, during severe exertion, is not usually noticed by the fit athlete, but irregularity of the pulse during recovery or at rest may be sufficiently noticeable to concern the athlete. Irregularity of the heart rate may be caused by strong vagal tone with sinus arrhythmia or even a "wandering pacemaker" in which the sinus node is inhibited and atrial or nodal pacemakers take over. Even 2nd-degree heart block (with Wenckebach phenomena) can result from this strong vagal tone, causing missed beats, followed by a large jolt. The most frequent cause of that symptom is ventricular ectopic beats, which are surprisingly common in athletes. Ventricular ectopic beats may occur at rest or only during recovery from exercise and are often then associated with a sinus arrhythmia. In the vast majority of cases, they are of no significance and usually are not noticed, but the jolting postectopic beat may reach the athlete's consciousness. Ectopic beats have obtained a sinister reputation through their association with ischemic heart disease in postmyocardial infarction disorders, where they may herald ventricular fibrillation. No such risk is attached to the subject with an otherwise normal (healthy) heart, and the vast majority of athletes with ventricular ectopic beats can be assured that they are usually normal findings.

pancreatitis, acute. A severe inflammation of unknown cause involving the pancreas, an organ located in the upper portion of the abdomen behind the stomach. Some individuals suffer recurrent attacks of the disorder, which is one of the most painful diseases that afflict humans. Pancreatitis typically develops after a heavy meal or the ingestion of large amounts of alcohol but may appear at any time. The pain is located in the upper part of the abdomen in the midline or on the left side but frequently radiates through to the back and to the shoulder blades. The onset is relatively rapid, building up to peak intensity over a few minutes to a few hours, but it is not so abrupt as the onset of symptoms of a perforated ulcer. Loss of appetite is almost invariably found; nausea and vomiting may usually be present; diarrhea is rare. In severe cases prostation and shock may be prominent. The individual is frequently cyanotic and generally has a rapid pulse or a low blood pressure or both. Fever is usually present. Upper abdominal tenderness is almost always present. However, spasms of the abdominal muscles and rebound tenderness may be rather mild, because the stomach is interposed between the pancreas and the abdominal wall. Many individuals with pancreatitis have a history suggestive of previous gallbladder disease, including a possible intolerance for fried or fatty foods.

paroxysmal tachycardia. Term used for a disorder characterized by the sudden onset of a very rapid heart rate with generally associated symptoms of pounding in the chest, weakness, dizziness, and shortness of breath. The heart rate is often very rapid and perfectly regular. The pulses may be so weak that a stethoscope applied to the chest is required to count the rate. The individual may have experienced similar previous attacks.

patella. Patellar rupture or tendinitis, quadriceps rupture or tendinitis (jumper's knee), and fatigue fractures of the tibia have a high incidence in basketball. In tendinitis the pain may be perceived either during and shortly after activity or may be chronic. Forceful jumping may result in an avulsive fracture of the patella. Repeated stress to the knee joint may cause the infrapatellar fat pad or the synovial to become hypertrophied. Symptoms may include joint weakness or definite locking, joint effusion when acute, pain on the medial aspect of the knee, and tenderness distal and medial to the patella. A sudden joint stress, usually rotational, may cause some soft tissue to be pinched within the articular structures during jumping, defensive running, kicking, etc. That is most frequently seen in the knee, where the infrapatellar fat pad is nipped, resulting in a degree of effusion and possible hemorrhage. Intracapsular pinches are more common in sports than are cartilage injuries. In chondromalacia patellae, there is a state of constant erosion and fragmentation of the cartilage of the patella. Incidence is generally in young adults from 7 to 25 years of age. Genu recurvatum is the typical cause, such as hyperextension during single-leg stance and the push-off phase of gait. In sports the patella tendon may be subject to partial tears, complete rupture occasionally, peritendinitis, and local degeneration. Chronic strain has a high incidence in high jumpers and runners, as in basketball and track.

patella dislocation, acute. A disorder caused by violence against medial aspect of patella from forcible rotation of the femur on fixed tibia or lateral rotation of the tibia on fixed femur. Symptoms may be severe pain and disability. Signs may reduce spontaneously by straightening knee and may include hemarthrosis, swelling, tenderness along supermedial border, tibia in position of abduction, muscle spasm, or palpable defect along medial border of patella. Complications may be recurrent dislocation, osteochondral fracture of patella or lateral femoral condyle and chondromalacia of patella.

patella fracture. A fractured kneecap that is caused by indirect violence, as in the snapping of the patella over condyles from force applied to semifixed knee, sudden violent contraction of quadriceps mechanism, jumping or a fall from height, or a direct blow. Symptoms may be pain and disability. Signs may include hemarthrosis, swelling, ecchymosis, sulcus palpated between fractured segments, or false motion without crepitus. Complications may be nonunion, residual stiffness, and traumatic arthritis.

patella fracture, chondral. Fall onto flexed knee, recurrent subluxational forces. Symptoms may be persistent pain; locking or catching of knee; or disability. Signs may include swelling; hemarthrosis; tenderness, especially on rubbing patella against condylar groove with knee in complete extension, or pain elicited by flexion and extension of knee against resistance. Complications may be traumatic arthritis; residual joint dysfunction; or persistent disability.

patella fracture, osteochondral. Fall upon flexed knee; recurrent subluxational force. Symptoms may be persistent pain, locking or catching or disability. Signs may include swelling, hemarthrosis, tenderness, particularly on rubbing patella against condylar groove with knee in full extension, and pain elicited by flexion and extension of knee against resistance. Complications may be traumatic arthritis or residual joint dysfunction.

patella osteochondritis. It is caused by vigorous activity, as in running and jumping on hard surfaces or running up and down hills. The symptoms may be mild pain around the patella, and it may be bilateral. The symptoms are generally aggravated by activity. Signs may include tenderness and swelling located at the inferior or superior pole and leg extension against resistance, which may produce pain.

patella tendon strain. A strain of the kneecap tendon. It is caused by repeated jumping, a fall from height, stumbling. The symptoms may be an inability to extend the knee and pain localized over the front of the knee. Signs may be graded by degree of severity, such as hemarthrosis, general tenderness, subcutaneous swelling at the site of tendon injury just below the patella, patella displaced upward intact and not tender, and definite impression in tissue palpable below the patella. Complications could be chronic weakness.

pelvic injuries. Fractures of the pelvis are divided into stable and unstable types. Any pelvic injury may damage the contained viscera, and in that respect urethral damage is of particular importance. Injury to the bladder, bowel, and genitalia (male and female) may coexist. In serious fractures blood loss should be assessed by careful observation of pulse and blood pressure. Although pelvic fractures (with solution of the pelvic ring and some degree of displacement) occur in sports, they are very rare. They usually follow high-speed falls, as from a horse, bicycle, or racing car, particularly if the vehicle rolls upon and crushes the individual. They also may occur in football. Isolated pelvic fractures, particularly of the iliac crest, are relatively more common as a result of direct violence or as avulsion injuries caused by violent contraction of the trunk muscles. In young athletes avulsion or epiphysitis of the epiphysis of the iliac crest may occur. Progressive rehabilitation is the key to successful treatment, and return to full activity usually occurs.

peptic ulcer, perforated. Perforation is one of the complications that may occur with a serious peptic ulcer. The same processes that have ingested the lining of the stomach or intestine form the ulcer crater, which continues until the ulcer extends through the entire wall of the organ. The resulting perforation permits stomach acids, food, and other intestinal contents to enter the abdominal cavity. Those substances cause an intense chemical irritation of the peritoneum and may initiate a severe infection. The individual usually has a history of peptic ulcer, however, though about 20 percent of those with perforated ulcers do not have prior symptoms. At the time of perforation, one generally suffers the abrupt, almost instantaneous onset of severe upper abdominal pain, which is sharp and continuous and may spread over the entire abdomen. The pain is usually followed shortly by the vomiting of recently ingested food or bile or both. The person appears quite sick and generally gets progressively worse for the next 12 to 24 hours. The abdomen is diffusely tender, but pain is more marked in the upper quadrants. Spasm of the abdominal muscle is often prominent, particularly in the upper abdomen. Bowel sounds usually disappear shortly after the perforation, followed by distension of the abdomen owing to intestinal paralysis. A perforated ulcer is a severe emergency.

periosteum. Bone surfaces are covered with a thick layer of fibrous tissue in the deeper layers in which blood vessels run. That layer is called the periosteum. The nutrition and growth of the underlying bone depends on the integrity of its blood vessels. The periosteum also has osteogenic properties and has the ability to produce new bone, e.g., in the repair of fractures. The periosteum does not cover the articulating surface of the bones in synovial joints. It generally has a good nerve supply and is very sensitive.

periostitis. An inflammation normally associated with joint injury, especially with that of the knee. It is the result of a violent muscle strain that damages the periosteum. If the strain is severe enough to detach the periosteum, a degree of hematoma may develop. The bruised joint is usually swollen and extremely tender, and movements are restricted.

peritonitis. Peritonitis is inflammation of the peritoneum, and it is a very serious disease. The peritoneum is a serous membrane that covers the surface of most of the abdominal organs to form the visceral serosa and the lining of the abdominal wall as the parietal layer. In addition to those parts of the peritoneum, there are more complex double layers of membrane that separate the abdomen into areas and spaces and in some cases aid in supporting the organs and holding them in place. Peritonitis has, in the past, been a dreaded complication following infection of 1 or more of the organs that the peritoneum covers, generally the appendix. The frequency of peritonitis has been greatly reduced by use of antibiotic drugs. However, it still occurs and can be very dangerous.

peroneal nerve contusion. Direct blow over the head of fibula. The symptoms may be pain over the upper fibular region along lateral aspect and a tingling sensation down the lateral side of the leg and dorsum of the foot. Disability may occur. Signs may include paresthesia or hyperesthesia of the dorsum of the foot and outer side of the leg, foot drop, and inability to dorsiflex the foot or extend the toes, with local tenderness. Complications may be permanent foot drop and equinus contracture of the ankle.

peronei strain and inflammation. The peronei tendons pass behind the lateral malleolus. They are best palpated during active eversion and plantar flexion. The peronei are the primary foot everter and help in plantar flexion. An aseptic tendon inflammation is often involved. If stenosis of the tunnel in which the tendons run occurs, the peroneal tubercle will feel tender and thick. Tenderness may also suggest bursitis or a fracture of the styloid process in a severe sprain. When the strain is associated with peroneal tenosynovitis or tendovaginitis, it may be characterized by acute tenderness, pain, motion, restriction, swelling of the sheath, and a probably squeaking crepitus on joint movement and possibly ecchymosis.

phlebitis. Inflammation of a vein with marked pain, considerable swelling, and involvement of the entire vein wall. A blood clot may form, causing the dangerous condition called thrombophlebitis, with the possibility of a piece of clot becoming loosened and floating in the blood as an embolus. If it reaches the lungs, as it does too often, sudden death from pulmonary embolism may be the result.

pityriasis rosea. A disease that is possibly of viral origin. A herald patch 3 cm to 5 cm in diameter is the first sign, followed in 7 to 10 days by a maculopapular rash limited to the trunk and the proximal portions of the extremities. The lesions are generally oval, brownish and scaly. Their long axis normally follows the lines of skin cleavage. Pruritis is common but not severe. The disease lasts from 6 to 12 weeks. When pityriasis occurs in athletes, they should wear T-shirts and may continue to play. There is no treatment other than oral medication, and activities need not be restricted.

plantar fasciitis. One of the most common injuries among long-distance runners. Long- and middle-distance runners may be susceptible to the condition owing to the many foot strikes during running and the hard surfaces usually encountered. The plantar fascia is a densely fibrous connective tissue that runs from the plantar surface of the calcaneus to the base of the proximal phalange. The fascia itself consists of 3 bundles, of which the medial bundle is the thinnest and the most injury prone. The plantar fascia has been described as the "bowstring" of the foot. It plays an important part in the stability and propulsion of the foot during the gait cycle. The foot supinates during the last portion of the stance phase of the gait. During that time the plantar fascia plays an important part in locking the rear foot, aiding in its supination, and locking the midtarsal joint for the propulsive phase of the gait. The most common cause of plantar fascia pain is overuse, running on hard surfaces, inadequate shoes, and structural problems, such as rear-foot varus, tibial varum, forefoot varus, and equinovarus deformities. Pes cavus is probably the most common foot type to develop plantar fasciitis. In a cavus foot the toes assume a "clawed" position. The digits dislocate dorsally on the metatarsal heads, and the fascia becomes tight from excessive stress. It usually tears at the medial insertion into the calcaneus. In severe cases the fascia can even detach the periosteum. That eventually will lay down new bone and spur fibrocartilaginous deposits in the calcaneal area. The inflammation projects downward into the soft tissue and distally along the course of the fascia.

plantaris rupture. The major muscle in the back of the calf is the gastrocnemius, which travels from the Achilles tendon to the back of the femur and aids in the flexing of the knee joint. Buried beneath that massive muscle is a long, thin muscle called the plantaris, which is joined at the back of the knee and ankle through its own tendons.

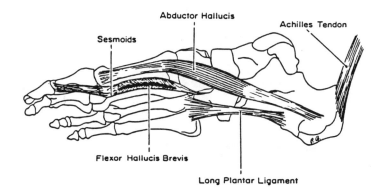

Sesmoids

Abductor Hallucis

Achilles Tendon

Flexor Hallucis Brevis

Long Plantar Ligament

The plantaris muscle is basically a "pushing off" muscle that comes into use when the foot is planted and pushed off abruptly in a forward or lateral position or direction. Often the long tendon (connecting the lower end of the muscle to the heel) will rupture during an excessive pushing-off maneuver or when the leg is braced to meet an oncoming force. That usually occurs at the point where the tendon and muscle blend together, just below the bulge of the calf; and when it does, it will feel as though the person has been whipped with a hot poker across the back of the calf. Extreme pain generally follows. The individual may not be able to put the heel down and may be forced to limp around on the ball of the foot for some time. As the rupture heals and the pain dissipates, the foot will remain in a heel-up position until either the taut tendon and muscles are restretched manually or stretched by the individual through appropriate exercises. Plantaris rupture is usually not a serious injury but can be quite disabling for several weeks if it is not attended to immediately.

plantaris strain. A forcible stretch, as in running, jumping, or excessive unaccustomed activity. The symptoms are generally in the calf on running and jumping: sudden sharp pain deep in calf or, if the pain is severe, disability. Signs may be graded by degree of severity: tenderness about 10 inches below the knee on the lateral side or in the middle; nodules possibly palpable in the calf, pain elicited by dorsiflexing foot, and plantarflexion unaffected. Complications may be calcification of plantaris and thrombophlebitis.

pleurisy. An inflammation of the thin membrane that covers the lungs and inner chest wall. The inflammation normally originates in the lung as part of some other process, often pneumonia, but occasionally it may be caused by a virus infection of the pleura itself, a bruise of the pleura caused by injury or an irritation resulting from pulmonary embolism. The inflammation produces a sticky exudate, which roughens the pleura of both the lung and the chest wall. When the 2 surfaces rub together during respiration, the roughness causes acute irritation. If the 2 surfaces stick together, the condition is called adhesion. Infection of the pleura may also cause abnormal flow of pleural fluid. It may accumulate between the 2 layers in such large amounts that the lungs may be compressed and there is an inability to obtain enough air. Viruses occasionally cause infections limited solely to the pleura. The disorders are of short duration and are not severely disabling. They are, however, rather uncomfortable, particularly at high altitudes or in similar situations in which the victim is required to breathe more rapidly and deeper than normal. The primary symptom, usually the only symptom, is pain with respiration. The pain is usually a rather sharp, stabbing sensation, limited to a small area on 1 side of the chest. Deep inspiration usually elicits a particularly severe twinge. Physical signs may be slight or absent. Motion on the affected side may be somewhat limited, and a few wheezes or rales may be heard over the involved area. Pleurisy unaccompanied by another disease, though painful, usually clears up in 3 or 4 days.

pneumonia. Bacteria and viral pneumonia are usually due to infections of the lung tissue, notably the alveoli. Persons weakened by fatigue, exposure, or disease elsewhere in the body are particularly susceptible. An inflammation of the alveoli may be caused by a *Diplococcus* known as the pneumococcus, although pneumonia may also be caused by a streptotoccus, a staphylococcus, or a virus. Any or all of those pathogens may be carried (all the time) by a healthy person in the mucosa of the upper respiratory tract. If the person remains in optimal health, the pathogens are kept under control (in small numbers) and may be carried for an indefinite period with no ill effect. However, if the individual's resistance to infection is lowered, the pathogens then may invade the tissues and work their damage. Exposure to inclement (cold and damp) weather for long periods of time, alcoholism, malnutrition, a severe injury, or other debilitating or weakening condition may cause a susceptible reaction to pneumonia. There are 2 main kinds of pneumonia, as determined by the method of lung involvement and other factors. Lobar pneumonia, in which an entire lobe of the lung is infected at 1 time, is 1. The organism usually is a pneumococcus, although other pathogens also may cause the disease. Bronchopneumonia is the 2nd type, where the disease process is scattered here and there throughout the lungs. The cause may be a staphylococcus or a virus. Bronchopneumonia most often is secondary to an infection from some other agent that has lowered the individual's resistance to disease. That is the more common form of pneumonia. The alveoli fill with infected fluid, impairing the exchange of carbon dioxide and oxygen. The respiratory rate and pulse rate generally increase. The fever associated with infection may increase the body's need for oxygen as the infection itself uses up the supply of oxygen. If a large amount of lung is involved, the oxygen lack combined with the toxic substances may cause death. Pneumonia should always be taken seriously. Its symptoms usually vary with the causative organism and the severity of the infection. All pneumonias usually cause a fever of more than 102°F (oral) and a rapid pulse or respiratory rate or both. Bacterial pneumonias are often ushered in by 1 or more shaking chills, followed by a high fever. The individual appears quite sick and may be very weak. Coughing is generally a prominent symptom of all lung infections. The cough may be dry at first but usually becomes productive (with mucus) after 1 or 2 days. The sputum, which is usually green or yellow (sometimes rusty), is usually thick and mucoid and frequently has an appearance resembling pus. The signs of the disease are limited to the area of the lung. The overlying pleura is often involved in the infection, and when only the pleura is inflamed, stabbing pain or breathing may be severe. Not infrequently pleurisy is an early and sometimes first indication of the underlying infection.

pneumothorax. On occasions, a broken rib may be displaced and puncture the underlying lung. Air may then enter the pleural space through the injury, causing the lung on that side to collapse. The tear in the pleura often allows air to enter, but not to escape from the chest, thus building up a considerable pressure in the involved pleural space (tension pneumothorax). As a result, the lung is further collapsed and respiration is severely impaired. The individual usually has received a severe, nonpenetrating blow to the chest, which may be followed by respiratory distress. Pain and tenderness are generally present over the fracture, but chest wall instability or flailing is usually absent.

pneumothorax, traumatic. A collapsed lung. It is caused by a direct sharp blow in back of the chest area, causing a tear of the pleura at its attachment to the large bronchi, a penetrating wound. Symptoms may include pain in the chest; shortness of breath on exertion; prostration in severe cases, especially in penetrating wounds. Signs may be diminished chest excursion on the affected side, hyperresonance with decreased or absent tactile fremitus and breath sounds, tracheal shift, tachycardia, and shock in severe cases. Complications may include hemothorax, serious respiratory disturbances, continual bleeding, or infection.

position sense. Receptors located in the muscles, tendons, and joints relay impulses that aid in judging the position and changes in the location of parts with respect to each other as well as informing the brain of the amount of muscle contraction and tendon tension being used. Those rather widely spread end organs (known as proprioceptors) are aided in that function by the semicircular canals and related internal ear structures. Information received by the receptors is generally needed for coordination of muscles and is important in such activities as walking, running, and many more complicated skills (e.g., playing a musical instrument). Those muscle sense end organs may also play an important part in maintaining muscle tone and good posture as well as in allowing for the adjustment of the muscles for a particular kind of work or sport to be done. The nerve fibers that carry impulses from the receptors enter the spinal cord and ascend to the brain in the back (posterior) part of the cord. Syphilis and certain other diseases may involve the posterior part of the spinal cord, causing degeneration and loss of position sense and giving rise to a condition known as "tabes dorsalis." The lower part of the body usually is affected first, with the result that the individual gradually loses not only position sense but also muscular coordination. Certain activities, such as walking—which because of those 2 faculties heretofore could be accomplished without the aid of sight and with hardly any thought at all—now become difficult (particularly in the dark) because the individual cannot see how he or she plants his or her feet. As the disease progresses, the individual may lose the ability to walk.

posterior tibial tendon dislocation. A violent twist of the ankle such as from falling into a hole or a direct blow on the extended leg with the foot either in everted position or propped on an object. The symptoms may be severe pain in the ankle or leg and disability. Signs may include: tendon riding out over medial malleolus, restricted ankle motion, swelling, or tenderness behind medial malleolus. Complications may be recurrence and persistent disability.

postural hypotension. Common to most conditioned runners. Differs from the idiopathic variety because it is most severe when postural changes occur from sitting to standing rather than supine to standing. When the athlete is supine, adequate pooling of blood in the lungs allows the next heartbeats to raise the suddenly lowered cerebral artery pressure to normal levels. When getting out of bed after a rest, he or she thus does not have postural hypotension. When sitting, the athlete has pooling of blood in the lower abdomen. Upon standing, there is no blood in the lung bed, and one may feel dizzy for 1 to 2 seconds. After a long run, however, the athlete more nearly resembles the individual with idiopathic postural hypotension, for he or she generally has wide open vascular channels, which allow pooling until the vessels contract. If the well-trained athlete is immobilized immediately after running, he or she may faint. The period of syncope is usually brief if the subject falls supine or prone so that the heart receives blood once again to perfuse the brain. Sitting in an automobile immediately after running is generally hazardous, since syncope may occur. The person is usually strapped upright (with belts) and is thus unable to slide into a prone position. In those circumstances the pooling effect may continue, and arrhythmia may develop. Walking or mild exercise during the cooling down phase will generally prevent that.

power. The rate of doing work (power) is determined by the rate at which energy can be released within muscle tissue. The type of contraction (isometric, isotonic, eccentric, or concentric), resistance, duration, quantity of repetitions, and the number of exercise bouts are generally important in any exercise program. But the most important power factor appears to be the fact that the contraction force developed by a muscle must be close to maximum if improved changes are to be expected. Low-repetition, high-resistance exercises generally develop short-term power in muscle mass. High-repetition, low-resistance exercise develops endurance, long-term power, and muscle tone. To produce the necessary energy, the body utilizes an aerobic (oxygen) pathway and an anaerobic (nonoxygen) pathway. To maintain life, the primary factor is generally the continuous and adequate flow of oxygen and nutrients. When oxygen demands exceed the supply (oxygen debt) during and following prolonged exertion, lactic acid generally accumulates within the muscle tissues and encourages fatigue. Usually the greater the exercise intensity, the greater the lactic acid accumulation. Following maximum exercise, it may take an hour or longer to attain resting levels. Oxygen debt must be repaid rapidly, such as through an increased breathing rate. Aerobic power may be essentially determined by cardiorespiratory function, intrinsic physical fatigue factors, duration and nature of the physical activity, possible genetic factors, extra demands on temperature regulations, and intrinsic environmental conditions, such as altitude, temperature, and humidity. Maximum aerobic power depends on the efficiency of the total cardiorespiratory system in the oxygen intake, transport, efficiency, and utilization rates. The greater the work accomplished, generally the greater the oxygen consumption, the faster the breathing rate, and the faster the heart rate.

protein in energy use. Whenever muscles are working hard or said to be active, they not only expend energy but also increase their rate of wear and tear. During hard training, to increase strength and power, there is generally an increase in the size (mass) of the muscles and in the total body weight. The increase in size of the muscles is in part due to a general increase in the diameter of the individual's fibers from additional proteins and some fats. Muscle fibers contain 20 percent protein, and therefore any increase in the size of a muscle will generally mean an increase in the total body protein. During vigorous activities the daily intake of protein must be increased from a normal level of 60 g/day to 120 g/day. That additional protein is metabolized to allow for the increase in the total body protein. It also provides for a greater rate of repair following the increased amount of breakdown of muscle tissue generally caused by the increased level of work. The need for additional protein has been recognized by athletes and their trainers as a vital part of high performance training. After metabolism, protein is excreted mainly as urea and uric acid, both of which are nitrogen-containing substances. The amount of nitrogen excreted must therefore be balanced by an equivalent amount of nitrogen taken in as protein. When that occurs, the individual is said to be in nitrogen balance. However, the amount of protein re-required to maintain nitrogen balance generally depends to some extent upon the amount of fats and carbohydrates in the diet. If they are not supplied in sufficient amounts, some of the proteins must then be metabolized to provide the needed energy. Proteins provide the necessary amino acids from which body proteins can be synthesized. Therefore, the amino acid content of the protein intake must therefore be considered. Protein foods may be graded according to the amounts of the essential amino acids they contain, which gives a measurement to the biological value of the food. Proteins generally cannot be stored in the body. Because of that, they are (relatively) poorly metabolized. Since they are required for the most effective gain in strength during hard training, drugs have been increasingly used to assist in protein metabolism. Such drugs, known collectively as anabolic steroids, have been used in clinical medicine for a long time. They have had value in convalescence after wasting illnesses. When athletes have taken anabolic steroids together with a high protein diet, they have experienced considerable increase in body weight generally, and the effects of strength-training program often have been dramatically increased.

psoriasis. A skin disease consisting of erythematous macular or papular lesions that develop a thick, silvery scale. The most common sites are the scalp, ears, eyebrows, elbows, knees, gluteal creases, genitalia, and nails. It may be a chronic, lifelong disease with exacerbations and remissions. It is not contagious and should have no effect on sports participation.

pulled elbow. A distal subluxation of the radial head that occurs in children, usually after judo or wrestling. A longitudinal pull on the forearm pulls the head of the radius out of the annular ligament. There is local tenderness and inability to supinate the forearm. The child classically holds the arm in pronation and supports the affected side in flexion with the contralateral arm. Manipulative supination reduces the radial head, usually with a "click."

pulled muscles. Term applied to rupture of muscle fibers of the quadriceps high up in the thigh, the hamstrings, or the calf muscles. It occurs generally in sprinters during extreme effort and to a lesser extent in runners at longer distances. The extent of the injury varies from a few damaged fibers to a very considerable tear demanding surgical intervention. The cause is probably an aggravated imbalance between the protagonist and the antagonist group of muscles, that is, a failure of 1 group to relax when the other group contracts. In that way rupture may occur at any situation between the muscle origin and insertion.

pulmonary edema. Potentially fatal, pulmonary edema becomes a risk between 8,500 feet to 12,000 feet, especially when exertion is prolonged in cold weather. It usually develops within 36 hours of reaching the new altitude. The picture may be one of rapid flooding of the lungs. It is usually initiated by severe exertion. Typical clinical signs may be those of intense acute dyspnea, loose cough, hemoptysis, nausea and vomiting, X ray evidence of intense pulmonary congestion, and an ECG indicating right ventricular strain. The lung congestion is often encouraged by the increased total blood volume, the increased left ventricular pressure resulting from diminished oxygen to the myocardium or the peripheral arterial vasoconstriction resulting from carbon dioxide washout, increased pulmonary capillary permeability, pulmonary venous constriction resulting from low alveolar oxygen pressure, or pulmonary hypertension resulting from previous exposure. Hospitalization is often required for bed rest, oxygen, and prevention of secondary infections.

pulmonary emphysema. An anatomic alteration of the lung, characterized by abnormal enlargement of air spaces distal to the terminal nonrespiratory bronchiole, which may be accomplished by destructive changes of alveolar walls. Increased size of air spaces generally arises from hypoplasia, atrophy, overinflation, or destruction. The description of emphysema generally depends upon the location of the disease. In panlobular emphysema all clusters of alveoli in a region of the lung are equally involved to a greater or lesser extent (the disease is generalized for that particular segment, lobule, lobe, or lung). In centrilobular emphysema, those alveoli directly contiguous to a respiratory bronchiole are most often affected. A respiratory bronchiole is the 1st order of bronchiole into which alveoli open; it is the earliest division of the airways in which gas exchange may take place. When panlobular emphysema results in selective parenchymal and vascular destruction of the lower lobes, individuals generally have shortness of breath at an early age. Loss of elasticity is the underlying defect in emphysema. Total elastin and collagen in the lungs of individuals with emphysema is normal; it is the loss of normal architecture and the resultant loss of airway support that generally leads to air trapping, ventilation and effusion abnormalities, and shortness of breath. The appearance of lungs with widespread emphysema demonstrates heterogeneity with large holes, small holes, and intermixed areas of compacted and normal lung. In emphysema airways are no longer held open by the tethering effect or normal elastic tissue and thus easily collapse. Capillaries are "pinched off" if not destroyed completely, and gross inequalities in matching of ventilation to blood flow occur.

pulse. The ventricles pump blood into the arteries regularly from 50 to 80 times a minute, depending on a person's level of cardiovascular conditioning. The force of ventricular contraction starts a wave of increased pressure that begins at the heart and travels along the arteries. That wave is called the pulse. It can be felt in most of the arteries that are relatively close to the surface, particularly if the vessel can be pressed down against a bone. At the wrist the radial artery passes over the bone on the thumb side of the forearm, and the pulse may be easily obtained here. Other vessel areas sometimes used for obtaining the pulse include the carotid artery in the neck and the dorsalis pedis of the toe of the foot. Normally, the pulse rate is about the same as the heart rate. But if a heartbeat is abnormally weak, it may be lost and thus not detected as a pulse motion. The pulse rate may be affected by various factors, such as: (1) it is generally somewhat faster in women than in men; (2) muscular activity levels may influence it; (3) during sleep, the pulse may slow down to 50 or 60 a minute, while during strenuous exercise the rate may go up to well over 100 a minute; (4) if a person is in optimal health and good condition, the pulse does not generally remain rapid, despite a continuation of exercise; (5) strong emotional disturbances may also increase the pulse rate; (6) in many infections the pulse rate increases with the increase in temperature; (7) excessive amounts of secretions from the thyroid gland may cause an increase in the pulse; (8) with aging and in some diseases, the blood vessels may lose some of their elasticity, causing an increase in the arterial blood pressure and pulse rate, since the walls can no longer stretch readily to accommodate so much of the heart's output during a systole.

punch-drunk syndrome. The term "punch-drunk" is derived from the fact that the individual exhibits the signs of a person who has had a little too much to drink. He or she may slur their speech and may be unsteady, fatuous, euphoric, sometimes quarrelsome, and even aggressive. Memory and intellect may be impaired, and moral sense may be lost. In advanced cases there is generally a coarse tremor, rigidity, or ataxia. The neurological features have generally been ascribed to petechial hemorrhages in or near the brain stem. It has also been suggested that diffuse neuronal destruction can result from the cumulative effects or minor repeated trauma. Cumulative head trauma is often found in many boxers fighting professionally or as sparring partners for 5 years or more. It is often expressed as a punch-drunk syndrome and sometimes referred to as dementia pugilistica or progressive post-traumatic encephalopathy. The early symptoms have generally been described as mental confusion and a slight unsteadiness of gait. Progressively, the individual may develop 1 or more of the following: leg dragging, jerky response, hesitant and slurring speech, hand tremors, head nodding, and the expressionless facial features of Parkinsonism, vertigo, deafness, euphoria or aggressiveness, and marked mental deterioration. It has been estimated that more than half of all boxers with 5 years' experience or more develop some degree of undesirable mental and emotional changes obvious to close associates. While a frequent point of impact in boxing may be the chin, the greatest damage is probably produced by concussive forces transmitted to the area of the brain stem at the base of the skull. That may also be true from blows to the side of the head resulting in sharp lateral or rotational shearing near the atlanto-occipital joint. With a knockout blow to the head, brain damage may result from the blow itself or just as easily and more seriously from the fall to the floor or canvas. Subdural hemorrhage, areas of diffuse small hemorrhages within the brain, cerebral edema, or thrombosis of superficial and deep vessels may result.

quadriceps strain. A strain caused by excessive forcible use or stretching of the quadriceps femoris. It is characterized by momentary incoordination, especially on fatigue, and contraction suddenly arrested by outside forces. The symptoms generally are stiffness, pain localized over front of thigh, and disability. Signs may be graded by degree of severity: muscle spasm, inflammation, swelling, followed by impaired function, ecchymosis that may be remote from damaged tissue, or possibly palpable defect. Complications may be muscle hernia, formation of cyst, and scar tissue.

R

racket players' pisiform. A condition brought about by using a racket with a wrist-flicking motion that initially gives rise to pain on the ulnar side of the hand at the base of the hypothenar eminence. It is due to stretching of the piso-triquetral joint capsule with ensuing instability of the pisiform. Chronicity produces a secondary chondromalacia in the joint.

real tennis (court tennis or royal tennis) injuries. The origins of the game lie in medieval France, where it was started by French priests as a handball game played in cathedral cloisters. That accounts for the shape of the court with its sloping roof and pillared openings and the wooden hatch. It gave its name to the word *tennis,* which derives from the French *tenez* or "attention" called by the server. Similarly *deuce* relates to the French *a deux* or "two," indicating 2 points to be played. As with tennis, running and cutting produce a crop of ankle and knee ligamentous injuries and sometimes ankle fractures. Falls can damage the wrist, elbow, or shoulder, and wielding a racket may produce rotator cuff injuries and inflammations. The elbow can be the site of common extensor origin strain or lateral epicondylitis. Stooping for the ball can give rise to back pain and wear in facetal and intervertebral disk joints.

rectus femoris strain. Changes of stride while one is running, uncoordination of muscles while one is running, fatigue, and improper warmup before vigorous leg exercise may lead to this malady. Symptoms may be acute pain, anterior aspect of thigh, and disability. Signs may be graded by degree of severity: swelling, ecchymosis, tenderness localized over anterior aspect of thigh and midline, palpable defect possible, inability to extend affected thigh, or pain elicited by active contraction of quadriceps group. Complications may be recurrence and persistent disability.

reflex action. The neuron is the anatomical or structural unit of the nervous system; reflex action is the physiological or functional unit on which all nervous activity is finally built. By definition a nervous reflex is an involuntary action caused by the stimulation of an afferent (sensory, ingoing) nerve ending or receptor. The structural basis of reflex action is the reflex arc. In its simplest form, it consists of a receptor, a sense organ that receives a stimulus from the environment, and an afferent nerve fiber (a dendrite). The fiber conveys the impulses set up in it to its cell body in a reflex center in the brain or spinal cord. Here a synapse occurs between the processes of the afferent neurons and the body of the efferent or motor neurons, the efferent nerve fiber (or axon) of which transmits impulses for the appropriate action to an effector organ.

In most reflex arcs in man, the afferent and efferent neurons are linked within the brain or spinal cord. Here a synapse occurs between the process of the efferent neuron and the body of the efferent or motor neurons, the efferent nerve fiber (or axon) of which transmits an impulse for the appropriate action to an effector organ. In most human reflex arcs, the afferent and efferent neurons are linked within the brain or spinal cord by at least 1, and often by more than 1, connector or association neuron. The knee jerk that clinicians test is 1 of the few examples of a 2-neuron reflex arc in people. Here the receptor is the muscle spindle in the muscle attached to the patella at the knee. When the tendon is sharply tapped, the muscle is stretched and the muscle spindle stimulated. Nerve messages pass into the spinal cord in the afferent neuron, which synapses with the efferent or motor nerve cell situated in the spinal cord. Outgoing impulses are generally transmitted to the muscle to cause it to contract in a familiar twitch. Reflexes form the basis of all central nervous system activity. They occur at all levels of the brain and spinal cord. Some reflex acts rise to consciousness. Links occur within the central nervous system between the reflex centers concerned and the higher centers, and we are made aware of what is happening. Others occur without our conscious knowledge, such as those involving stomach movements or alterations in the size of the pupil of the eye.

renal injury. Both kidneys are situated high in a retroperitoneal position on the posterior abdominal wall. Both may be prone to damage from direct blows sustained in the loins. Those injuries are variable. They may be minor with bruising only, or they may result in actual rupture of the kidney tissues. The signs of such trauma may be pain occurring over the region of the kidney, followed by hematuria. Any such case requires observation and urological investigation.

respiration. Normal rates of breathing vary from 12 to 25 times per minute. The term hypernea means "overbreathing" owing to abnormally rapid respiratory movements. Apnea means "temporary cessation of breathing." It may be compensatory, following forced respiration. In some fevers the respiratory rates may increase in direct proportion to the increase in temperature. In other cases there may be no correlation between the respiratory rates and the temperature. Breathing is generally controlled by the respiratory center of the brain, which is located in the stem portion (called the medulla) immediately above the spinal cord. From the neck part of the cord, the nerve fibers continue through the phrenic nerve to the diaphragm. Unlike the heart, the diaphragm does not continue to function if it is cut off from its nerve supply. If a single nerve is cut leading to the diaphragm, that side is generally paralyzed. The diaphragm and the other muscles of respiration are usually voluntary in the sense that they can be regulated by messages from the higher brain centers. It is possible for a person to deliberately breathe more rapidly or more slowly or to hold his or her breath and not breathe at all for a time. Usually a person breathes without thinking about it, while the respiratory center in the medulla does the controlling. That center is generally governed by variations in the chemistry of the blood. If there is an increase in carbon dioxide in the blood, the cells of the respiratory center are usually stimulated. When that happens, they send impulses down the phrenic nerves to the diaphragm. The following is a list of terms designating various abnormalities of respiration. They are not specific diseases but are the symptoms of disease or some other injurious condition. (1) Anoxia, which means "lack of oxygen." Certain tissues, such as the brain, may be permanently damaged because of an oxygen lack. (2) Asphyxia, a term indicating an increase in carbon dioxide (or monoxide) in the blood vessels and tissues and accompanied by an oxygen deficiency. It is synonymous with suffocation. (3) Dyspnea, which means "difficult or labored breathing." (4) Cheyne-Stoke respiration, which is a type of rhythmical variation in the depth of respiratory movements found in certain critically ill or unconscious individuals. (5) Suffocation, which refers to any stoppage of respiration. (6) Cyanosis, which refers to a bluish color of the skin and visible mucous membranes caused by an insufficient amount of oxygen in the blood.

respiration mechanics. The function of the lungs is to generally provide oxygen to the body and to dispose of or exhale carbon dioxide. During inspiration the chest is expanded by the muscles in the chest wall. Simultaneously, the muscle in the diaphragm contracts, pulling that structure downward. Air is drawn into the lungs by the negative pressure created through the bellows action of the chest and the diaphragm. Expiration is essentially a passive action involving releasing air and no muscular contraction. Lung tissues are usually stretched by the expansion of the chest during inspiration. When the muscles relax at the end of inspiration, the chest wall and diaphragm are generally pulled back into their original positions by the elasticity of the lungs. Each lung is enveloped by a thin membrane called the visceral pleura. Another membrane, the parietal pleura, lines the inner surface of the rib cage. The space between those 2 layers of pleura is called the pleural cavity. Normally, the lungs fill the entire thorax so that the 2 layers of pleura are in intimate contact with each other. If the chest wall is perforated or if the lung is punctured, air enters the pleural space. The elasticity of the lung may cause it to collapse, extruding or pulling more air into the pleural space, depending on the site of the opening. Subsequent expansion of the chest cavity may serve only to pull air in through a hole in the chest into the pleural cavity, but it does not generally expand the lung itself. That condition is known as pneumothorax. At high altitudes where great demands may already be made on pulmonary function, the resulting loss in pulmonary capability may well prove fatal.

respiratory infections. The chief importance of a cold in the athlete is that it may initiate a more serious secondary infection. There is no known reliable method of preventing colds. Athletes who are overly fatigued and not properly conditioned seem to be more susceptible to catching colds. Vitamins may not generally have any value as cold preventatives. If a cold lasts more than a week, there may be suspicion that a secondary infection has occurred in the sinuses. Sinus infections are a common condition with many people and a major cause of chronic partial disability in athletes. Most cases of sore throats wih a cough and increased sputum production in young persons are usually secondary to the infected sinus drip coming down the back of the throat. Posterior cervical lymph nodes may also be enlarged and tender. Two red streaks may be seen running down the posterior pharynx, 1 on each side. Frontal headache is almost always present and may be very severe. A sore throat may be a symptom of sinus infection, but in some cases the throat infection is primary, usually caused by a streptococcus. Bronchitis is usually secondary to an infection in the sinuses in its acute form. Chronic bronchitis is frequently associated with asthma in younger individuals. There are many strains of influenza, and their behavior is almost as varied as their numbers. Young people are seldom seriously affected by the "flu" but may be disabled for a week or more.

respiratory system. Every cell requires oxygen for combustion to provide the energy for its activities. The oxygen is generally conveyed to the cells by the blood, which also removes the carbon dioxide produced as a waste product of combustion. The interchange of oxygen and carbon dioxide between the blood and the tissues is called internal respiration. The main function of the respiratory system is to replenish the blood with oxygen and to remove the carbon dioxide from the blood. The interchange of gases that occurs in the respiratory system between the blood and the atmospheric air is called external respiration. The organs composing the respiratory systems are the nose, the pharynx, the larynx, the trachea, the bronchi, and the lungs.

rib, broken. A severe blow to the chest may break 1 or more ribs, but they are enmeshed by muscles so that they do not generally need to be splintered or realigned, as is usually necessary with other broken bones. Other than producing discom-

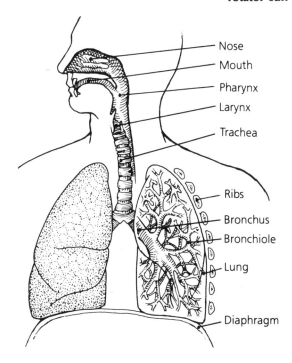

Anatomy of the respiratory system

fort, most rib fractures can interfere with movement of the underlying lung. Fluid and secretions may then collect in the immobile segment of the lung, producing congestion or even pneumonia. Very rarely, a broken rib may be displaced by the force producing the fracture. The displaced bone end may puncture the lung or, if it is low in the chest, be associated with kidney, liver, or spleen injury. A broken rib should be suspected after any blow to the chest followed by pain and tenderness over the area of the injury, particularly if the pain is aggravated by deep breathing.

Rocky Mountain Spotted Fever.   A disease caused by a bacterialike organism, *Rickettsia rickettsii,* which is transmitted to man by the bite of a tick (principally *Dermacentor andersoni* and *D. variabilis*). Some 3 to 14 days after the bite, mild chilliness, loss of appetite, and a general run-down feeling may appear. Those symptoms are generally followed by the onset of chills, fever, headache, pain in the bones and muscles, sensitivity of the eyes to light, and confusion. Between 2 and 6 days after onset of the disease, a red rash may appear on the wrists and ankles and spread over the entire body. The rash may be present on the palms of the hands and the soles of the feet. It may consist of small, red spots. They may be actually hemorrhages penetrating the skin. In severe cases large blotchy red areas may appear all over the body. The fever generally lasts about 2 weeks. The individual usually has the appearance of being seriously ill without obvious cause. The disease could be of potential concern to mountain climbers and campers.

rotator cuff tears.   Cuff tears involve the supraspinatus, infraspinatus, subscapularis, and teres minor, mainly used for elevating and abducting the shoulder. Cuff tears are more common in mature athletes with some preexisting fraying of the cuff, secondary to use. The attenuated insertions of the rotator cuff are usually torn while the fleshy

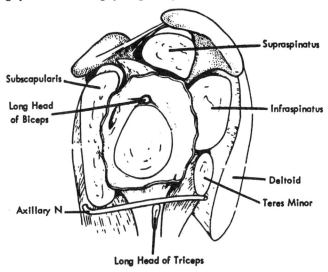

Subscapularis

Long Head
of Biceps

Axillary N

Supraspinatus

Infraspinatus

Deltoid

Teres Minor

Long Head of Triceps

The rotator cuff.

parts remain intact. Degenerative changes are not usually a factor in the injury process in athletes. Tears may be partial or complete. There are 4 mechanisms for rotator cuff damage: (1) Throwing. The velocity of the whirling head of the humerus is applied to the anterior capsule with subsequent labrum loosening, subluxation, and rupture of the capsule and subscapularis. (2) A direct fall onto the shoulder may tear the capsule and cause a fracture of the humeral tuberosity. The displaced fragment can distort the normal overhanging arch leading to subacromial bursitis and interfering with shoulder mobility. (3) A vertical thrust through an extended limb can be transmitted to the capsular structure. Normally the arm is held in abduction and flexion during a fall, and the forces are transmitted through the bony structure. When the arm is kept by the side, the soft tissues suffer most; such an accident occurs in skiing because skiers tend to hold the poles close to the body. (4) Cuff injuries accompany shoulder dislocation. A sudden force, such as might be encountered in tackling or lifting weights, creates a tear. The athlete will complain of pain in the shoulder, particularly when it is abducted to about 90 degrees. There will be difficulty in performing any activities with the hand above the head, but there is little discomfort below that level. The athlete may also complain of pain when he or she is turning on the shoulder at night and often adopts a position of sleeping away from the painful shoulder. With a complete tear examination usually shows a tender area over the anterior superior aspect of the shoulder.

rugby union and rugby league injuries. These are impact sports in which an oval ball is handled and kicked. The scrum is a minor penalty situation. Rows of players face each other—the front row being locked together with the opponents and the 2 sides try to push their opposition backward. The ball is put into that group of players and is moved out to the rear of the group when it can be picked up. Injuries are of the "impact" type and can be to any part and can be serious, ranging from head injury and concussion to the fracture of any bone and dislocation of even major joints. Trampling can cause serious abrasions and lacerations as well as damage to deeper tissues. Tackling and tugging can result in dislocation and fractures of the fingers. Wrist injuries following falls are quite common, as are injuries to the clavicle and elbow. The collapse of the scrum because of the nature of the interlocking that occurs can cause severe hyperflexion injuries of the neck and produce fracture and dislocation of the cervical spine with cord damage and permanent tetraplegia or paraplegia. The relative weight and maturity of opponents is most important, and much more care is now being taken not to mismatch teams of players, especially to avoid immature youngsters playing against adults. In addition, indirect injuries common to all running sports—particularly damage to the knee, ligamentous and meniscal, and to the ankle—are very common. Ligamentous and meniscal knee injuries are frequently seen.

runner's cramps. The most familiar muscle cramps are those that occur in the lower leg and foot. They may be common in any sport that involves a lot of running and are generally brought about by 2 major causes, a precipitating cause and an underlying cause. The precipitating cause may be the fatigue and overloads experienced by the calf and foot muscles during extended running. The underlying cause is generally that the lower extremities naturally receive the least amount of fresh oxygen from the heart. That is well illustrated by the fact that some nonathletic people with poor blood circulation (caused by a circulatory disorder) often suffer from leg and foot cramps when they are doing nothing more than lying in bed or sitting at their desks. Nonathletic individuals with poor circulation quite often do not get enough oxygen in the muscles of their lower extremities. As lactic acid accumulates in the inactive muscle tissues, even less oxygen becomes available. Suddenly, and for no apparent reason, the muscles go into spasm and cramps ensue. In the athletic person with poor circulation, cramps may occur just as readily during an athletic activity. Here, however, they may be additionally provoked by stress on the muscles. They generally occur less frequently in people who have good peripheral circulation and who do not smoke.

runner's knee. Chondromalacia of the patella. Attributed to an erosion or irritation of the undersurface of the knee cap or patella. Pain from runner's knee is usually felt under the knee cap and is often first noticed when one is running down hills or walking up stairs. In those situations the flexed knee generally pulls the knee cap against the knee joints with added force. As the condition progresses, pain may even be present when one is running on the flat. A grating sensation is often felt with knee motion and stiffness around the knee occurring after periods of rest. If we take a functional look at the cause of runner's knee, we see that the patella is firmly suspended by the quadriceps tendon and muscles above the patellar ligament from below. The patella itself is v-shaped and fits into a similarly shaped groove on the knee joint. When the knee is flexed and extended, the patella glides up and down. That function gives mechanical advantage to the quadriceps muscles to extend the knee. Injury generally arises when the foot pronates excessively. Pronation of the foot usually causes internal rotation of the leg and knee. Under those abnormal conditions, the suspended patella rides on the outer shelf of the V-shaped groove and may cause chondromalacia, or runner's knee. The triad of chondromalacia, tendinitis, and ligament strain may all be present at the same time in the runner's knee syndrome. Ligamentous strains, however, are more prevalent in sports requiring quick movements in a side-to-side fashion. That motion generally puts a greater twisting force on the knee joint. The 3 main reasons athletes develop soft tissue strains around the knee are (1) lack of proper conditioning for the activity, (2) unnatural activities leading to unusual stresses, and (3) inherent musculoskeletal weaknesses. When vigorous activity is attempted without adequate preparation, the muscles are generally too weak to effectively stabilize and coordinate the specific (knee or other joints) motion. That state may put excessive stress on muscle tendons and ligaments that are responsible for maintaining joint stability. The unusual stress generally results in fatigue and damage to soft tissue structures. Participation in sports that require unnatural body movements may cause knee injury. Musculoskeletal weakness in the feet and legs is often a major contributor to overuse knee injuries. When faulty foot mechanics throw the leg and thigh bones out of alignment with every step, the supporting tissues cannot maintain stability without some signs of fatigue.

running injury prevention. In running, attention to 4 general principles of injury prevention is essential as a first step in reducing the rate or severity of injury. They include matching of participant to the sport; specific training and conditioning; modifying, if necessary, running terrain or surface; and using appropriate running equipment. While running is generally an effective technique of aerobic fitness training, certain people constitutionally are often ill-matched for the sport. There are those who, because of limited flexibility in their hips or foot abnormalities, are unable to run distances without experiencing many of the problems that may arise. The risk factors as mentioned are training errors, including abrupt changes in intensity, and duration of frequency of training. These are important problems encountered in running injuries. Proper attention to slow progressive training and conditioning is probably the best single way of preventing the serious running injuries. In addition, supplemental muscle strengthening and flexibility training is generally important. The runner may develop imbalances, consisting of relatively weak anterior abdominal muscles, relatively strong and tight quadriceps or thigh muscles, and relatively strong and tight calf muscles with a matching weakness of the muscles in the front of the leg and the back of the thigh. Supplemental exercises to increase the flexibility of the tightened muscles and increase the strength and flexibility of the weakened muscle is important in the general prevention of running injuries. There is increasing research on the impact qualities of different running surfaces. Excessive running on hard surfaces (such as asphalt or concrete pavement) may contribute to shin splints and the onset of overuse running injuries, back problems, and in some cases brain damage. Wearing of good-quality padded running shoes may reduce some of the potential risks associated with aerobic running on hard surfaces. Running on the beach (hard sand, grass, or dirt), may be a good alternative.

ruptures. Owing to the great tensile strength of the normal Achilles tendon, femoral or calcaneus fractures invariably occur before the tendon ruptures. However, that may not be true when excessive force is applied to a previously injured or diseased tendon. The cause is usually traced to overuse, direct violence during stretch, or a poorly placed injection. A bronchial or tracheal rupture may show signs of air leakage along the mediastinal tissue planes, seen as vertical lucent streaks adjacent to mediastinal shadows. A gastric air bubble displaced medially may point to a splenic hematoma. Blunt trauma may cause superior or anterior dislocation of the lower ribs, and lower rib fractures may be associated with diaphragmatic, splenic, or hepatic rupture. In diaphragmatic rupture the hemidiaphragm takes on an abnormal contour, which sometimes can be seen on the standard posterior-anterior full chest view. Most diaphragmatic ruptures occur on the left side, as the liver generally offers considerable protection during a blunt blow on the right. In retinal hemorrhage and choroidal ruptures, retinal edema and bleeding usually occur in the macula or temporal area, and resolution usually occurs in a few weeks without radical treatment. A choroidal rupture generally appears as a whitish circumscribed area near the disk in ophthalmoscopy because the herniation allows underlying sclera to be viewed. Several examples of sports deaths have been attributed to blunt trauma to the abdominal area. The most common fatality is generally that of rupture of the spleen as well as intrasplenic or subsplenic hematoma and retroperitoneal hemorrhage. Rupture of the splenic capsule may produce severe hemorrhage, often from what may be considered minor trauma. It may even rupture spontaneously following infectious mononucleosis. Although the pancreas is generally quite protected, blunt injuries to it in sports have been reported with some serious consequences. Injury may also likely be due to crushing forces against the spine. Symptoms may be dramatic or subtle. There may be epigastric tenderness and pain, often radiating to the back or left scapula, moderate shock, mild muscle resistance, and signs of hemorrhage.

S

sacroiliac injuries. Sacroiliac dislocation creates direct trauma from behind or behind and laterally. Symptoms may be local pain and inability to stand, sit, or turn over in bed, with local tenderness, especially on compression of the pelvis or manipulation of the leg. There could also be a persistent disability. Sacroiliac sprains may be frequent, especially when weights are lifted. Heavy loads or severe blows may rupture some associated ligaments and subluxate the joint. Pain may be local or referred. The individual generally assumes the characteristic posture with a flattened lumbar area, trunk inclined away from the lesion, guarded gait, and limited spinal motions, especially spinal flexion because of hamstring tension. Jarring the spine may cause a sharp localized pain in the affected joint.

sartorius strain. A strain caused by excessive forcible muscular action, as in running or jumping. Symptoms may be local pain over anterosuperior spine of ilium and along anterior aspect of thigh and disability. Signs may be graded by degree of severity: swelling and tenderness near anterosuperior spine of ilium and pain elicited by passive external rotation of leg and by flexion of abduction of thigh. Complications may be persistent disability and recurrence. That often mild but persistent disability is often seen with "squatting" football linemen and occasionally in oarsmen. Discomfort may be aggravated by abduction and extension, and it may be eased after warmup.

scalp injury. Scalp contusions are apt to be circumscribed or localized (producing a hematoma of the scalp) and may sometimes be accompanied by brain concussion. A depressed skull fracture may be falsely suspected because most of these types of blood pools are depressible in the center and offer the sensation of indentation of the skull. In scalp lacerations, associated with compound fractures, the prevention of sepsis leading to meningitis is generally the principle aim in emergency care. The subarachnoid space is usually protected by the skin and galea and in certain areas by the temporal and occipital muscles, the pericranium, bone, dura, and arachnoid. The deeper the penetration of the wound, generally the greater the chance of meningitis and thus the necessity of greater care in preventing infection.

scuba diving. Abnormal accumulation of carbon dioxide is unusual except for the scuba diver. The word *scuba* is an acronym from Self-Contained Underwater Breathing Apparatus. The sport, requiring highly specialized training, is exceptionally demanding. Thus such activity is generally a contraindication if the individual is not in good physical shape or is suffering from breathing problems or even a mild infection or disorder. The equipment itself contains a large variety of potentially dangerous hazards; thus it must be maintained in excellent condition. During deep dives special problems arise from sustaining thermal homeostasis, physiologic alteration of gases, changes in renal circulation, psychosomatic reactions to stress, and alterations in bacterial population characteristics. Two major dangers in deep dives are generally the fact that nitrogen absorption may lead to euphoria, resulting in recklessness, and the fact that too rapid an ascent may quickly lead to decompression sickness (the bends).

self-produced injuries.   Injuries of various kinds may occur as the result of body activity, without the intervention of any outside agencies at all. The basic force producing such injuries is generally muscular contraction, which may cause damage in some circumstances without being itself in any way abnormal. A powerful contraction of the peroneus brevis may avulse the base of the 5th metatarsal. More frequently, however, such injuries are due to some unbalanced or abnormal body movement. They may also be caused by some action that, while not unbalanced, is abnormal and, therefore, throws too much strain on the body tissues. An example is the sudden movement of the low back requiring extreme rotation and lateral flexion, which is necessary when the so-called shut-face technique is used in striking a golf ball, which may cause various low back disorders of traumatic origin.

sesamoid bone injuries.   The most common sesamoid injury occurs in the prehallux or accessory navicular. In an eversion injury with a tight posterior tibial tendon, an avulsion force is applied to the accessory bone, and it is pulled away from its attachment to the navicular. In sesamoiditis, pain beneath the 2nd metatarsal head can be due to a problem with the medial or lateral sesamoid. There may be a history of landing on the ball of the foot. Occasionally a cleat, such as in soccer or baseball, underneath the ball of the foot can create enough irritation to produce problems in articulation between the sesamoid and the 1st metatarsal head. The athlete complains of pain in the ball of the foot, especially in running activities that involve sprinting. Examination reveals tenderness beneath the 1st metatarsal head, tenderness that may be localized enough to be attributed to either the medial or the lateral sesamoid. The medial sesamoid under the 1st metatarsophalangeal joint is subject to trauma when the toe is in forced dorsal flexion and a blow is applied to the ball of the foot. The mechanics of the injury resemble that of patellar fracture, in which the combination of tension on the patella and a localized blow fractures the bone. That injury can be extremely painful, since it prevents the athlete from running on his toes. Bipartite sesamoid is a congenital condition in which the medial and occasionally the lateral sesamoid will show transverse separation of the 2 segments at the midline. That must not be confused with fracture, which is much less frequent. The symptoms are ordinarily those of accompanying metatarsal arch strain, and the bipartite sesamoid is found coincidentally and usually is of no significance.

Sever's disease.   Some young athletes 9 to 11 years of age frequently have heel pain after excessive running. The pain is generally localized over the insertion of the Achilles tendon into the apophysis of the tip of the calcaneus. The condition, called Sever's disease, is an example of disruption of a tendon-cartilage interface. In X rays the apophysis generally appears fragmented because of irregularities in the ossification process. The heel pain usually responds well to rest.

shin splints.   An ailment common to many people who involve themselves in running sports, but it is generally most frequently seen among joggers. It is usually an ailment of the anterior tibial muscles of the lower leg, 3 long thin muscles that travel along the front of the leg, from below the knee to the foot, and function to lift the foot and, through their tendons, the toes. Shin splints are basically a form of cramps, in that they develop in a similar manner. When an individual runs, especially on hard surfaces and after having not done so for some time, the stresses on the unconditioned shin muscles may be great. As they fatigue, they generally build up an oxygen debt and may

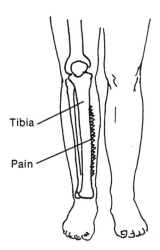

Tibia

Pain

accumulate large amounts of lactic acid. When the debt becomes too much, the muscles often go into spasm. The only difference between shin splints and ordinary cramps is that, instead of going into acute spasms, the shin muscles usually develop milder and smaller but recurrent spasms. They generally become very hard, and when the area is touched, it is often difficult to tell the difference between the muscles and the lower leg bone. As they become hard, they generally act to squeeze off the veins, causing further engorgement and distention of the muscles. The best way to deal with shin splints is generally to rest the leg until the pain and muscle hardness have disappeared, which generally takes 1 to 2 weeks.

shock. The most common cause of shock is generally sudden reduction in the volume of the body's blood, usually as a result of severe injury, trauma, or bleeding. All the constituents of the blood (blood cells and serum) are lost by hemorrhage. However, the volume of blood may also be reduced by other disorders in which only the fluid portion of the blood is lost. Large volumes of serum may be poured out from the damaged tissues following a severe burn. Dehydration resulting from fluid losses, caused by severe vomiting or diarrhea, as frequently occurs with cholera, may cause a reduction in blood volume, which is fatal if untreated. When the blood volume is reduced, regardless of cause, the arteries in the skin and muscles generally constrict, tending to direct the available blood to the vital organs. At the same time, the heart generally begins pumping at an increased rate in order to circulate the remaining blood faster and enable a smaller volume of blood to carry the required amounts of oxygen and nutrients to the tissues. When those mechanisms can no longer compensate for the derangements in blood volume, shock usually results. If untreated, severe shock eventually becomes irreversible, regardless of therapy, and the victim generally dies. Shock can also occur in other disorders in which there does not appear to be a definite reduction in blood volume. Severe infection or heart attacks are often associated with shock. A period of shock of varying duration is generally characteristic of the terminal stages of any fatal disease. Mild shock often results from loss of 10 to 20 percent of the blood volume. The individual generally appears pale, and his or her skin feels cool to the touch, first over the extremities and later over the trunk. As shock becomes more severe, sweating generally appears. The individual usually complains of feeling cold and is often thirsty. A rapid pulse and reduced blood pressure may be present. Moderate shock often results from loss of 20 to 40 percent of the blood volume. The signs of mild shock may be present and become more severe. The pulse is often fast and weak or "thready." In addition, the blood flow to the kidneys is generally reduced as the available blood is shunted to the heart and brain, and the urinary output declines. A urinary volume of less than 30 cc (1 oz) per hour is generally indicative of moderate shock. Severe shock often results from loss of more than 40 percent of the blood volume and is generally characterized by signs of reduced blood flow to the brain and heart. Reduced cerebral blood flow generally produces restlessness and agitation, often followed by stupor, confusion, and eventually coma or death or both. Diminished blood flow to the heart may produce abnormalities of the cardiac rhythm.

shoulder capsulitis. Excessive postinjury immobilization generally leads to muscle atrophy and loss of capsule elasticity, a predisposing factor to capsulitis. Lack of joint movement often fosters retention of metabolites, edema, venous stasis, and ischemia leading to fibrous adhesions and trigger-point development. Shoulder capsulitis is often the result of a sprain attended by a spontaneously reduced subluxation or of prolonged overuse. Joint pain is usually aggravated by movement. Tenderness and other symptoms may be generalized with the whole joint area rather than being localized. Motion limitation may be considerable in adhesive capsulitis (frozen shoulder) when the head of the humerus is "glued" to the glenoid cavity.

shoulder girdle. The shoulder girdle is composed of the clavicle anteriorly, the scapula posteriorly, and the humeral laterally. The shoulder girdle is a very loosely constructed mobile mechanism of bones, muscles, and ligaments designed to give great mobility to the upper extremity with only sufficient stability to provide a proper foundation for the muscular activity of the upper extremity. The skeletal connection of the shoulder girdle to the trunk is extremely tenuous and consists only of the relatively insecure articulation of the inner end of the clavicle against the sternum and the first rib. Injury of the girdle structure may start as a "pain in the shoulder." Acromioclavicular dislocations or separations can be easily palpated; fractures of the clavicle are not only easily palpable but also usually visible. The shoulder is an extremely complex mechanism, and anything affecting 1 portion is bound to have an effect on the other components. That is particularly pertinent because of the function of the upper extremities and more particularly in relation to the throwing arm. The integrity of the sternoclavicular joint is maintained by the ligamentous structures that bind the inner end of the clavicle to the sternum and the first rib. There is little inherent bony stability in the articulation. Contusion in that area does not happen frequently because, generally, the athlete has been trained to protect the anterior part of the neck and chest by keeping his chin down. In football, shoulder pads provide the necessary protection. The most common injury to the sternoclavicular joint is sprain caused by forces that thrust the shoulder sharply forward. The portion of the clavicle lying between the coracoclavicular ligament attachment, which coincides with the beginning of the distal portion of the clavicle, and the proximal expansion leading to the sternoclavicular joint is designated as the shaft of the clavicle. Since the clavicular shaft is subcutaneous, it is subject to contusion. The injury is ordinarily readily recognizable because of local swelling. Hematoma formation occasionally occurs in the area and also infiltration of blood into the skin and subcutaneous tissue. Fracture of the clavicle is a frequent athletic injury, much more likely to occur in the preadolescent or adolescent youngster than in the adult. In the adult, ligament injury at either the inner or outer end of the clavicle is more likely to occur than in the youngster. Since there is no "built in" bony stability between the acromion and clavicle, the entire integrity of this joint is maintained by ligamentous support. A sprain of the ligaments is caused by anything that forces the acromioclavicular joint through a range of motion beyond its normal capacity. Various forces may cause injury to the acromioclavicular joint. The most common is a downward blow against the outer end of the shoulder, driving the

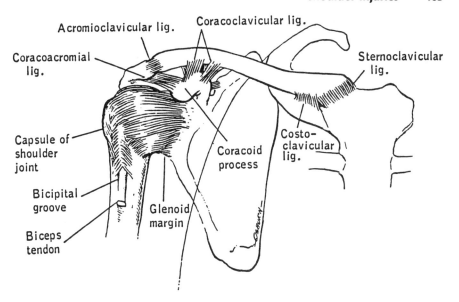

Acromioclavicular lig.   Coracoclavicular lig.

Coracoacromial lig.

Sternoclavicular lig.

Capsule of shoulder joint

Costo-clavicular lig.

Coracoid process

Bicipital groove

Glenoid margin

Biceps tendon

Anatomical drawing showing the ligamentous structures about the shoulder girdle.

acromion forward, the clavicle remaining upward. Another is traction on the arm, pulling the shoulder away from the chest wall and causing true lateral displacement of the acromion. The majority of such injuries occurring in football consist of falling on the outstretched hand or flexed elbow with the arm flexed forward 90 degrees and in a neutral lateral position.

shoulder injuries. Painful shoulder is a common complaint among athletes, particularly as age advances. The pain occasionally extends into the upper arm when the shoulder has been abducted from 45 degrees to 120 degrees. There is usually no pain with full abduction or with the arm completely at rest at the side. The syndrome can be produced by several different lesions, all of which cause pain by trapping a tender structure between the acromion process and the tuberosity of the humerus. Tears of the capsular soft tissues and repeated sprains can result in pericapsulitis with a limitation of all ranges of shoulder movement; in the extreme a "frozen shoulder" results. Sometimes an associated hand stiffness is found. Cervical spondylosis, brachial neuralgia, and tennis elbow may also be present. By far the greatest number of shoulder dislocations are anterior, being common in high jumpers and water pole, wrestling, judo, and football players. The condition occurs with an extension force to an abducted, externally rotated arm, as in a "hand off" in rugby. Acromioclavicular dislocations are usually produced by a fall on the tip of the shoulder but may occur when the shoulders are pinned to the floor in wrestling. In subluxation the superior and inferior capsule is torn, but the main stabilizing ligament, the coracoclavicular ligament, remains intact. Dislocation of the shoulder is a problem in sports injuries because recurrence is not uncommon in fit, young athletes who again put stress on the shoulders, and surgery necessarily imposes a restriction on shoulder mobility often with a lowering of sporting performance. Primary dislocation may have associated damage to the capsule or labrum at the glenoid rim. There may also be a defect in the posterolateral aspect of the humeral head. Both factors militate against stability. Posterior dislocation of the shoulder is caused by a forced internal rotation of the abducted arm or by a blow on the shoulder in boxing.

Several problems involving the supraspinatus tendon can create pain. A minor tear can cause pain without loss of power. A calcium deposit within the tendon will become surrounded by an inflammation, which takes up space and causes impingement through the arc of abduction. That particular cause is often acute and can be extremely uncomfortable. Another lesion of the supraspinatus tendon is an inflammation secondary to degeneration of tendon fibers. Another cause of pain in the area is an incomplete fracture of the tuberosity of the humerus or contusion of the bony prominence of the humerus. All create swelling, which obliterates the acromiohumeral space with abduction.

sinusitis.   An infection of 1 of the sinuses of the skull. The sinuses are located close to the nasal cavities and in 1 case near the ear. The sinuses are open spaces within the bone, lined by a thin mucous membrane similar to that of the nose and connected with the nose by narrow canals. Infection may easily travel into these areas from the mouth, the nose, or the throat along the mucous membrane lining, and the resulting inflammation is called sinusitis. Long-standing, or chronic, sinus infection may cause changes in the epithelial cells, resulting in the formation of tumors. Some of those growths have a grapelike appearance and may cause obstruction of the airpath. The tumors are called polyps. Sinusitis is generally caused by an obstruction of the canals that drain the sinuses, usually as a result of a swelling of the mucous membrane around the opening because of a cold or an allergy. Mucus may collect within the sinus and become infected, and the infection may spread to the surrounding tissues. Sinusitis, although sometimes painful, is rarely disabling by itself. However, complications may occur, particularly the spread of the infection to the bones of the skull or to the brain itself, resulting in meningitis or a brain abscess. Such complications usually follow chronic sinusitis, which a physician should generally treat. Acute sinusitis usually accompanies or follows a cold. The most prominent symptom may be a headache, which may be located in the front of the head, "behind the eyes," or occasionally in the back of the head. A purulent discharge frequently drains into the nose and back into the throat, where it may be swallowed, the so-called postnasal drip. Fever may be absent, and tenderness may be present over the involved sinus. Infection in the maxillary sinuses may produce pain or tenderness in the teeth of the upper jaw.

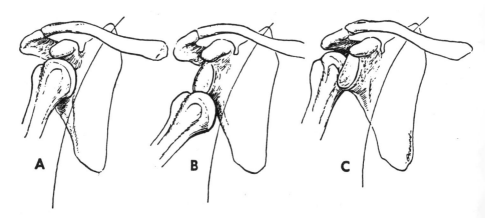

Dislocations of the shoulder. (1) Typical subcoracoid dislocation. (2) Subglenoid dislocation. (3) Posterior dislocation.

skater's ankle. The ankles are supported and moved by muscles around the joint, and when they are weak, the result may be a tendency of the ankles to bend excessively from side to side. Most incapacitating ankle injuries, especially when there are no bone fractures involved, usually take the form of moderate to severe sprains. They generally result from episodes in which a great sudden stress has been applied to the anterior talofibular ligament (on the outer aspect of the ankle) or to the medial deltoid ligament (on the inner aspect) through a turning in or out of the side of the foot as it strikes the ground. Such episodes generally occur when the foot strikes an uneven surface during walking, jumping, or running or when it strikes the ground already turned in or out after jumping. In either case the weight of the body is usually concentrated on the affected ligaments, and as the force overpowers the ligament's maximum checkrein capability, the ligament tears, either partially or wholly. Complete tears (or ruptures) of the ankles' side-supporting ligaments generally require corrective surgery to restore proper ankle function. Because most severe ankle sprains generally come about through the foot turning inward under the ankle, it is usually the anterior talofibular ligament that is most often damaged and weakened. What follows may generally be a chronic tendency of the ankle to collapse inward, whenever the foot strikes an uneven surface.

skier's heel. The ankle, in addition to its inner and outer aspects, relative to ankle sprains, has another important dimension. That is the backside, which is called (in formal anatomy) the tendo calcaneus or, in general medicine, the Achilles tendon or Achilles heel. Since distress in that area most often occurs in skiers, it has become known as "skier's heel." The tendo calcaneus, or Achilles tendon, is a long, thick, rounded tendon which can be felt at the back of the ankle and which attaches the muscles in the rear of the calf to the calcaneum, or heel bone. Those muscles, gastrocnemius (which is a flexor of the knee), and the soleus, which along with the gastrocnemius as the principal flexor of the ankle, share the Achilles tendon in common. Like the flexor and extensor tendons in the elbow, the Achilles tendon may be strained and become inflamed as a result of repeated overloads. Unlike the extensor tendon in the elbow, though (because it is such a long tendon), it may also have frequent tendency to tear, or rupture. It is for that reason it is called the Achilles tendon, after the hero of Homer's Iliad, the great warrior of the Trojan war whose only weakness manifested itself when his tendo calcaneus was cut. Ruptures of the tendon frequently occur among skiing enthusiasts and usually have a combination of precipitating and underlying causes. The most obvious are the strains and stresses placed on the tendon during a day of skiing. In no other sport is the Achilles tendon generally required to endure such continual overloads. Corollary causes may be the nature of the principal maneuvers of skiing and the design and construction of the ski boot. The principal maneuver of skiing is the turn. In order to make one, the skier must abruptly jerk his heels upward and then down again. At the same time the boot is normally constructed in such a way that the forepart of the foot is virtually immobilized. Thus, the forces and stresses of the constant movement of the lower limbs in skiing are generally not distributed throughout the foot, as they are in other sports. They concentrate and terminate in the ankle, which is usually bound tightly into the boot by virtue of its design, at least in the lateral aspects. The only part of the ankle really free to move is the part that permits the individual to raise and lower the heel. That part is mostly the Achilles tendon, therefore, that most of the forces are concentrated in and terminate there. Put all those causes together and add to them fatigue factors in the Achilles tendon and calf muscles that accrue from hours of repeated and constant strains of turning, edging, and trying to keep one's skis parallel, and there is an ideal set of conditions for the rupture or at very best the partial tear and inflammation of the Achilles tendon.

skiing injuries. High-speed direct trauma is usually the most important cause of head injury. Cervical disk lesions are common, particularly in the middle-aged holiday skiers when preexisting degenerative disease may be activated by unaccustomed minor trauma. Almost any type of injury may result from collisions or lateral falls onto hard icy surfaces, but 2 injuries are quite common, dislocation of the shoulder and the ski pole fracture. The former often occurs in falls during slalom racing when the outstretched hand becomes fixed in the soft snow as the body continues to descend down the slope. The shoulder is generally abducted, extended, and dislocated. Ski pole fracture often occurs in the outstretched hand that has hold of the ski stick. The metacarpals are usually affected, either a fracture of the 3rd and 4th or more usually an adduction injury of the 1st metacarpophalangeal joint. The most common injury to the trunk is the aggravation of an existing lumbar disk lesion. Cervical disk injuries are more likely to occur in the older skier who only skis occasionally. Other trunk injuries are usually the result of collision. In knee injuries the injuring force is generally abduction, but there may also be some rotation. Fifty-six percent of all torsion injuries to the lower limb result in a knee injury; of those, 30 percent are associated with ankle strains and 8 percent with an injury to the opposite knee. The most common knee injury is generally a partial tear of the deep fibers of the medial collateral ligament between their attachments to the femur and the meniscus. The only common form of direct trauma to the lower leg may be lacerations from the edge of the opposite ski. By far the most common skiing injury is generally a fracture of both leg bones caused by rotational forces. Ankle injuries are almost always a result of rotational force. In the unsupported lower limb, a rotational force applied to the foot will usually produce an injury at the ankle joint. If the force is applied slowly, the ligaments are likely to tear first, but if the force is applied rapidly, the bones of the ankle mortise are most likely to fracture. Approximately half the ankle injuries seen are fractures, and only half are strains. Internal rotation injuries are more common than external. Plantarflexion injuries almost never occur. Some of the ligaments guarding the talotibiofibular joint may be involved. Subcutaneous rupture of the tendo Achilles just above the level of the boot may be another injury of importance, because of the disability that may follow incorrect treatment. Injuries to the foot are made up of a collection of many different lesions, from lacerations and punctures to rotational and fatigue fractures.

skin diving. Carried out by taking a deep breath and then going under water. Underwater swims for distance and spear fishing are competitive forms of such diving. With training, individuals can cover distances of 60 yards to 70 yards and can descend to depths greater than 75 feet. Preliminary hyperventilation may lead to hypocapnia (washing out of carbon dioxide) and hyperoxia (excessive oxygenation) of the blood. Exercise then generally alters this state gradually to hypercapnia and hypoxia, but not exactly in step. In spear fishing, the hyperoxia may be increased by the rise in ambient pressure. That may suppress the response to slight hypercapnia; in fact, the best divers can all tolerate raised blood CO_2 levels. However, as the ambient pressure decreases during ascent to the surface, the hyperoxia rapidly falls and may become hypoxia (depending on time and oxygen consumption), and once again unconsciousness may supervene.

skull. Name given to the bones that make up the skeleton of the head. The only bone of the skull that is movable is the mandible or lower jaw. The rest of the bones are firmly joined together at immovable joints called sutures. The skull is divided into an upper boxlike portion called the calvarium and a lower irregular portion that constitutes the skeleton of the face. The calvarium contains the brain. It is made up of 8 bones: 1 frontal bone, 2 parietal bones, 2 temporal bones, 1 occipital bone, 1 sphenoid bone, and 1 ethmoid bone. The facial skeleton is made up of 14 bones: 2 zygomatic bones, 2 maxillae, 2 nasal bones, 2 lacrimal bones, 1 vomer, 2 palatine bones, 2 inferior nasal conchae, and 1 mandible.

skull fractures. Common in sports played on a hard surface and in those utilizing a ball or club. They are generally classified as: (1) closed, or simple, fractures, which do not involve a break in the overlying skin or membrane; and (2) open or compound fractures, which involve a tear in the covering adjacent to the fracture. Linear skull fractures may be simple or compound. Signs of a simple linear fracture are generally pain, swelling over the fracture line, and discoloration. X-ray studies may reveal a "crack" in the skull. Depressed skull fractures usually occur when the head is struck by an object such as a golf club and the skull is pushed onto the brain. Those fractures may be compound or simple. When they are compound, emergency surgery is generally indicated for debridement and removal of bone fragments from the brain. Skull fractures in the bones at the base of the skull generally cause discoloration around the eyes and nose or over the mastoid and may be accompanied by leakage of cerebral spinal fluid into the ear (otorrhea) or the nose (rhinorrhea). They are not usually visible on X-ray film. Concussion is generally a syndrome in which there is an immediate impairment of neural function following a blow to the head. That deficit is usually noticeable in the degree of consciousness but may also involve memory, visual disturbances, and equilibrium problems. In 3rd-degree concussions there may be unconsciousness for more than 5 minutes and moderate retrograde amnesia. Multiple concussive blows to the head, like those received in boxing, may result in a combination of symptoms from involvement of the pyramidal, extrapyramidal, and cerebellar pathways. The common symptoms may be slurred speech, dull face, slowness of movement and mentality, and tremor. Cerebral contusion is a bruising of the brain. When a small area of the brain is involved, it is often difficult to distinguish from a concussion, and no permanent effects occur. In more severe contusions cerebral edema with brain swelling generally results in increased intracranial pressure. If a generalized contusion with bruising of the brain stem occurs, decerebrate rigidity usually follows and the individual may die or have a permanent deficit after a long illness.

skull wounds, closed. Except for a possible bruise or contusion, there is generally no obvious external damage in closed wounds. Injury may be to the brain itself or to the pia mater or arachnoid meninges. Rupture of blood vessels in the pia may be particularly important in closed injury. Blood spilled onto brain cells is usually treated as a foreign substance that disturbs the functioning of those tissues. Blood collecting within the cranium generally exerts pressure against the brain. If there is no skull fracture or if skull fracture is such that the integrity of the dura is not disturbed, the cranium may be unyielding. If the skull is depressed or displaced inwardly, it may exert direct pressure on brain tissues even without formation of a hematoma. Frequently, a fall upon the back of the head will cause much more internal damage than a blow to the anterior head with a fist.

skull wounds, open. Open wounds of the head are generally classed according to whether or not the integrity of the dura mater is disturbed. Two classes are seen: (1) Nonperforated dura mater. The wound may be no more than a laceration of the scalp which, although not to be taken lightly, may not be serious. There may be 1 or more fractures of the skull, but the dura is not usually perforated. In either case possible internal damage is likely to be or become more serious than that of the scalp and skull. If the skull is fractured, it will usually hold in the same manner as a closed injury against the pressure of any hemorrhage that may occur within the cranium. (2) Perforated dura mater. With the skull and the dura opened, the meninges may be exposed to environmental air and pathogenic invasion. When the delicate meninges are open, the brain itself may be exposed. The skull may be fractured in such a way that it is no longer a closed vault, or part of it may be torn away, and brain tissue may protrude through the opening. In regard to symptoms, the individual may be either conscious or unconscious. Signs may be intracranial pressure and internal damage, if any, and are generally the same as for a closed injury. Lacerations of the scalp often bleed profusely because the blood vessels, which are quite numerous, do not constrict and retract like those of other areas of the body. Scalp lacerations may gape open because the scalp, when intact, envelops the skull quite tightly. The severely fractured skull may be malshaped, yielding, and minus parts.

slipped disk. Back disorders generally evolve from the combination of weak outer back muscles and strains to those muscles and then go on to develop into recurring, deeper muscle strains as the larger supporting muscles tend to lose their ability to support the spine fully. The progressive weakening of the back may eventually work its way down to the spine itself, so that the vertebrae of the spinal column, especially in the most weight-bearing lumbar region, may undergo slight but significant changes in their relationships to each other. That in turn generally places unaccustomed strains on their ligaments. As the ligaments weaken, the vertebrae and all their parts may experience further relational distortions. Once that condition is reached, it usually takes only a minor twist or strain to unleash a whole new kind of havoc, the slipped disk. A "slipped disk" neither slips, nor is it a disk. The affliction is in reality a complete breakdown of an intervertebral joint in the spine, for that is what a disk is. A slipped disk can and often does occur in the neck or cervical region of the spine, but the most frequent site is generally in the lumbar region. That is because this portion of the spine generally bears most of the upper body's weight.

snow blindness. The surface of the eye (cornea and conjunctiva) absorbs ultraviolet radiation just as the skin does. Excessive exposure may result in sunburn of those tissues, producing snow blindness (photophthalmia). Any source of high-intensity ultraviolet radiation, including sun, ultraviolet lamps, and electric welding equipment, may produce photophthalmia. During the actual period of exposure, there may be no sensation other than brightness to warn the individual. Symptoms may not develop until as much as 8 to 12 hours after exposure. The eyes initially feel simply irritated or dry but, as symptoms progress, may feel as though they are full of sand. Moving or blinking them generally becomes extremely painful. Even exposure to light may cause pain. Swelling of the eyelids, redness of the eyes, and excessive tearing may occur. A severe case of snow blindness may be completely disabling for several days.

soccer syndrome. In soccer, the common "scissors" kick frequently leads to instability of the sacroiliac and symphysis pubis joints. Groin pain may be aggravated during full stride, jumping, and in the stretching motion of kicking with power. Also in soccer players and jockeys, a periosteal reaction may be noted at the origin of the adductor muscles (gracilis syndrome).

soft tissue injuries. Generally refers to all of the body tissues except the bones and specialized organs of the head and trunk. From the standpoint of traumatic injuries, the most important of those tissues are generally the skin (and its underlying layer of fatty tissue), the muscles, the blood vessels, and the nerves. The amount of bleeding from a wound may depend upon the size, number, and type of blood vessels that have been severed. Arterial blood is generally under high pressure, approximately 2 pounds per square inch, which causes profuse bleeding following damage to an artery of significant size. The pressure in veins is usually only about 1/20 that in the arteries, so venous bleeding is generally much less severe. Blood spurts from the end of a severed artery in rhythm with the heartbeat, a feature of arterial injury that may be easily recognized. That sign should be identified, because a large amount of blood may be lost in a short time from arterial bleeding. Application of local pressure is generally 1 of the most effective means of controlling bleeding. The severed vessels need to be collapsed, obstructing the flow of blood and permitting clots to form. Venous bleeding may be easily controlled because the walls of the veins are easily collapsed, and the clots that occlude the vessels are rarely forced out when the normal pressure is released. The thicker walls of the arteries make them more difficult to compress, and the higher blood pressure tends to dislodge clots that may be forming.

somatic nervous system. The somatic nervous system is often directly involved in many ways in athletic activities and in the ailments and injuries that may occur. The somatic nervous system usually carries commands from the brain to the muscles and enables them to contract, thereby producing the movements desired to be made. The nervous system has 2 basic kinds of nerves: the sensory nerves, often called "receptors," and the motor nerves, often called "effectors." The sensory, or receptor nerves, generally receive stimuli from within or without the body and instantaneously transmit those sensations back to the brain center. There the sensations are usually interpreted again instantaneously and acted upon by the appropriate stimulation of the motor, or effector, nerves. Each normal body part has a sensory and motor nerve that connect to the brain through the complex network of nerve branches and subbranches. The nervous system may also be the source of pain. When nerves are damaged, it may be the source of physical weakness or disability.

speed. The ability to move the body or any 1 of its parts rapidly. Because speed is generally directly related to muscle power (power = force/time), it is essential for athletes who are involved in running, jumping, throwing, or striking. How fast the athlete can run or move depends on several factors, many of which are genetically determined: characteristics of the nervous system (how many muscle fibers for each nerve ending), the arrangement of bones and the attachment of bones by ligaments and tendons, and adequate muscle strength. But speed primarily depends on the muscle's fiber type. Every muscle in the body contains 2 distinct types of muscle fibers, commonly called fast-twitch and slow-twitch fibers. Fast-twitch fibers are generally characterized by high anaerobic capacity, rapid contraction, short fatigue time, and the ability to generate a relatively large force. Slow-twitch fibers have high aerobic capacity, slow contractile rates, long fatigue time, and the ability to generate a relatively low force. Biochemically, fast-twitch fibers are best suited for sprintlike activities, and slow-twitch fibers are advantageous in endurance events.

speed, power, and organism. An organism obtains both speed and power from muscular contractions. The skeletal muscles will shorten when contracting against a submaximal load; the degree of shortening may vary inversely with the magnitude of the load applied. Initially, the muscle may contract without shortening (isometrically) until it has developed a tension equal to the load applied; thereafter, it will contract and shorten (isotonically). In that manner, a load will usually be reached that equals the maximum isometric tension of which the muscle is capable. In that instance, no shortening can occur, and the whole contraction is isometric. Thus, maximal isometric tension of a muscle is generally known as the muscle strength and is usually measured in practice with a dynamometer. When a muscle contracts isometrically, it will expend energy, but, paradoxically, it will generally do no mechanic work because no joint movement occurs. In movements of the whole or part of the organism, there must be joint movement, and, therefore, there must be a shortening of the muscles (prime movers) that bring about the movement. In the movement of any mass—be it the whole body, or part, or an object propelled by the body—power may be developed.

spinal cord. The spinal cord lies within the vertebral canal. It is continuous above with the medulla oblongata. A central canal contains cerebrospinal fluid and connects with the ventricles of the brain. Thirty-one pairs of nerves take origin from the cord: 8 from each side of the cervical section, 12 from the thoracic, 5 from the lumbar, 4 sacral, and 2 coccygeal nerves on each side leave the foot of the cord as a leash of fibers forming the cauda equina. The spinal cord shows enlargement in cervical and lumbar regions. Those areas contain the neurons that give rise to the nerves for the

172 • spinal cord injuries

arms and legs. Unlike the cerebrum, the white matter, containing the nerve fibers traveling to and from the brain and linking various parts of the cord with each other, is on the outside; the gray matter, containing the nerve cell bodies, lies deep in the substance of the cord surrounding the central canal. In cross-sections of the cord, the gray matter appears roughly H-shaped. The posterior horns of the H contain neurons that synapse with ingoing (afferent) fibers whose cell bodies lie in posterior root ganglia just outside the cord. The anterior horns of the H-shaped gray matter contain the cell bodies of lower motor neurons, i.e., the nerve cells whose axons carry outgoing (efferent) motor signals to cause contraction of voluntary muscle. Just after leaving the cord, the anterior motor nerves join the posterior or sensory fibers entering the cord to form the spinal nerves. The anatomical spinal nerves, therefore, contain both motor and sensory fibers. They travel to all parts of the trunk and limbs. In the thoracic and upper lumbar segments of the cord, small additional lateral horns, protrusions from the middle of the H-shaped gray matter, contain nerve cell bodies from which sympathetic nerves arise for distribution to viscera and blood vessels.

spinal cord injuries.   About 6 percent of spinal cord injuries occur within sports. Most injuries generally are caused by extreme flexion where subluxation, fracture, and dislocation may be associated. Hemorrhage may occur at the site with the same reaction as brain injury (liquefaction, softening, disintegration). Congenital fusions and stenosis may predispose a child to spinal cord trauma during a sporting activity. There are direct and indirect classes of injuries, such as direct injury to the cord and to the nerve roots, or both may be caused by impact forces or shattered bone fragments. The cord may be crushed, pierced, or cut. That type of injury is generally an open wound. An indirect injury to the cord may be caused by the disturbance of tissues near the spine by violent forces, such as falls, crushes, or blows. Such an injury, which is normally closed with respect to the spinal column and cord, is usually of a lesser degree than direct injury. It takes the form of concussion, hemorrhage, or edema of the cord. The cord may cease to function below the site at which the force was applied, even if the cord itself received no direct injury. Such dysfunction may be temporary or long-standing. Injuries to the spinal column in which the cerebrospinal fluid is rapidly depleted may be fatal. If the cervical cord is injured, there may be loss of sensation and flaccid paralysis. The lower limbs may exhibit a spastic paralysis. If the space in which the spinal fluid flows between the spinal cord and the surrounding vertebral column is either compressed or enlarged, severe headaches may occur. A spinal cord concussion is generally a direct blow to the spine. Symptoms may be clinical syndrome characterized by immediate and transient impairment of neural function, pain in the back, numbness and weakness of extremities or trunk, or interruption of normal bladder and bowel function with recovery. Signs may be transient with recovery: paresis, paralysis, and abnormal tonus of extremities, loss in any or all sensory modalities to the level of lesion, but usually no pathologic reflexes. A spinal cord contusion is generally a direct blow to the spine with structural alteration of the spinal cord, often characterized by extravasation of blood cells and tissue necrosis with edema. Symptoms may include weakness or paralysis of extremities and trunk, numbness of extremities and trunk to level of lesion; and bladder and bowel dysfunction. Signs may be partial or permanent impairment of neural function, paresis, paralysis of extremities and trunk, varying degrees of sensory modality loss consistent with extent and level of lesion, and hyperflexia with pyramidal tract signs.

spinal fractures, compression.   Forcible flexion spinal injury. The cause may be a blow on the head, as from diving in shallow water or a fall from a height onto the feet. Symptoms may be local pain, with nerve root compression; numbness; radicular pain in chest and extremities; unilateral or bilateral injury; spinal cord compression; weakness or paralysis, perhaps numbness in trunk and extremities; and bladder and bowel dysfunction. Signs may include percussion that elicits radicular pain or local pain over spine, accentuated on any movement; possible radicular hypesthesia or muscular weakness; in extreme cases, tetraplegia, areflexia, bladder dysfunction, and partial to complete sensory impairment, pathological reflexes. Complications may be possible subsequent neurological deficit, as spine may be somewhat unstable.

spinal fracture, dislocation. The cervical type is caused by forcible flexion, lateral or rotary twisting of head and neck, or a blow to head, as in diving; the thoracic, by forcible flexion, as in wrestling; the lumbar, by a fall from a height, landing on the buttocks. The symptoms may include local pain without neurological deficit if the problem is a simple spine lesion; radicular pain, numbness, and weakness in upper extremity if there is root involvement. The dislocation is often associated with spinal cord injury with symptoms appropriate to level of lesion. Signs may be variable from none to complete neurologic deficit according to the level and degree of nerve injury or tenderness on percussion if limited to a simple spine lesion. Complications may be permanent tetraplegia or paraplegia.

spinal injuries. Ligamentous sprains and pulled muscle fibers are common spinal problems but rarely inconvenience the athlete for more than a week or so. However, backache caused by a prolapse of an intervertebral disk or a bony abnormality of osteoarthrosis of the facet joints is generally more refractory to treatment and may thus be responsible for longer periods of incapacity than simple sprains and contusions. Even direct kicks and blows to the spine rarely damage the vertebral bodies, disks, and appendages. A more serious problem is a collision at running speeds, as in football, which adds to the normal momentum and generally produces a twisting force. That force generally causes shearing of the posterior ligamentous complex and possible dislocation and fracture-dislocation of the facet joints and intervertebral disk damage. Sprains are quite common in all athletic competition, especially in weight lifting and javelin throwing. New tennis players with a poor serve can often develop backstrain. Fractures and dislocations of the spine may be divided into stable and unstable, the latter being associated with serious disruptive bony or ligamentous instability and thus more likely to involve the spinal cord or peripheral nerves. Compression, hyperextension and a combination of flexion and rotation are the movements that generally cause cervical spine injuries. Compression injuries may occur in diving into shallow water, exercising on the trampoline, high jumping, or pole vaulting. Hyperextension injuries may occur in football with a tackle from behind or when the chin is in collision with the knee or the ground. Wrestling also has a proportion of lateral rotational injuries to the neck. Forced flexion, shearing forces, and hyperextension tend to cause thoracic, lumbar, and thoracolumbar injuries. Forced flexion is often common after falls at high speeds (e.g., motor cycle and horseriding accidents), but the posterior ligaments may remain intact. However, with shearing forces, such as may occur when the body is thrown and twisted at the same time, a slice of bone may be sheared off the top of 1 vertebra and the posterior facets fractured. That is generally a very unstable fracture because of the extensive disruption of soft tissues, which usually cause a swelling within an hour or so, but a palpable gap between the spinous process is generally found in the lumbar fascia at once. Hyperextension injuries may occur with a tackle from behind or with a collision at high speeds. The principal fracture is generally that of the laminae.

spleen injury. The spleen is an organ situated posteriorly under the diaphragm. It may be very susceptible to direct trauma and is often associated with fractures of the 9th and 10th ribs, which lie behind it. Trauma generally results in a rupture of the splenic capsule with hemorrhage. Such ruptures may occur with the most minor injury or even spontaneously, such as when the athlete has been suffering from an unsuspected infectious mononucleosis. Initially, the athlete may feel abdominal pain in his or her left upper quadrant, with the discomfort being felt behind the left shoulder tip, from referred diaphragmatic irritation. The hemorrhage, if increasing, may result in spreading generalized abdominal pain and increasing abdominal rigidity. Signs of bleeding may be present, becoming more obvious with increasing blood loss. Initially, the athlete will generaly develop pallor and tachycardia. Any drop in blood pressure may be a late phenomenon. Most athletically trained cardiovascular systems are generally highly efficiently trained units, and circulatory collapse, as shown by hypertension, may be a late manifestation. When there is significant shock, urgent resuscitation is generally necessary, followed by immediate surgical splenectomy. Occasionally, the injury may not be sufficient to cause a complete disruption of the spleenic capsule, and a spleenic hematoma may develop. Because that may occur at any time from 1 to 2 weeks after the injury, in all cases where damage to the spleen is suspected the athlete should be kept under hospital observation until the danger period is past.

spondylosis.   A break in the continuity of the pars interarticularis of the neural arch, almost always in the lumbar spine. Previously considered to be a congenital defect, it is now generally believed to be a stress fracture since this is not the usual site of fusion of ossification centers. It has not generally been found to occur at birth. There may be an increasing incidence with age. One suggested mechanism is that movement between adjacent articular facets may produce a pincer effect on the area. It may be asymptomatic or produce localized pain in the back. However, if there is nerve root pressure, it is much more likely that there may be an associated disk protrusion rather than nerve pressure from the fibrocartilaginous mass that binds this fracture together. When the condition is bilateral, there may be a high risk of spondylolisthesis, such as the upper vertebra slipping forward on the one below it. Other potential causes of spondylolisthesis include laxity of posterior structures without bony defect. In athletes it is probably a stress fracture that may occur among soccer players, oarsmen, weight lifters, and javelin and hammer throwers. Although it may be asymptomatic, it usually produces lumbar pain in the buttocks and legs.

sprain.   An injury to a ligament generally resulting from overstress, which causes some degree of damage to the ligament fibers or their attachments. A ligament is generally designed to prevent abnormal motion of a joint, while permitting normal functional motion. Fundamentally, abnormal motion to a degree beyond the power of a ligament to withstand it will generally cause a sprain. That may be contrasted with a direct blow over a ligament, which may cause a contusion. As abnormal forces are applied, the ligaments may become tense and then give way at 1 or the other of its attachments or at some point in the substance of the ligament. If the attachment pulls loose with a fragment of bone, it is called a "sprain fracture," but the mechanics are the same. The location of the damage will generally depend upon the weakest link in the chain of the ligament, which may be within the ligament itself or at 1 of its attachments, possibly at the site of an area of previous damage. The extent of damage generally depends upon the amount and duration of the force. If the abnormal force is arrested or terminated promptly, there may be little actual functional loss to the ligament and only a few of its fibers involved. If the damage is more severe, so that there is actually more disruption of ligament fibers, there may be considerable functional loss. Where the ligament is completely torn, all function may be lost. One-third of all sports injuries involve ligaments and are classified as sprains. The likelihood of a sprain increases with the "violence" of the sport. Sprains are more common in contact sports, such as football and wrestling, and are generally more frequent in team sports. The location of the sprain is frequently a function of the demands of the specific activity, such as running and jumping sports, which produce ankle sprains; jumping, cutting, start and stop sports affect the knee; sports using the upper extremities for support (i.e., gymnastics) may produce injuries of the wrist, elbow, and shoulder. Loss of joint stability is generally the basis for grading sprains. Sprains are usually divided into 3 groups: mild (Grade I), moderate (Grade II), and severe (Grade III). A Grade I sprain normally involves "overstretching" or microscopic tearing of ligaments, but not to the extent that there is an increase in the instability of the joint involved. Grade II sprains may involve partial overt tearing of the ligament with at least some ligamentous continuity remaining. Thus there is generally an increase in stability but not to the point of total laxity. In Grade III sprains there is generally a total loss of ligamentous continuity. The joint is usually more lax, and there will be no solid end point on testing for stability. Most ligaments serve multiple stabilizing functions, such as the medial collateral ligament of the knee, which generally prevents medial or valgus openings of the joint (primary function) and excessive rotation and anteroposterior motion (secondary function).

sprain, sternoclavicular. Sternoclavicular joint sprains are generally classified according to the severity of injury. They are often overlooked in the early stages after injury,

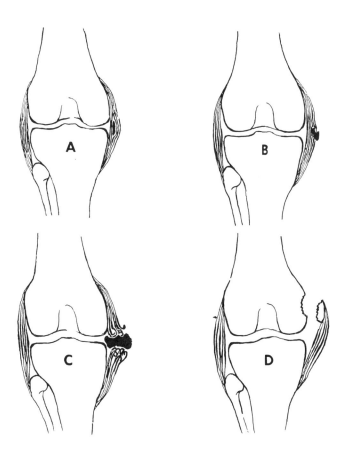

Knee joint, showing various types of sprain. (1) Grade 1 (mild) sprain, in which only a few fibers of the ligament are separated. (2) Grade 2 (moderate) sprain, in which greater tearing of the ligament occurs. (3) Grade 3 (severe) sprain, in which the ligament is ruptured. (4) sprain-fracture. The ligament has torn loose a piece of bone rather than rupture itself.

because the pain is frequently felt out on the medial or distal clavicle. The athlete with a sternoclavicular injury characteristically turns his or head away from the side of injury. Palpation over the sternoclavicular joint will generally indicate an acute area of tenderness, and a prominence may be observed. Instability may be detected by grasping the proximal clavicle between the thumb and index finger and forcibly pushing it in an anterior-posterior manner and then in an upward direction. The injury usually results from force being applied to the lateral aspect of the shoulder.

stasic eczema. Venous insufficiency may arise in the ankles or lower legs as a result of tight ankle wraps or binding from high shoes. The result is generally congestion, brownish pigmentation, and later scaling and weeping. Repeated injury may lead to edema and phlebitis. Chronic scratching may lead to secondary infection and, if left unmanaged, cellulitis, with or without ulceration developing. Varicose veins, ulceration, thrombophlebitis, and secondary infection are always a potential threat.

stenosing tenosynovitis (deQuervain's Disease). Pain on the radial side of the wrist without a history of injury may be caused by stenosing tenosynovitis. The short extensor tendon and the abductor tendon to the thumb pass through a tunnel across the radial styloid on their way to the base of the thumb. With overuse of either the thumb or the wrist, those tendons may become inflamed, producing a space problem with the tunnel. Thus motion of the thumb or wrist will create pain. Examination reveals tenderness and swelling.

steroids. As the use of amphetamines among athletes has decreased, the use of the so-called muscle building drugs has generally increased. Anabolic steroids ordinarily produced in the male testicle and adrenal cortex have been manufactured synthetically. Some athletes have seized on the use of anabolic hormones for sports involving muscle power, including shot put, hammer, discus, javelin, weight lifting, boxing, and football. The drugs apparently are widely used. With the increasing emphasis on winning and the rewards associated with victory, many athletes may be persuaded by a coach, a manager, an athletic trainer, or even a physician to use anabolic hormones. There is little doubt that their use generally leads to larger-appearing muscles. That effect is largely the result of both salt and water retention plus the additional fatty tissues (marbling) in the muscle fiber. The salt and water retention, one of the many undesirable side effects of the drugs, may be associated with a propensity to produce hypertension. A host of other complications have been reported, including hepatitis, jaundice, and cancer of the liver. There may be additional side effects in males, such as loss of sexual drive, altered spermatogenesis, testicular atrophy, and, from the use of preparations containing female hormones, gynecomastia. Acne, hirsutism, and permanent deepening of the voice may be expected side effects in females. The administration of anabolic hormones to immature athletes may result in early maturation, closure of the epiphyses, and short stature. Most investigators agree that the use of anabolic steroids generally results from the concomitant increase in caloric intake, fluid retention, increased muscle work in training, improvement in the basic skill, and a potential placebo psychological effect. When the use of anabolic agents is discontinued, there is often a reported water weight loss of diuresis, and only minimal associated loss of strength.

stitches. Crippling but temporary abdominal stitches are acute unilateral (usually on the right) pains on inspiration in the area of the lower ribs and upper abdominal quadrant. They are not generally a state of asphyxiation but are usually associated with windedness. Disability may arise in that air hunger may be combined with increased pain on deep inspiration. The "spell" usually subsides in 3 to 5 minutes. Attacks generally occur during running, especially downhill. Running on a full stomach often appears to be an aggravating factor.

stomatitis. A generalized inflammation of the oral mucosa. Canker-sore lesions of the mouth are generally associated with systemic disease, vitamin C or riboflavin deficiency, drug allergy, denture irritation, or a visceral-reflex nature. In athletics stomatitis can usually be traced to a poor-fitting mouthpiece, as in football or boxing, which may cause the gums to become red, swollen, and sore and the tongue to become large and thick. Salivation is usually marked. A football helmet's chin strap may exert considerable pressure upon an ill-fitted mouthpiece.

strain. Damage to some part of the unit (muscle, tendon, or the attachment), occasioned by overuse (chronic strain) or overstress (acute strain). There may be mild (1st degree), moderate (2nd degree), and severe (3rd degree) strains of the unit. The strain generally occurs at the weakest link of the muscle tendon unit at a given time. Under a given stress, the tendon may rupture, and the muscle tendon junction may give way, or the damage may be to the muscle itself or to its bony attachment. Chronic strain from overfunction may cause fatigue of the muscle and its sequelae, muscle spasm, myositis, and ischmia. It may also result in irritation at the musculotendinous junction or tenosynovitis along the course of the tendon or inflammatory reaction at the tendon attachment. Acute strain may be the result of a single violent force applied to the muscle, such as the violence of the sprinter coming out of the blocks when his or her muscles contract violently against the resistance of the block. It may be the result of resistance to a force, such as muscle contraction, or when a violent force is applied that is greater than the unit's ability to withstand. That is exmplified by the strain to the biceps brachii, which may result from trying to support with a flexed forearm a weight that is greater than the biceps unit will tolerate. In a mild strain the degree of strain generally causes no appreciable disruption. Pathological changes are generally confined to a low-grade inflammatory process with swelling, edema, and some discomfort on function of tendon or muscle. There may be neither discernible loss of strength nor any restriction of motion. In severe strain, rupture of any component of the unit is usually the result of violent contraction against firm resistance. It may be preceded by damage to a lesser degree that has improperly healed. The tendon may give way or separate at the muscle junction, or the muscle itself may rupture. When the forces applied are greater than the strength of the unit, something must give.

strength, dynamic. If the explosive efforts are to be repeated in rapid succession (as in sprinting), the stored energy of adenosine triphosphate is generally replenished by the breakdown of creatine phosphate to creatine and phosphate radicals. That usually involves dynamic strength. Performance limits may be imposed on the 1 hand by the forces resisting acceleration and sustained movement, and on the other hand by the cumulative power of the 2 phosphagen-splitting reactions and the total store of phosphagen energy within the active muscle fibers.

strength, explosive force. The effective power of a single strenuous (violent) effort generally depends upon the factors similar to speed in that the total time required for a sprint even includes the lag in initiating the body movement, the rate of acceleration to peak velocity, and the potential subsequent loss of speed as the event continues. However, it generally depends in particular upon the force-velocity characteristics of the active muscles. The proximate basis of movement within the muscle fibers is the chemical coupling of 2 long chain proteins, actin and myosin, using energy stored in the phosphate bond of adenosine triphosphate. The observed response depends upon the rate of chemical coupling, the number of actin and myosin filaments per fiber, the number of fibers activated, and the leverage that can be exerted. The results of all those factors may be opposed by the dynamic viscosity of the part.

strength, static. Important in events such as weight lifting. It usually varies with the total number of active muscle fibers and their individual cross section; thus, unless a muscle is "diluted" by fat and connective tissue, there is generally a rather consistent relationship between the potential force and the dimensions of a given muscle. Physiological tests may measure some of the performance dynamics of a group of muscles. Some forms of weight training may produce marked gains of measurable strength without muscle hypertrophy. In such circumstances it may be possible that the contraction has been dispersed over a wide range of muscle fibers, possibly with more complete relaxation of antagonists. Central inhibition of the contraction may also have lessened so that individual fibers can sustain a more continuous titanic effort. The endurance of maximum static contraction is generally quite brief (20 to 30 seconds), and it is unlikely that glycogen reserves are exhausted so rapidly. The tolerance limit is generally imposed by the interaction of motivation with pain and exhaustion, and that may be consequent upon accumulation of acid metabolites in the active tissue. However, the fatigued muscle may initially show poor relaxation, and that normal compliance in the recovery period may suggest that an immediate depletion of intramuscular phosphagen stores may also be involved. The capacity to sustain repeated and prolonged but submaximum static contractions is generally important in certain sports. Tolerance of repeated sustained static contractions may be improved by specific strengthening of the active muscles, since they then contract at a small percentage of maximum voluntary force.

stress fracture.   Produced by too much activity too soon or by too much activity all at once. With the increasing involvement in sports activities by nonathletes, the nonconditioned participant is exposed to the same hazards of injury as is the trained athlete. However, he is ill-equipped physically to withstand the forces to which the weekend activities will expose him. In conditioned athletes the condition happens when the athlete has run or hiked more or farther than usual. There is an onset of a vague ache in the midportion of the foot, which becomes painful with continued activity. Examination usually reveals tenderness in the region of the 2nd or 3rd metatarsal shaft and occasional swelling. If the symptoms have been present for several weeks, thickening of the metatarsal cortex may be palpable. The greater incidence of stress fractures in female athletes also represents a lack of conditioning and proper training techniques rather than a true predisposition to injury. Stress fractures occur when the rate of bone breakdown from activity (a normal process) is greater than the rate of bone formation (repair). The pain of a stress fracture that is typically restricted to a specific area may often be relieved with rest.

stretch injury.   A type of injury to the nervous system caused by overstretch of the nerve, such as overstretching of the peroneal nerve after rupture of the lateral collateral ligaments of the knee. In severe cases the ligament injury may screen the nerve condition so that it may not be recognized until later. The symptoms will vary with the seriousness of the injury. If there is a complete avulsion of the nerve, there will be immediate and complete loss of function, whereas if the nerve is stretched but not torn, there will be hemorrhage and shock to the fibers but function will be more slowly and less completely lost. Whenever there has been complete loss of function of a nerve, a decision has to be made whether or not surgical exploration is necessary.

stroke.   A term applied to a group of diseases in which the blood supply to the brain may be disturbed. The most common of the disorders are hemorrhage, which may destroy much of the brain, and clotting of a blood vessel, which may cause the death of the tissue supplied by that vessel. Strokes usually result from restricted blood supply, often caused by arteriosclerosis (hardening of the arteries), which is associated with high blood pressure (hypertension). It is a condition that often occurs in elderly people. Although many persons survive strokes, frequently with surprisingly little disability, the prognosis is still generally serious. The onset may be quite variable. Headaches may or may not be present. Other symptoms that may be transient can include weakness of an arm or leg and weakness over one-half of the body; vague, unusual sensations, such as tingling, "pins and needles" feelings, or numbness; visual disturbances, such as blurred vision or partial blindness; and difficulties with speech, both in speaking and understanding the speech of others. Personality changes, such as combativeness, indecisiveness, or irritability, may occur. With more severe strokes, headaches are generally present. Unconsciousness may follow fairly quickly and rapidly progress to a deep coma in which the individual does not respond to any stimuli. Breathing is usually noisy and may be very irregular (Cheyne-Stokes respiration). Paralysis is often present, most usually affecting 1 side of the body. It may also include the face as well as the extremities. The paralysis may involve the entire body and is often difficult to evaluate in the presence of a coma.

subdural hematoma.   Bleeding or swelling, which accompanies injuries to any organ or tissue, leading to compression of the brain within its rigid covering and frequently producing damage and dysfunction quite out of proportion to the size and severity of the original injury. A minor hemorrhage, which would not generally be of any significance with a wound anywhere else, is often sufficient to cause death when it occurs in the skull. Occasionally, a blow to the head, although not severely injuring the brain at the time, breaks some of the blood vessels around it. Blood from the torn vessels pours out into the narrow space (between the brain and the skull) and produces a clot, which then compresses the brain. Death may generally be the final outcome in untreated cases or in those in which the treatment is obtained too late. The speed with which the clot develops generally depends on the number and size of the blood vessels that have been damaged. It may also be affected by a person's level of cardiovascular well-being, as evidenced by the speed at which the blood vessels close down (vasoconstriction) in the area of injury. Following severe injuries, the evidence of bleeding may become apparent within a few hours. In other cases signs of injury may not appear for 2 or 3 weeks or occasionally even longer. The prognosis for the individual correlates fairly well with the speed with which the hematoma becomes evident. An acute subdural hematoma, which develops within 24 to 48 hours, generally carries a very poor prognosis. A chronic subdural hematoma, which may develop 2 to 3 weeks after the injury, carries a much more favorable prognosis. An epidural hematoma, a similar disorder, usually follows a fracture of the skull. The clot may be located between the bone and its covering fibrous membrane, but the effect on the brain is generally the same. The damaged blood vessels producing an epidural hematoma are usually medium-sized arteries rather than the smaller veins that produce a subdural hematoma. Therefore, signs of an epidural hematoma usually come on faster and are generally more severe.

subtalar varus.   In this condition the subtalar joint, in its natural position, has the calcaneus in a varus position. That may be 1 of the most common foot disorders in runners and is thought to be either a congenital or hereditary deformity. Clinically, the sagittal plane of the posterior surface and the plantar surface of the calcaneus are often inverted to the weight-bearing surface when the foot is in its neutral position. When the plantar surface of the calcaneus is in an inverted or varus position relative to the floor and if there is enough motion available at the subtalar joint for pronation, the calcaneus may evert enough to reach a vertical position with its sagittal plane, and thus the foot may reach the floor. If there is no motion available at the subtalar joint for the foot to pronate, the calcaneus generally remains inverted in a varus position. That is usually an uncompensated rear-foot varus and is normally rare among runners. When there is sufficient motion in the subtalar joint for the foot to reach the transverse surface, that probatory motion is generally an abnormal or excessive pronation, but it is usually needed to bring the foot flat on the floor. During running the forces needed to cause that pronation come upward upon the lateral plantar aspect of the foot. Those forces may cause an unequal push on the lateral side of the foot, and thus pronation may be accomplished. When the force upon the foot tends to be equal, both medial and lateral, the foot is usually lying flat on the floor and the calcaneus is vertical (but the subtalar joint is abnormally pronated from its original position). All that motion generally occurs while the foot is in contact with the floor during the 1st 75 percent of the stance phase of gait. At heel lift, the foot usually starts to supinate but may never get back to the normal supinated position. The foot is a mobile adaptor on heel contact and a rigid lever during propulsion. In this foot the metatarsal and phalanges are often unstable. Runners with such a foot type may develop a shearing force on the outside of the foot, and multiple lesions or plantar keratomas may occur. That mobile foot type is often susceptible to metatarsalgia and foot pain. Extreme heel wear may be seen on the outside heel of the running shoe. The individual may complain of how fast the shoes wear down.

sudden death.   Most sudden fatalities occur with head and cervical spine injuries. They are usually due to severe external forces, such as being thrown from a vehicle or struck by a heavy ball or stick. Certain speed sports (motor car and motorcycle racing) and airborne pursuits (hang gliding and ordinary gliding) have some inherent dangers that may be difficult to eliminate. Swimming, which is basically a safe pursuit, is often associated with a high mortality rate from drowning (owing to the large number of participants). Sudden death, attributable to a person's being unaccustomed to strenuous physical activity, especially in middle age, may be precipitated by ventricular fibrillation or myocardial infarction.

sunburn.   Variation in sensitivity to sunlight between individuals is often considerable. Blue-eyed redheads and blondes are more generally susceptible to sunburn than are brunettes. Sensitivity to sunlight may also be increased by a number of drugs and other substances. Excessive exposure to ultraviolet radiation of 2,900 to 3,200 Å may damage the tissues of the superficial skin layers. An exposure of 30 minutes often produces redness of the skin along with slight swelling. More prolonged exposure may cause pain and blistering. In severe cases chills, fever, or headache may develop. Sunburn of the lips is often followed by painful herpes simplex infection (fever blisters and cold sores), which may cover most of the surface of the lips. There is considerable evidence to support a theory that continued excessive exposure to the sun may be an important cause of skin cancer. Tanning results from the skin's trying to protect itself by producing considerably more than the usual amount of dark pigment (melanin). That increase in pigmentation may also have the effect of reducing the ability of the body to profit (such as vitamin D conversion) from the desirable smaller amounts of sun available during other parts of the year. A moderate amount of exposure to the sun enables the skin to convert certain substances into vitamin D, the so-called sunshine vitamins.

sunstroke.   Caused by high outside temperature. It differs generally from heat exhaustion in that 1 of the heat regulators is usually affected, namely, the sweat glands. Dehydration often begins a chain of events that terminates in decreased blood supply to the skin and diminished secretion of perspiration. As a consequence, the body temperature may rocket up to a level that may be fatal. The victim of sunstroke generally exhibits many of the symptoms of heat exhaustion (i.e., dizziness and fainting), but there is generally a significant difference in that there is often an absence of perspiration, and the skin may be dry and flushed. Sunstroke is usually an extremely serious emergency. The most important 1st-aid measure is to lower the body temperature (especially the head); otherwise permanent brain damage can result.

surfers' ear.   Hyperostosis of the external auditory canal that occurs in surfers and may cause deafness. It may be due to repeated barotrauma produced by punching through heavy surf.

surfers' knobs.   These are exostoses of the tibial tubercle and the dorsum of the tarsus and the metatarsals caused by the trauma of spending hours kneeling on a board while one is paddling out to catch a wave. Knobs are less common nowadays with the introduction of the lighter smaller board, which most surfers paddle.

stork view.   An anteroposterior X ray of the pelvis taken with the subject standing 1st on one leg then the other. In cases of pubic instability, seen particularly in football when it will cause severe localized pain, a "step" will be clearly seen between the 2 superior pubic rami at symphysis level.

sweating.   Heat dissipation generally depends on the efficient vaporization of sweat, and sweat production is usually proportional to the rate of energy expended. With high energy expenditures, sweating approaches 1 liter/m^2/h, which may result in a 5-liter sweat loss of an average-sized person (160 lbs) during a 3-hour marathon. A warm environment may further increase sweat volume. Despite fluid intake during a race, sweat may produce a 12 percent reduction in body water and 8 percent reduction in body weight. Greater than 2 percent weight loss from exercise-induced sweating generally places severe demands on the thermoregulatory and cardiovascular systems. Sodium, potassium, chloride, and magnesium concentrations in sweat vary considerably from person to person and are usually influenced by sweat rate and heat acclimatization. Sweat is generally hypotonic, and the ions lost are principally sodium and chloride. As the sweat rate rises with increasing energy expenditure, the sodium and chloride in sweat usually increases; potassium and magnesium may remain about the same, and calcium often decreases.

swimmer's cramps.   The mechanics of swimmer's cramps is often similar to that of leg-and-foot cramps in the runner, with oxygen debt generally playing the leading role. It is possible that some of the muscles involved may be different. After food is ingested, the involuntary stomach and intestinal muscles usually get busy processing it through the gastrointestinal system. The individual generally has no conscious control over those muscles, yet while digesting and breaking down the food in the stomach, they must work quite intensely. To lend them support, the blood supply system generally (automatically) diverts blood and oxygen from other parts of the body to the gastrointestinal area. In regard to swimming, if an individual enters the water shortly after eating, with the involuntary stomach muscles working overtime, oxygen debt may develop in both the legs as well as in the stomach muscles. When one swims, the breathing is intermittent or irregular. One generally takes breaths at longer intervals. That generally reduces the intake of oxygen, further adding to its debt. The body will usually demand payment either in the stomach first or in the legs or both. And when payment is not forthcoming, the muscles of the stomach or legs, whichever is suffering the greater starvation, will often respond with cramps. Stomach cramps will generally bend a person in half with pain, and the individual will often feel as though he had been hit with the blunt end of a ramrod. Leg cramps, usually in the calf, will generally lock the leg with equal force and pain. The best way to overcome that situation is to remember that cramps are generally caused by an oxygen debt in the affected muscles, usually brought about by a temporary insufficiency of oxygen in the bloodstream. The task, then, is to get more oxygen into the system by squeezing fresh blood into the cramped area (with the hands) and by taking deep breaths of fresh air.

swimmer's ear.   Swimmer's ear is not generally an infection, but it is often secondarily infected by the time it is first seen by a physician. It is an eczema of the ear canal generally caused by retention of water in the ear following bathing, showering, or swimming. The most common secondary invader may be *Pseudomonas aeruginosa*. It may be an extremely painful condition. Middle ear infections can result typically from infected materials being forced through the Eustachian tube into the middle ear.

Swimmers and divers are generally more exposed to the infections but will not usually get them if upper respiratory infections are treated promptly.

swimmer's shoulder. The most important factor in the production of this lesion is generally in the form of arm recovery necessitated by the front crawl. At the end of the propulsive stroke, the arm usually ends up at the side of the trunk with the hand by the thigh, the shoulder being fully adducted and in a position of mid-rotation. The hand is usually then lifted from the water, the scapula forcefully retracted, the shoulder rapidly and externally rotated and then abducted. As the arm comes to a position level with the head, the shoulder is generally partially internally rotated, which usually brings the arm level with the shoulder and in the correct position to start the next downstroke. That movement is often helped to some extent by body roll. The majority of variations of the front crawl stroke may have derived as a result of attempts to accomplish the recovery of the arm with the minimum effort with maximum of comfort and relaxation and with the possible elimination of the roll. Despite variations, recovery generally remains an extremely awkward movement and places considerable strain on the scapular muscles, abductors, and rotators of the shoulder joint, especially for the 1st few degrees of movement when they may be acting in a position of maximum effort yet minimum efficiency. The majority of swimmers suffering from painful shoulders usually have 1 or a combination of 2 main lesions, minor sprains of the muscle of the glenohumeral and interscapular groups, and supraspinatus tendonitis.

swimming, heat regulation. Swimming often poses a special heat regulation problem since evaporation heat loss is generally curtailed and most body cooling must occur by convection or conduction or both. The temperature range of pool water for competitive events is not standardized and has been found to vary from 20°C to 32.2°C (68°F to 90°F). In a study made of the influence of pool water temperature on swimming performance, optimal performance for the 50-meters dash was generally obtained in water temperatures between 28.9°C to 34.4°C (84°F to 94°F), whereas endurance swimming (1,500 meters) was best performed in water between 23.3°C to 26.1°C (74°F to 79°F). As the temperature of the pool water begins to approach that of the body, performance in the 1,500-meter event generally deteriorated. It may be possible that the larger volume of blood in the skin overextended time necessary for conductive and convective cooling, partially depleted the blood supply available to the working muscles, and thus the performance fell off as a result. In the shorter event, improved performance in warm water is probably associated with an optimal "core" temperature for peak performance (warm-up). If the water is near freezing, 0°C (32°F), mere survival generally becomes a problem because of large convective and conductive loss.

swinger's wrist. Refers to many forms of athletic activity, such as those in which one holds a racket, bat, or club and strikes a ball with it. It may also occur in tennis players and may be a common hazard of golfing. Swinger's wrist generally arises for pretty much the same reasons that tennis elbow comes about, although it may be a markedly different kind of disorder. It comes from an overload at the wrist at the moment of force or impact. The chief cause is generally a faulty swing and is often aided by underdeveloped forearm muscles. Swinger's wrist is generally an alteration of the normal articulation and an inflammation of the radio-ulnar joint. It is not the main wrist joint but that joint between the 2 forearm bones at the wrist that generally enables them to move against one another during various motions of the wrist itself. The condition may be caused in tennis by hitting the ball with the wrist in an ulnar-deviated position, with a faulty backhand stroke, the same stroke that generally brings about tennis elbow. When a tennis player consistently hits a backhand when the ball is far in front of the body, the weight is generally on the forward foot, and the elbow is usually high and bent, tennis elbow will often develop. What usually follows is that the player may continue to play without correcting the swing, but now, favoring the elbow, he or she will begin to hit the ball short so that most of the force and excess stress is transferred to the wrist. Since the stroke is habitually faulty, before onset of tennis elbow, the power of the stroke would come from the forearm-elbow regions of the arm. After the onset of tennis elbow and its attendant pain, the stroke's power must be generated in the forearm wrist region. That means there must often be an excessive snapping of the wrist at impact, with the radio-ulnar joint already in an extreme state of stress because of the faulty position of the arm in the elbow position. Repeated shocks may be driven into the overstressed joint, tearing fibers in its menicus or cartilage and causing inflammation around its attachments to the bone. It also may occur frequently in the wrists of golfers who have a tendency to let their club heads hit the ground before they hit the ball.

syncope.   Fainting, or syncope, during exercise may be a classical warning of heart disease, since it generally indicates a low fixed cardiac output that cannot increase to compensate adequately for the increased vascular bed that opens up on exercise. It may also indicate a dysrhythmia precipitated by exercise or even coronary insufficiency. The more common causes of syncope on exertion are aortic and pulmonary stenosis and hypertrophic obstructive cardiopathy, all of which generally have definite physical signs and may cause sudden death on exertion. Although syncope during exertion may be a serious symptom, it also may occur in normal, fit athletes after strenuous exertion. Many of the athletes generally appreciate that, and it is often 1 of the reasons cyclists and runners keep moving at the end of a race. That prevents the pooling of blood in the lungs, which may result in cerebral ischemia and thus syncope. Syncope, unassociated with exertion or after exertion, is generally more frequent during recovery from or incubation of an infection or when one is in a state of severe fatigue and the cardiovascular reflexes may be more sluggish. Alcohol usually has the same effect.

synovial hernia (ganglion).   A condition generally involving the tendon sheath and sometimes the joint, which may result from a defect in the fibrous sheath of the joint or tendons that permit a segment of underlying synovium to herniate through it. In the athlete it usually follows a mild strain, although it may also be degenerative in nature. The irritation accompanying the herniation generally results in continued secretion of fluid so that the sac gradually fills up and enlarges. As a rule, the synovial hernia will generally appear as a small, discrete, sometimes extremely hard nodule lying directly over the tendon or the joint capsule. The consistency of the tumor may vary from that of bone to that of a soft, fluctuant, obviously liquid mass. Certain areas of the body have a particular predilection for synovial hernia, notably the wrist.

systolic murmurs.   Aortic stenosis may be present as a congenital abnormality besides the more common type of degenerative stenosis that develops often in late middle age. Minor abnormalities of the aortic valve (a biscuspid valve) are generally present in about 2 percent of the male population, often giving rise to a systolic murmur, and may later result in stenosis or incompetence of the valve. Significant stenosis will generally manifest itself by a prolonged weak carotid pulse, but there may be no associated increase in heart size or hypertrophy on the ECG with the congenital variety. Sudden death may occur with tight aortic stenosis on strenuous exertion.

T

talotibial exostoses. A chronic condition that may cause pain and disability when the athlete bears weight on the leg with the foot in dorsiflexion as he or she drives off it. It probably occurs more frequently in athletes than is generally recognized, since in most cases it does not generally cause symptoms. It often occurs as the result of repeated impingement of the anterior portion of the talus against the leading edge of the tibia. As the bone builds up on both sides, the contact may become painful. Although prolonged rest with no weight bearing on the leg will usually relieve the symptoms, successful treatment is generally accomplished only by surgical removal of the exostoses.

talus fracture, neck. Fall onto foot, with the talus crushed between the tibia and calcaneus with shearing force. Symptoms may be pain and disability. Signs may include the forefoot displaced slightly upward and inward on the heel; marked swelling and tenderness at the front of the ankle; deep palpation of sharp proximal edge of distal fragment; with posterior displacement of body, marked swelling beneath Achilles tendon. Complications may be traumatic arthritis, chronic disability, or aseptic necrosis of talar body.

target heart rate. At any level of health and fitness, a training effect is achieved when aerobic exercise produces a pulse that is 70 percent to 85 percent of the maximum expected (age dependent) heart rate. Thus, instead of measuring the oxygen consumed, the pulse rate may be more important for measuring to determine if the exercise performed is generally of sufficient intensity to improve cardiovascular fitness. That relation has led to the concept of the target heart rate, which is that rate, adjusted for age, that must be achieved to improve aerobic capacity and conditioning and develop cardiovascular fitness. The maximum heart rate and the target rate generally decrease with age. But that decrease is usually slow, and the target rate will be relatively constant during the early stages of a fitness program. As fitness is achieved, higher intensity and duration of the exercise will be required to produce the target heart rate. Mesuring the pulse rate is generally an excellent way of preventing excessive demands on the heart. If one exercises much below 70 percent of his or her maximum expected heart rate, only a limited training effect generally occurs. Exercising above 85 percent may be generally safe for a younger person but dangerous for an elderly individual. It has been generally recommended that a training program should aim toward a specific goal. To calculate one's target heart rate, first determine the maximum expected rate by subtracting one's age from 220. Then multiply that number by 70 percent. That is generally a reasonable target for most individuals. Thus for a 40-year-old subject, the target heart rate would be 70 percent of 180 (220 minus 40), or 126. The relatively well conditioned 40-year-old might aim for a slightly higher rate; the less well conditioned subject should probably start at a target rate a bit lower. The aerobic activity chosen should generally be performed at an intensity so the target heart rate can be maintained from 20 to 30 minutes 3 or 4 times a week.

tarsal navicular fracture. Forces transmitted upward from the forefoot through the cuneiform bones, compressing the navicular between those bones and the head of the talus; a fall onto the ball of foot; excessive forcible dorsiflexion or torsion of the foot. Symptoms may be pain in the region over the navicular or inability to bear weight. Signs may include medial fragment being palpable on anterior border of foot and foot tending to be held in eversion, and pain elicited by inversion or dorsiflexion of foot. Complications may be nonunion, traumatic arthritis, and persistent stiffness and pain.

temperature homeostasis. Stored body heat generally helps one to tolerate brief exposures to cold. When the environment begins to cool, heat is usually conserved by vasoconstriction of the subcutaneous vessels. That is the first physiologic defense, usually taking place from 88°F to 75°F air temperature, but it may be greatly impaired by alcohol intake. During exposure to cold, physical efficiency generally ebbs if the core temperature falls only 2°F. That loss must be replaced either by voluntary effort (exertion) or involuntary effort (shivering). Radiant heat loss may be a distinct factor in unheated shelters and after sunset. Conduction heat loss through contact with cold equipment or the ground may also contribute to the problem when protective clothing is not adequate. In prolonged sports events, subcutaneous arterial vessels further constrict to direct more blood to the active muscles, superficial veins constrict to improve venous return, maximum oxygen intake is only slightly increased, tissue viscosity may increase, and blood pressure may increase (which increases cardiac work). Heavy clothing not only adds to the metabolic burden from its weight but also may produce excessive sweating during strenuous physical activities, which may contribute to excessive heat loss through evaporation. Evaporation may also increase with sweat-laden or rain-soaked clothing. Regardless of the cause for the moisture loss, the body spends 580 kcal of heat for the evaporation of each liter of water.

temperature sense. Heat and cold receptors have separate nerve fiber connections. Each has its type of end organ structure peculiar to it, and the distribution of each generally varies considerably. A warm object will stimulate only the heat receptors, while a cool object affects only the cold terminals. More heat receptors are found in the lips than in the hands, so that the lips are more sensitive to heat than are the hands. As in the case of other sensory receptors, continued stimulation results in adaptation; that is, the receptors adjust themselves in such a way that one does not generally feel a sensation so acutely if the original stimulus is continued. For example, the initial immersion of a hand in hot water may give rise to an uncomfortable sensation; however, if the immersion is prolonged, the water will not feel as hot as it did at first.

tendinitis. Tendons connect the contracting muscles to the bone that is being moved. They have a sparse blood supply and metabolism but, owing to compactly aligned collagen fibers, have a high tensile strength. Tendons have limited elasticity, and loss of that with age predisposes to injury. Most tendons have a fibrous sheath containing synovial fluid as a lubricant, which allows free sliding movement. The body's 2 largest tendons, the Achilles and the patellar, do not have such a sheath and present slightly different medical problems. Because of repetitive activity, the tendon eventually breaks down, producing inflammation that causes pain and tenderness. A few sports that are associated with overuse injuries, and the sites of injury involved, include: swimming, shoulder rotator cuff; tennis, elbow; throwing sports, shoulder; crew, forearm musculature; running, lower leg (Achilles tendon) and foot (metatarsal bones); basketball, patellar tendon. Calluses develop on the hands of gymnasts as protection from friction against the bars and ring. Peroneal tendinitis, inflammation of the peroneal tendon, can occur from excessive eversion activity, a single incident, or a series of repeated incidents. Continuing to run in worn-down shoes is often a predisposing factor with the athlete complaining of pain over the lateral border of the foot and ankle. If he or she complains of a feeling that something is slipping out of place, subluxation should be suspected. A previous ankle sprain is usually part of the history. Examination reveals tenderness along the peroneal tendon, particularly at the insertion of the base of the 5th metatarsal. Resistance to eversion of the foot re-creates the pain.

The patellar tendon can become inflamed and tender, usually owing to an overuse syndrome. Recurrent forces probably produce microfailure of the collagen bundles, and the pain with inflammation follows. That occurs in the jumping athlete (jumper's knee), who complains of pain over the tendon, difficulty in jumping or running, and pain with many of the prescribed exercises. The fat pad may even become inflamed and contribute to the symptoms. Evaluation reveals tenderness and swelling along the patellar tendon, usually concentrated along the upper portion of the tendon but not necessarily. In the chronic case, a nodule of scar tissue, often very tender, can be palpated within the tendon or near its insertion site into the patella.

Bicipital tendinitis occasionally results from rupture of the transverse ligament that holds the tendon in the bicipital groove. The tendon then subluxates with overhead activity. The symptoms of bicipital tendinitis, whether caused by overlying cuff disease or associated with tendon subluxation, are essentially the same. Pain is localized in the proximal humerus and the shoulder joint. Resistive supination of the forearm aggravates pain since the bicep's primary function is supination.

tendons. The special significance of tendons is generally in their role of attaching muscle to bone. The tendons of the body are numerous and occur in many sizes, from very short and compact to very long and slender. Each tendon provides power and

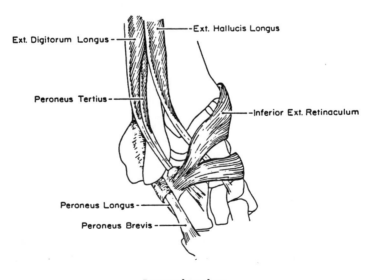

Peroneal tendons.

motion from the muscle out of which it grows to the bone to which it attaches. Because of that function, tendons may become the source of many problems in athletic endeavors, for when a weak or unconditioned muscle is overextended, it may stretch 1 or more of its bone attachments (tendons) or even cause them to separate partially from the bone, thus producing inflammation and pain. Tendons are generally dense, tough, and relatively inflexible. They are neither muscle nor bone, but a stiff cord or band of fibrous tissue. Although the word *tendon* derives from the Latin verb meaning "to stretch," its name is misleading because tendons do not have an unlimited stretch capacity; most ailments involving tendons occur when they are abnormally stretched. Tennis elbow is probably the most frequent manifestation of a tendon's inability to bear much stretching.

tendon injuries. Acute tendon injuries are divided into partial and complete. In young people muscles are generally ruptured more than tendons; in older persons, the reverse is often true. A tendon may rupture either during normal activity or during abnormal physical stress. The avulsion of a tendon from its insertion into bone is almost always traumatic, as is usually a rupture at the musculotendinous junction. Rupture generally occurs within a tendon only if it is abnormal, either from intrinsic degeneration or from wearing and fraying from friction. Bicipital tendinitis (golfer's, baseball, and tennis shoulder) may be difficult to differentiate from partial tears of the long head of the biceps. Both conditions generally respond to rest, analgesics, and general exercises. The tendon of biceps may be displaced from the intertubercular groove. Tears of the triceps may occur in throwing, especially the javelin. The quadriceps tendon usually ruptures transversely just proximal to the patella. Rupture of the patellar tendon usually occurs at the inferior border of the patella. The fine tendon of the plantaris may rupture as it passes down the medial aspect of the Achilles tendon. The symptoms may mimic a partial tear of the Achilles tendon, but palpation of the latter does not reveal local tenderness and the athlete is generally able to stand comfortably on the toes. Occasionally, the Achilles tendon tears at the musculotendinous junction, or the medial or lateral head of the gastrocnemius may be partially ruptured. Repeated kicking in soccer may produce a tenosynovitis chiefly affecting the dorsiflexors of the toes. Any contact sports with body checking may cause strain of the above tendons with possible swelling and bruising being localized at the affected tendon sheaf. In displacement of the peroneal tendons, the tendons may be displaced from their normal position on the posterior surface of the lateral malleolus and may lie obliquely over the lateral 3rd of the distal surface of the fibula. Since their fulcrum or pull may be lost, their mechanical efficiency is usually impaired. The Achilles tendon may rupture close to the musculotendinous junction or near its insertion into the calcaneous. Areas of collagen degeneration may be found in the tendon bundles.

tendon ossification. It is not unusual for cracks to occur in the cortical bone at points of tendinous insertion, and the adjacent fibrocartilaginous region and the tendon itself may be invaded by osseous tissue and include bone marrow elements. Compact bone may then be found to extend for up to 2 or 3 cm along the tendon. Those lesions do not generally cause pain or interference with function per se but may be apt to fracture, in which case pain generally persists until the ossicle is excised.

tendon ruptures. Ruptures of the Achilles tendon are a relatively common injury, the majority of cases occurring in the older athlete. Rupture usually occurs during strenuous activity, most always without any premonitory pain or tenderness. Occasionally, rupture may occur because of direct violence, for example, a kick on the heel while the triceps muscle is actively contracting. The theoretical strength of the Achilles tendon in an optimally healthy state is usually far in excess of any load that can be applied to it by physiological circumstances, and the conclusion that rupture may be the result of degeneration of the tendon is in some cases supported by histological evidence.

Rupture usually occurs approximately 3 cm above the insertion of the tendon into the os calcis. There may be a sharp pain and a feeling of a thud, which often prompts the individual to feel that somebody has shot him in the heel or kicked him. Subsequently, pain is not generally a prominent symptom, but there may be weakness in the ankle with a typical flat-footed gait.

tennis elbow.   Lateral epicondylitis, the medical name for tennis elbow, means that the outer epicondyle of the elbow is generally inflamed. There are 3 principal factors in tennis and, to a lesser degree, in other racket sports that generally create the conditions that lead to tennis elbow. The 1st is often the force of the speeding ball as it meets the opposite speeding racket. The 2nd is the dissipation of that force through the arm. And the 3rd is the ability of all the structures in the arm to satisfactorily dissipate that force. The first 2 factors are invariable; they almost always exist in tennis. The 3rd variable usually depends on 2 further factors: (1) the point at which the ball is hit in relation to the arm; and (2) the ability of the muscle of the arm, especially the forearm muscles, to absorb excessive stresses that arise from faulty ball-arm relationship at the moment of impact. The 2 factors are more often present in recreational tennis players and are generally the primary cause in the development of tennis elbow. The constant hitting of a tennis ball in an awkward or improper way, coupled with an unconditioned forearm extensor muscle, will usually produce some form of tennis elbow over time. It may also frequently result when only 1 of the factors is present, particularly when that factor is weak or unconditioned extensor muscles. Most expert players usually do not suffer from tennis elbow, because by playing as frequently as they do, they continually train and condition their forearm muscles to absorb some of the overloads occasioned by faulty stroking, before the loads and stresses can reach the epicondyle area. Generally, the underlying cause of tennis elbow is a weak or unconditioned forearm musculature.

tennis toe.   A chronic complaint of pain in 1 or more of the longer toes that is frequently associated with hemorrhage, usually horizontal, under the toenails. The cause, seen in several sports, is generally felt to be sudden stops, quick changes of direction, and severe forward motion of the body, which propels the long toes against the front of the inside shoe. If the hemorrhage is longitudinal, the disorder may easily be confused with the splinter hemorrhages associated with subacute bacterial endocarditis after a recent illness. Other contributing factors may be the narrow, hard-toed European tennis shoes that have improved traction soles. When the tennis player jams a big toe into the front of the sneaker, the result may be the rupture of the small blood vessels beneath the toenail, which may produce discoloration, swelling, or pain. When enough vessels are ruptured, the nail will generally lose its blood supply, die, and often months later fall off, making further activities quite uncomfortable until the nail has had a chance to grow back.

tenosynovitis.   Inflammation of the synovium surrounding a tendon. The inflammation is usually due to strain from unaccustomed overuse, but it may be attributable to a direct blow and infection. The results generally include reaction of the normally avascular synovium with increased blood supply, invasion by inflammatory cells, oversecretion of synovial fluid, and increases in fibrin content, often causing sticky adhesion between the tendon and its surroundings. The exact manifestations vary greatly, depending upon the tendon involved. The first manifestation is generally pain on function, which may progress to the point of constant pain even at rest. Crepitation may be frequently present. As the tendon slides up and down, it usually adheres to the synovium causing so-called snowball crepitation, which may be felt by placing the fingers over the involved tendon while it slides up and down. As the condition progresses, the adherence between the tendon and synovium often becomes more firm and may finally result in complete loss of the gliding capacity of the tendon within its sheath. Under ordinary circumstances and with proper care, the tenosynovitis will usually subside completely and normal function may return. In certain cases, however, complications may occur because of the severity of the condition, inadequate treatment, or the anatomical characteristics of the area involved. The complications may cause severe or permanent disability.

thermal hemostatis. The mechanical efficiency of performance is generally poor even in a well-conditioned athlete. Theoretically, it is around 13 percent of anaerobic work and 25 percent for aerobic performance. Generally, the high proportion of the chemical energy (used by the athlete) must thus be dissipated as heat. In runners high efficiency values (up to 40 percent) are sometimes encountered. In those cases the expectations of thermodynamics are apparently exceeded because a part of the energy of descent is absorbed by the stretching of elastic tissue. In that way a store may be provided that can be used in making the next stride. Intramuscular temperature generally increases rapidly during the 1st 5 minutes of activity. The general body temperature usually continues to rise for at least 15 minutes, but if effort continues, a plateau may be reached. That reflects, in part, the increase of thermal gradient generally associated with the rising core temperature, in part the onset of copious sweating, and in part a progressive increase of subcutaneous blood flow. With sustained effort, equilibrium may largely depend upon evaporation of sweat. The endurance athlete can generally tolerate very high core temperatures; values of 40°C to 41°C have been recorded from marathon runners even under temperate conditions. The immediate effect (of a rise in local muscle temperature) is to generally improve physical performance through a reduction of muscle viscosity and a dilation of intramuscular blood vessels. With sustained activity in a hot environment there may be a progressive reduction of central blood volume as well as the cardiac stroke volume. If the environment is extremely hot and humid or heat loss is impeded by attractive but impermeable team garments, cardiac output may fall to the point where the cerebral circulation can no longer be maintained. Heat collapse has usually occurred. If cutaneous and renal flow also fail, fatal hyperpyrexia may supervene. Cumulative loss of mineral ions over several days of competition may also lead to cramps, muscle weakness, or neurasthenia.

thermoregulation. Of the chemical energy involved in muscle contraction, 75 percent to 80 percent is generally transformed into heat with a rise in muscle temperature. Distribution by the bloodstream and conduction to neighboring tissues may disperse that muscle heat throughout the body. The resulting rise in body temperature is often related to the use or increase in metabolic rate involved in the muscle work. When the active muscle mass is large (as in walking or running) and exercise is intense, there may be an 8- to 19-fold increase in the resting metabolic rate. The core temperature of the body may increase 1°C to 1.5°C in 20 to 30 minutes. Two physiologic regulatory mechanisms are usually available to humans to prevent an excessive rise in core temperature: (1) an increase in blood flow to the skin so more heat may be transferred from core to periphery, and (2) increased production by the sweat glands so there may be greater evaporation from the surface of the skin. The degree of thermoregulatory stress generally depends not only on the metabolic rate but also on the climatic conditions, of which air temperature is just 1 component. Other factors are humidity in the air, radiant heat (mostly solar), and air movement. The athlete's clothing also may affect heat stress. The most common factor on the athletic field is usually the relative humidity of the environment. As long as the skin is warmer than the environment, heat will generally be dissipated by convection and radiation. If surrounding objects are cooler than the skin, thermal conduction will usually be another avenue for dissipation of heat. Generally the warmer the environment, the less cooling by convection, radiation, or conduction. When ambient temperature exceeds skin temperature, there may be an influx of heat into the body. Then the only means of heat dissipation left may be the evaporation.

thigh injuries. Sports injuries and related disorders of the thigh include contusions, abrasions, strains, contractures, vascular abnormalities, and occasionally femoral fractures. Pain may be related to the above, such as the lumbar spine, hip, or from below, such as the knee, ankle, and foot. Minor mat court or grass abrasions of the thigh may be seen in sports that do not require protection. They are easily managed if precaution is taken against secondary infection. The most common bruise of the thigh is generally the result of an interior blunt blow. The classic injury is often the "charley horse," a blow to the front of the thigh during active contraction of the main body of the quadriceps. Even if complex rupture of the rectus femoris does not occur, muscle damage tends to be quite extensive with marked intramuscular bleeding. Occasionally, bruising over the bony prominence (greater trochanter, lateral femoral condyle) may be associated with grazing of the skin (mat burn and grass burn). In such cases healing may be delayed because of a secondary infection that generally requires a greater amount of treatment. Muscle strains in the thigh generally involve either the hamstrings or the quadriceps group. Psoas (or iliopsoas) strains may be characterized by pain on exercise and deep tenderness in the groin. The pain may be made worse by external rotation of the hip in extension. In chronic cases calcification may occur. Hamstring tears may involve the semimembranosus, semitendinosus, or biceps (long head), and although they are simple to treat, recurrence is generally common. Bicipital tendinitis is occasionally seen and is sometimes difficult to differentiate from strains of the lower muscle fibers or sprains of the lateral ligament of the knee. Differentiation in the latter case may be made because pain is not produced by "springing" the knee. In many contact sports the most common injury to the thigh may be a contusion. It may be the result of a direct blow usually to the anterior or anterolateral aspect of the thigh. While many thigh contusions are not usually serious and do not generally lead to any prolonged disability, a severe blow to the thigh may often lead to a condition known as myositis ossificans traumatica. Strains of the musculature in the thigh may be found frequently in track athletes as well as in other athletes engaged in running activities. Generally the frequent type of injury is the one to the hamstring muscles. It may also be seen in the rectus femoris on the front of the thigh. The degree of severity is often indicated by the amount of pain and disability that is present immediately following the injury. Fractures of the femoral shaft are generally rare in sports. They are usually identified by the presence of swelling deformity, tenderness or palpation over the fracture site, and crepitation on motion as well as significant disability and inability to bear weight.

thoracic injuries. Injuries to the thorax, abdomen, and perineum occur usually in the contact sports as a result of direct trauma. In most cases the injury may be only a minor one and can be dealt with easily. Sports injuries, however, may lead to serious problems and can even be fatal. The chest consists basically of a bony cage, generally designed for the protection of underlying major organs, the heart and lungs. That leads to the classification of injuries of that region into superficial and deep. In superficial injuries external injuries to the chest are common. Bruising and hematoma are frequently experienced. Muscle strain, especially to the pectoral muscle group, is generally a disabling condition. It usually results from direct muscular effort, when a characteristic tearing pain may be experienced. That may be followed by tenderness and swelling. Breast injuries are not common. In female athletes such injury may lead to a localized hematoma with damage to breast tissue, producing an area of fat necrosis. It generally presents a painless hard lump in the breast for some weeks or even months after the traumatic incident. As a result of a direct blow or rotational strain, rib fractures may be a common problem. Along with rib damage, a more specific type of

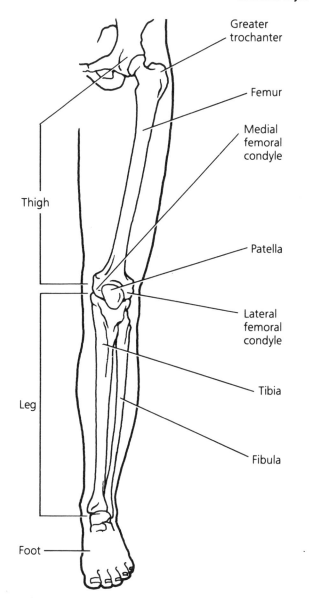

The lower extremity, consisting of the thigh, leg, and foot.

injury involving the chest wall may occur when abnormal forces have been applied to the costochondral junction. Lung injuries may be the result of a direct blow, with a contusion showing on a chest X ray as an area of consolidation. Usually it results in hemoptysis, which generally clears quickly. It still may need a period of clinical observation. Other cases of hemoptysis may be found in those sports demanding forceful pulmonary exertion. That often is thought to result from vascular engorgement leading to the rupture of small subendothelial blood vessels. Regarding pleura, injuries may be potentially serious, the most common being a pneumothorax. It usually results from a puncture of the lung by a fractured rib. It may also result spontaneously during exertion because of the rupture of a lung at a site of unsuspected pathology. Often this is due to an emphysematous bulla. Serious respiratory problems may occur as a result of a direct blow to the larynx, which can also produce laryngeal hemorrhage and edema with increasing respiratory distress. The blow may be severe enough to fracture the laryngeal cartilage. Heart or great vessel injury may result from trauma to the chest. Such a condition, if due to a direct penetrating lesion, may be obvious while others result from contusion, which may be asymptomatic and not easily diagnosed.

thrower's elbow. Thrower's elbow can also be a form of tennis elbow. Although the pain and inflammation generally occur on the inside of the elbow in the ailment, the mechanics and causes of the condition are similar to those of conventional tennis elbow. Thrower's elbow, because it occurs mostly in baseball pitchers and football passers, is an inflammation of the inner epicondyle of the elbow. The underlying causes are similar to the underlying causes of lateral epicondylitis, even though the precipitating causes may be different. The only significant difference between the 2 lies in the fact that because the ulnar nerve (1 of the major nerves of the arm) passes much closer to the inner epicondyle than to the outer, medial epicondylitis may be infinitely more painful and debilitating than lateral epicondylitis. The flexor muscles and their attachment to the medial epicondyle are generally the chief causes in medial epicondylitis. For that reason the ailment may occur in tennis players as well as in those who use their arms to throw. The affliction generally comes about through repeated excessive strains and overloads on the flexor muscles and through the continual unrelieved trauma they create at the site of their terminal attachment to the elbow, the medial epicondyle. In weekend tennis players, medial epicondylitis may not be nearly so common as lateral epicondylitis, but it is generally considerably more devastating when it does occur. The stresses may become compounded in pitchers who throw curveballs and screwballs. A curveball usually requires sudden extension and supination of the wrist to impart spin, followed by equally abrupt flexion and pronation in the follow-through. The screwball's spin may be the reverse of the curve's; thus the stresses on the arm of the screwball pitchers are after hyperflexion and hyperpronation all the way through the motion of the arm as it releases the ball.

thrower's shoulder. A tendinitis of the shoulder that occurs mostly as an inflammation of either the tendon that connects the biceps muscle of the upper arm to the scapula of the shoulder or of the tendon that connects the muscles of the shoulder's rotator cuff to the humerus of the arm. In order to move a joint, the muscles that do so must generally cross the joint. That is, if they originate from below or above a joint, they must extend and connect beyond it in a direction opposite to their site of origin. The extensor muscle of the elbow originates in the forearm of the humerus. The attaching device is the extensor tendon. The quadriceps muscle originates in the thigh and crosses the knee, through its attachment to the kneecap, to connect to the bone below the knee. The attaching device is known as the quadriceps tendon. In both cases the muscles, by being so attached, may provide their respective joints with specific kinds of motion. That is also true of the biceps muscles of the upper arm in their relation to the shoulder. In order to move the shoulder forward, they must attach on the far side of the joint. It is the way in which they do so that is exceptional and provides danger for their connecting biceps tendon. The biceps muscles originate in the front of the upper arm and flow to both the elbow and the shoulder. Because the area over the forward aspect of the joint is so crowded—a maze of muscles coming from the chest, the top of the shoulder, and the back—there is simply no room for the bicep muscles to cross over the joint here, so nature devised an alternative. It routed the biceps muscles, or biceps tendon, directly through the shoulder joint. By so doing, nature solved a space problem but also created another problem. In no other joint of the body does a tendon actually enter and exit itself. The biceps tendon enters the joint through a groove at the top of the humerus. It pierces the synovial capsule, lies free within the joint, and then exits to attach to the upper rim of the scapula's socket. Because of its unique position and its role in 1 of the primary motions of the arm and shoulder, the biceps tendon may be subject to considerably more strain than are most other tendons of the shoulder. The strain usually occurs when one is throwing an object while off balance, when serving incorrectly in tennis, when rotating the arm and shoulder forward in a hard swimming stroke, and when performing rapid poling motions during skiing. In each case excessive weight is generally placed on the biceps tendon at its moment of optimal stretch through the fore-rotating motion of the shoulder. Repeated irritation of the portion of the tendon that lies in the groove generally causes inflammation and pain. Biceps tendinitis may follow with pain in front of the shoulder radiating into the arms.

thrust (speed and power). In many human activities the acceleration of the body as a whole or the acceleration that the body can impart to an external object may be very important. The thrust that a muscle may exert must therefore be considered. Thrust is a force, and therefore the maximum thrust that may be exerted is equal to the maximum isometric strength of a muscle. When the human body is being accelerated, the thrust of the legs is exerted against the ground and is exactly balanced by the reaction of the ground to the thrust. In the same way the thrust exerted upon an external object is exactly balanced by the reaction of that object. Thus, if a weight is being lifted at a uniform rate, the thrust of the muscles that may be used is exactly equal to the weight lifted. It is apparent that when a subject makes a vertical jump, he or she does mechanical work equivalent to the product of his or her body weight and the height jumped. The energy for the jump was mostly generated by exerting thrust against the ground. All energy generated during the thrust against the ground is generally dissipated by the time one reaches the top of his or her jump. The time during which the thrust takes place is of importance in a number of sporting skills. The long last stride of the high jumper allows a long time for the operation of the thrust of the jumping legs to obtain maximum velocity for the center of gravity. The arc of a golfer's swing and the point at which the club head strikes the ball dicatates the length of the period of contact between the club head and the ball and, therefore, the function of the thrust. On the other hand, a basketball player or a soccer player who, when jumping for the ball, needs to exert thrust for a long time may be beaten to it by another player who, being more powerful, is able to generate the necessary impulse for his jump from a shorter ground-contact time. The longer the limb, generally the smaller the fraction of the maximum weight that may be used to produce the greatest power output. Thus, it is apparent that both power and speed depend, to some extent, upon body type.

thumb and finger sprains. Very painful injuries. The proximal interphalangeal joint of the finger is frequently injured in athletics. Disruption of the capsule usually causes an anterior or posterior subluxation or dislocation. When there is also injury to the collateral ligament, initially deformity may not be present. Because the athlete seldom complains of pain and often feels that he or she is capable of continuing participation, the severity of the injury is often overlooked or minimized. A complete tear of the collateral ligament of the PIP (proximal inner phalangeal) joint may be a very disabling injury with persistent symptoms after injury and resultant stiffness and pain in the PIP joint. If allowed to go untreated, it may result in residual laxity and weakness in that joint with periodic resprains. Tearing of the ulnar collateral ligament of the thumb may require repair to prevent disability. The distal interphalangeal joint is the most frequently sprained in the body and most easily treated, normally.

tibia fracture, lateral condyle avulsion. Excessive forcible adduction of leg. Symptoms may be pain and disability. Signs may include swelling and hemarthrosis, tenderness over lateral tibial condyle, varus deformity possible, or abnormal varus mobility of leg inward. Complications may lead to persistent instability.

tibia fracture, medial condyle. It is caused by direct or indirect violence, a fall onto the feet with the leg bowed outward, and excessive forcible adduction of the leg. The symptoms may be pain and disability. Signs may include swelling, hemarthrosis, variable varus deformity, tenderness, possible broadening of the region below the knee, and abnormal varus mobility of the leg. Complications could lead to malunion and traumatic arthritis.

tibia fracture, shaft. The cause is direct or indirect violence through falling onto the feet from a height and excessive forcible torsion, as with the foot or thigh fixed while the other end is twisted. The symptoms may be pain and an inability to bear weight. Signs may include possible shortening of leg, possible deformity, rotation of foot, variable amount of swelling and tenderness, or pain elicited by compressing or rotating the foot with the knee immobilized or by pushing the foot upward. Complications could lead to malunion, nonunion, delayed union, tibiofibular synosteosis, impaired circulation or nerve supply to the foot.

tibia fracture, spine. Fracture of lateral tubercule, produced by sharp inner margin of lateral femoral condyle as the leg may be externally rotated and driven backward and flexed upon the femur; avulsion of tibial spine at anterior cruciate ligament attachment. The symptoms may be severe pain and variable disability. Signs may include swelling, joint effusion, abnormal mobility in anteroposterior plane or upon abduction stress, firm bony block limiting knee extension, or tenderness not localized over meniscus but beneath patellar tendon. Complications may be residual limitations of knee extension and recurrent effusion.

tibial varus (bow legs). A condition in which the lower portion of the tibia assumes a varus attitude as compared with the normal perpendicular attitude. It is seen mostly in male distance runners. Women runners are more likely to develop tibia valgus or "knock knees." The condition is not ideal, because the foot usually strikes the ground on the lateral side and there is often an excessive pronatory force exerted in order to bring about the calcaneus to a perpendicular position. The excessive pronation generally leads to runner's knee and overuse syndromes of the lower leg and knee area. Often there is irritation of the lower aspect of the Achilles tendon and calcium build-up on the outer heel area with bursae.

tinea corporis. *Microsporum canis, Trichophyton rubrum,* and *T. mentagrophytes* are generally the organisms most commonly responsible. The skin lesions are erythematous, sharply defined scaly patches, and are usually acquired through contact with infected persons. The border is generally dark with a clear center. Those areas may range from 10 mm to 500 mm. Ringworm is a common skin disease found on the extremities as well as on the body. The lesions should be well covered before athletes are allowed to participate in tumbling, wrestling, football, and basketball.

tinea cruris. Jock itch. The initial lesion, a scaly, erythematous patch on the inner aspects of the thighs, spreads rapidly. The border is sharp and scaly and may show vesicles. The organism usually involved is *Epidermophyton floccosum,* although other species and *Candida albicans* may cause the lesions. Jock itch should be differentiated from intertrigo, bacterial infection, and allergic dermatitis. All activities usually can be allowed.

tinea pedis. Athlete's foot. A common overtreated and overdiagnosed foot disease. It has been called the "plague of the gym." *Trichophyton floccosum, T. rubrum,* and *T. mentagrophytes* are the usual etiologic agents. The disease may cause tenderness, a foul odor, and severe itching. The most common areas affected are generally the skin of the 3rd and 4th interdigital spaces and the soles of the feet. Other areas of the foot may be involved. A secondary bacterial infection may occur, causing severe pain, swelling, and fever. Other complications may occur when one follows self-diagnosis. The individual may use irritating over-the-counter medications, causing contact dermatitis and further tissue irritation. Participation in sports should generally depend on the discomfort and the extent and severity of the lesions.

tinea versicolor. A superficial fungal infection often caused by *Malasezia furfur,* consisting of oval macules with a fine scale. The lesions may be present on the neck, chest, upper back, or shoulder. Treatment must be persistent, for recurrence in hot humid weather is common.

tissues. Although the basic structure of cells, as well as certain behavioral patterns, generally remains constant regardless of the type of cell, cells themselves vary enormously with respect to shape, size, color, and speciality. Tissues are groups of cells of the same type that have been brought together for a common purpose. Tissues are full of water. The cells of which tissues are made contain from 60 percent to 99 percent water. Gases, liquids, and solids dissolve in that water. Chemical reactions that are necessary for proper body function may be carried on much more readily in a watery solution. Substances that do not go into solution may be suspended in the various liquids of the body, many of which circulate and thus may be moved from place to place. Water is indispensable for cell life, and lack of water generally causes death more rapidly than the lack of any other dietary constituent. The solution of water and other materials in which the tissues are bathed is slightly salty. The substance is called tissue fluid. The insufficiency of tissue fluid is called dehydration, and an abnormal accumulation of that fluid may cause a condition called edema. The four main groups of tissues are (1) epithelium, which forms glands, covers surfaces, and lines cavities; (2) connective tissue, which hold all parts of the body in place; (3) nerve tissue, which conducts nerve impulses; and (4) muscle tissue, designed for power-producing contractions.

tissues, hard connective. The hard connective tissues are more solid and include cartilage and bones. Cartilage, usually called gristle, is a tough, elastic, and translucent material that is found in such places as between the segments of the spine and at the ends of the long bones. In those positions cartilage acts as a shock absorber as well as a bearing surface that reduces the friction between moving parts. Cartilage is found in other structures also, such as the nose, ear, epiglottis and other parts of the larynx. The tissue of which the bones are made (called osseous tissue) is very much like cartilage in its cellular structure. The bones of the unborn baby in the early stages of development are generally nothing but cartilage. However, gradually that tissue becomes impregnated with calcium salts. Since calcium is another word for lime, there is generally a continual mineral deposit until the bones develop their characteristically hard and bony state. Within the bones are nerves, blood vessels, bone-forming cells, and a special form of tissue in which certain ingredients of the blood may be manufactured. Like epithelium, it repairs itself easily. In connective tissue there may be an abnormal growth of cells that forms tumors.

tissues, soft connective. A group of connective tissues serving a number of different purposes. One group, the adipose tissue, stores up fat for use by the body as an energy reserve (food), a heat insulator, and as padding for various structures. Another kind of tissue serves as a binding between organs as well as a framework for some organs that are otherwise made of epithelium. Another form of that tissue that is particularly strong is built up of fibers and serves to support certain organs that are subjected to powerful strains. An example of that kind of tissue is a tendon. Soft connective tissue is used by nature to repair muscle and nerve tissue as well as to repair connective tissue itself. A large gaping wound will generally require a corresponding large growth of the new connective tissue, as will an infected wound. The new growth is called "scar tissue." The process of repair generally includes stages in which new blood vessels and nerve chords are formed in the wound area, followed by the growth of the scar tissue. An excessive development of the blood vessels in the early stage of repair may lead to the formation of so-called proud flesh. Normally, however, the blood vessels are gradually replaced by white fibrous connective tissues, which form the scar.

toe-in. Excessive toeing-in, especially in children, may be the result of excessive internal rotation of the tibia caused by a fixed point at either end of the tibia. Common points of fixation are generally at the malleoli in the ankle or at the tibial tubercle below the knee. The ankle mortise normally faces 15° externally, but in internal tibial torsion, the ankle mortise may face anteriorly or internally.

toe injuries. Pain in a foot during midstance may be caused by corns, calluses from a fallen transverse arc, rigid pes planus, or subtalar arthritis. Pushing off with the lateral side of the front of the foot is usually seen in disorders involving the great toe. Sharp pain in pushing off is often caused by corns between the toes or metatarsal callosities. Claw toes, usually associated with pes cavus, may feature flexed proximal and distal interphalangeal joints and hyperextended metatarsophalangeal joints. An early sign may be the formation of callosities over the dorsal surface of the toes, on the tips of the toes, and on the plantar surface under the metatarsal heads. A hammer toe generally presents flexion of the proximal interphalangeal joint and hyperextension of the metatarsophalangeal and distal interphalangeal joints. It usually is singular and associated with a callosity on top of the proximal interphalangeal joint. Predisposing factors may include forceful plantarflexion of the metatarsal, pes cavus, short metatarsal, forefoot valgus, trauma, or pronation imbalance. A mallet toe may be a distal interphalangeal joint flexion contraction that usually occurs in the smaller toes. Hallus valgus is a state of lateral deviation of the great toe, usually found in connection with a hypermobile pronated foot and the wearing of pointed toed shoes, often producing abuse to the medial aspect of the front toe. The 1st metatarsal becomes fixed in abduction and hallux subluxates laterally. In time, the abductor hallucis may become fixed in a lateral displacement beneath the metatarsal head. The muscle generally becomes ineffective in maintaining abduction. The most common sprain of this area may be that of the great toe, especially at the metatarsophalangeal joint as the result of forced plantar flexion or dorsiflexion. Sideward sprains are not generally common. Swelling may be severe, but bony tenderness or crepitus is usually absent. Disability may be severe because weight bearing is predominantly on the hallux. A chronic complaint may be the tennis toe, in which pain in one or more of the longer toes is frequently associated with hemorrhage, usually horizontal, under the toenails. The cause seen in several sports if felt to be from sudden stops, quick changes of direction, or the severe forward motion of the body, which propels the long toe against the front of the inside shoe.

traumatic arthritis. When trauma is the chief factor, an acute arthritis may be induced. The extent of the local reaction may be relative to the severity of the injury and the resistance of the tissues. Repeated injuries from excessive joint stress may cause pathologic reactions or produce derangements within the joint. Arthritis resulting from a single severe injury, especially improperly treated, may be indefinitely prolonged and result in chronic symptoms or permanent disability. Trumatic arthritis generally presents signs of pain, possible ecchymosis, and soft-tissue swelling or periarticular tissue that may be limited to effusion within the capsule or obliterate the bony prominence depending upon the severity of trauma, tenderness on pressure, and loss of function. Motion is usually limited because of pain, and there may be joint instability if the injury is sufficient to tear a tendon or joint capsule. Intra-articular fractures and fragments may be associated.

traumatic myositis. Myositis is an inflammation of muscle tissue, usually involving only the skeletal muscles. Contusion and trauma may cause an inflammation of the muscles, wherein the involved muscles become red, swollen, tender, painful, and almost of wooden hardness. That type of myositis usually subsides without any suppuration. Disease of muscle tissues may often be mistaken for disease of the adjacent joint, tendon sheath, or some type of neuralgia. Muscle pain is not generally localized subjectively with the same accuracy as is pain in the more superficial structures. Therefore, such vague localization requires careful examination. Functional use of a muscle may be painless if the inflammatory process lies entirely within the muscle sheath, but perimyositis may cause pain during function. myositis often causes pain only when the muscle is palpated or stretched.

traumatic myositis ossificans. A condition of heterotypic bone formation that may occur in collagenous supportive tissues, such as skeletal muscles, ligaments, tendons, and fascia following hematoma. It is commonly the effect of direct muscle bruising, especially repeated contusions, as seen in many of the contact sports, on the anterior aspects of thighs and arms. Connective tissue that surrounds the muscle may rapidly invade the traumatized area, and connective tissue may retain its embryonal ability to be transformed into more differentiated tissue. Following the primary interstitial myositis, there may be a transformation of the connective tissue into bone.

traumatic spondylosis. Chronic bending stresses may be applied to the pars inter-articularis in athletic activities that may vertically hold the spine in the lower lumbar area. That is often especially true when the spine is vertically loaded in the extended position. Such repetitive stresses occur during blocking by an interior lineman in football. A gymnast who lands on his or her feet with the spine extended generally loads the spine in a similar fashion. The same condition may occur in wrestlers and competitive divers. Those individuals initially have normal spines but begin to experience some pain during various sporting activities. The pain soon begins to persist even after the activity ceases. Initially the X rays are negative. However, if more sophisticated diagnostic studies are performed, there may be evidence of increased bone repair in the interarticular areas of the lamina of the lower lumbar vertebra. That generally indicates an impending stress fracture. A complete fracture may develop if the stress continues.

trick knee. There may be a number of precipitating causes, injuries to the ligaments or cartilages brought about by a variety of severe outside blows and stresses, lesser outside stresses that are usually compounded by weaknesses in the knee's supporting musculature, or spontaneous deterioration in the tissue of 1 or more of the knee's ligaments or cartilages. These are precipitating causes because they are generally events that initially cause a disorder in the knee joint. The underlying causes, those causes that permit a knee damaged by injury to become a chronic trick knee, reside both in and around the knee itself. Once a cartilage (meniscus) or ligament is damaged, it cannot repair itself, unlike many other tissues in the body. The reason it cannot is the fact that cartilages and ligaments are inert tissues that receive very little nourishment from the blood supply system. The only way they can be repaired is through surgery.

trigger finger. An entrapment syndrome produced by scar tissue compressing an extensor tendon, often a consequence of De Quervain's disease. Its incidence is relatively high in fencing. Squeezing action by the constricted sheaf tends to develop pealike mass distal to the thickening. It is most often seen in the thumb, but several fingers may sometimes be affected. Simple surgery usually remedies the situation.

tumors, benign. Benign tumors, theoretically at least, and depending on location, are not generally dangerous in themselves; that is, they do not generally spread (metastasize). Benign tumors usually grow as a single mass within a tissue, often lending themselves neatly to complete surgical removal. Some innocent tumors may be anything but innocent in their effect; they may grow within an organ, increase in size, and cause considerable mechanical damage. A benign tumor of the brain, for example, may kill a person just as a malignant one can. Ordinarily, however, benign tumors are not so dangerous. Here are some examples. Papilloma, which grows in the epithelium as projecting masses, such as a wart. Adenoma, which is epithelial, growing in and about the glands. Lipoma, a connective tissue tumor, originating in fatty (adipose) tissue. Osteoma, a connective tissue tumor originating in the bones. Myoma, a tumor of muscle tissue, rare in voluntary muscle but common in some types of involuntary muscle, particularly the uterus (womb). When found in this organ, however, it ordinarily is called a fibroid. Angioma, a tumor that usually is composed of small blood or lymph vessels and includes the type of discoloration known as the port wine stain or birthmark. Nevus, a small skin tumor of various tissues. Some are better known as moles; some are angiomas. Ordinarily they are harmless but may become malignant through irritation.

tumors, malignant. Unlike benign tumors, they can cause death no matter where they occur. The word *cancer* means "crab," and that is descriptive; a cancer usually sends out clawlike extensions into neighboring tissue. Not only does that happen often, but a cancer may literally spread its own seeds, which plant themselves in other parts of the body. The "seeds" are free cancer cells and may be transported everywhere by either the blood or the lymph system (a fluid related to the blood). When the cancer cells reach their destination, they immediately can form new (secondary) growths. Malignant tumors, moreover, grow much more rapidly than benign ones. Malignant tumors generally are classified in 2 categories according to the type of tissue in which they originate. (1) Carcinoma, a cancer originating in epithelium and by far the most common type of cancer. The usual sites of carcinoma are generally the skin, the mouth, the lung, the breast, the stomach, and the uterus. It is usually spread by the lymphatic system. (2) Sarcoma, a cancer of connective tissue of all kinds that may be found anywhere in the body. The cells are usually spread by the bloodstream, and it often forms secondary growths in the lungs. There are other types of malignant tumors, such as those originating in a nevus called melanosarcomas and those arising in the connective tissue that separates the nerve cells of the brain.

U

ulna fracture, olecranon. Elbow fracture. The cause is a direct blow, as in a fall onto the elbow; avulsion of the olecranon by violent contraction of the triceps muscle; or falling on a semiflexed and supinated forearm. Symptoms may be pain and disability. Signs include swelling, crepitus, gap between fragments, and inability to flex or extend the elbow.

ulnar nerve injury. The ulnar nerve is usually not injured in a posterior dislocation of the elbow. However, in a fracture involving the medial epicondyle, ulnar nerve injury occurs with some frequency. Contusion of the ulnar nerve is quite frequent because of its anatomic position at the elbow. As it traverses the inner side of the arm, it passes behind the medial condyle through a tunnel, the floor of which is made up of the ulnar groove of the humerus, the roof being a rather loose fibrous sheath. As the arm flexes and extends, the nerve slides up and down in the ulnar groove. In this region the nerve is subcutaneous and lies directly on the bone. Therefore, a direct blow may damage the nerve to a greater or lesser extent depending upon the strength and direction of the force applied. A direct blow causes immediate severe pain with a shocking sensation extending down to the ring and little fingers. This paresthesia is usually transient, disappearing after a few minutes or several hours depending upon the severity of the injury. Under ordinary circumstances no permanent injury results from ulnar nerve contusion, but occasionally there may be late sequelae. Ulnar nerve entrapment is a condition similar to carpal tunnel syndrome except that the ulnar nerve is involved. The athlete complains of pain along the base of the 5th finger with paresthesias of the 5th and ring fingers. In a long-standing problem there may be atrophy of the hypothenar musculature.

underwater problems. If air is prevented from entering freely any of the air-containing spaces of the body, a relative vacuum develops that may disturb or rupture the lining of such a space. Pain and bleeding into the sinuses, bleeding in the middle ear with rupture of the tympanic membrane, bleeding into the lung, and conjunctival hemorrhage from failing to breathe into the face mask while one is descending are all examples of such a mechanism. Gas in the intestinal tract and air under dental fillings may also expand painfully during descent. Prevention of "squeeze' involves avoiding diving when colds or other conditions impair free exchange during descent. Also a person should learn to not hold the breath during descent, thus allowing pressure to be equalized gradually. All those "squeezes" generally tend to correct themselves spontaneously, but repeated barotrauma may cause permanent hearing loss. At pressures as low as 1.6 atmospheres, the first symptoms of intoxication from nitrogen may be experienced. At 4 atmospheres most divers suffer from some loss of judgment, and at 125 feet euphoria is usually present. At 200 feet and below, there is generally serious danger of death owing to loss of consciousness or irrational acts, such as removing the face mask and mouthpiece. Pure oxygen may cause convulsions and unconsciousness at 2 atmosphere pressure in a closed circuit system. Carbon dioxide poisoning may appear when the partial pressure gives a concentration of 1 percent and will cause unconsciousness at or before a concentration of 10 percent. In closed circuit scuba the condition is often due to failure of the carbon dioxide absorbent, and in open circuit it is usually due to accumulation in the face mask. Anoxia may occur on ascending when overbreathing before descending has blown off so much carbon dioxide that the stimulus for breathing is temporarily lost. That may be the cause of "shallow-water blackout." When a diver is using compressed air as his or her supply, the air may have been contaminated during its compression with oil droplets, carbon monoxide, or pathogenic bacteria. If the air was very humid at the time of compression, the diver may get a mouthful of water with his first breath, start to choke, and then panic. A relatively small concentration of 0.1 percent carbon monoxide at sea level may cause poisoning at depth. Decompression sickness may be caused by the formation of nitrogen bubbles in body tissues. Being inert, the amount of nitrogen in the blood is directly related to the underwater depth reached and the time spent there. The critical ratio that causes the formation of large bubbles in the blood and tissues is reached when the partial pressure caused by nitrogen in the tissue is approximately twice that in the atmosphere. That ratio may be achieved when a diver ascends rapidly from a depth of 33 feet or more. On dives to 600 feet, bends may appear as low as 350 feet beneath the surface.

upper limb injuries. Apart from fractures of the upper humerus and scapula and dislocation or subluxation, the shoulder joint and its intimate structures are generally the site of a wide variety of painful conditions, all closely related. Fractures involving the shoulder joint are not very common in sports. They may include fractures of the surgical neck and greater tuberosity of the humerus and of the scapula. Dislocations of the shoulder joint occur frequently in the body contact sports and may also be seen in high jumpers, pole vaulters, water polo players, and riders. They may occur typically when an extension force is applied to the abducted externally rotated arm. Recurrent dislocation of the shoulder is often a particular problem to some athletes and may be the result of too energetic early mobilization following an initial acute dislocation. Painful shoulder syndromes include various injuries and degenerative conditions, all of which may be characterized by pain that is generally exacerbated by movement and that may provoke a greater degree of functional disability. The shoulder joint is peculiar in that its stability is derived entirely from the surrounding soft tissues, capsule, ligaments, and muscles. It must serve as a firm yet highly mobile base for all the various activities of the hand and arm. Any injury, therefore, which involves 1 of the supporting structures of the shoulder joint will invariably interfere with the mobility and efficiency of that joint. Capsulitis of the shoulder may result from a sprain in which the degree of violence is not sufficient to provoke more than a transitory subluxation. It may also follow excessive or unaccustomed use of the shoulder, particularly in implemental sports. The joint may be painful, particularly on movement, and in some instances limitation of movement may be considerable (frozen shoulder). Symptoms may be referable to the whole body of the joint area, and signs, particularly tenderness, may not be well localized.

urticaria (hives). Transient urticarias are generally caused by drugs, bites, stings, foods, and some infections. The cause of recurrent urticaria is often elusive but may be related to emotional upset. Hives may occur anywhere on the body and can be large or small. The lesion is a red papule, which may come and go quickly, with possible severe itching. Treatment consists of eliminating the cause when possible.

V

varicose veins. A condition in which superficial veins have become swollen, tortuous, and ineffective. It frequently is a problem in the esophagus, rectum, the spermatic cord in the male, and in the broad ligament of the uterus in the female. The veins that are generally found to be abnormally enlarged may be those that involve the saphenous veins of the lower extremities, the condition found frequently in people who spend a great deal of time standing. Varicose veins in the rectum are normally referred to as piles, or hemorrhoids. The general term for those enlarged veins is varices, the singular form being varix.

ventilation. The external ventilation attained by the exercising athlete may be very large, normally averaging 160 l/min BTPS. The respiratory frequency may remain relatively low, often being linked with the rhythm of the movement of activity. Thus, the oarsman with a stroke of 38/min takes 1 breath per stroke, while the cyclist with a pedal frequency of 100 may have a breathing rate of 50/min. Many athletes often show some development of both static (such as vital capacity) and dynamic lung volume (such as maximum voluntary ventilation). It is not generally uncommon to find that three-quarters of both static and dynamic lung volumes are utilized in maximum strenuous activities. Those are higher proportions than would be tolerated by the average sedentary person and undoubtedly contribute to some discomfort of the contestant. Thus, in the psychological sense at least, ventilation may limit the endurance athlete. In physiological terms, external ventilation is not a significant limiting factor. Usually up to a quarter of external ventilation is "wasted" in the dead space. During intense exercise that may be attributed mainly to "stratified inhomogeneity," that is, incomplete mixing of airway and alveolar gas. The slow respiratory rates of a well-trained athlete generally allow more time for that mixing to occur, but there is no appreciable alveolar ventilation, since the associated prodigious tidal volume causes expansion of the airway zone in which mixing must occur. The work of breathing imposes a 5 percent to 10 percent change upon oxygen delivery in maximum effort. However, respiratory work cannot be a limiting factor unless the oxygen delivered to be circulation by additional ventilation is less than the corresponding increment of oxygen consumption in the chest muscles. Under most conditions, ventilation may be adjusted to ensure a maximum uptake of oxygen by pulmonary capillary blood, without surpassing the "cross-over point" of diminishing oxygen returns. However, the margin between normal exercise ventilation and the cross-over point is usually not large, and hyperventilation from anxiety of a premature accumulation of lactate could conceivably cause an athlete to pass this critical point.

vertebral column. Forms the central axis of the trunk. It is composed of 33 irregular bones called the vertebrae, most of which are connected to each other by joints at which a small range of movement is possible. The large number of joints, however, normally results in a considerable range of movement of the column as a whole. The vertebral column has 2 main functions. The first is support. The weight of the head, the upper limbs, and the trunk is transferred to the vertebral column and from the vertebral column to the hip bones, and thus to the lower limbs. The second is protection. The vertebral column provides protection for the spinal cord and is divided into 5 regions: (1) The cervical region, consisting of 7 vertebrae; (2) the thoracic region, consisting of 12 vertebrae; (3) the lumbar region, consisting of 5 vertebrae; (4) the sacral region, consisting of 5 vertebrae, which in the adult are used to form a single unit, the sacrum; (5) the coccygeal region, consisting usually of 4 vertebrae, which in the adult are fused to form a single unit, the coccyx. Although the vertebrae all have certain structural characteristics in common, each region is different, and the vertebrae within each region differ in detail. A typical vertebra is composed of 2 parts, an anterior part called the body and a posterior part called the vertebral arch. The posterior surface of the body and the vertebral arch enclose a foramen called the vertebral foramen, through which the spinal cord passes.

vertigo. Implies a hallucination of turning or rotating either of the self or the surroundings. The fault is often anywhere from the middle ear (semicircular canals, labyrinthitis) to the brain stem through the 8th cranial nerve. Pallor, sweating, and nausea may be normally associated. A related hearing loss of sensitivity to noise may point to involvement of both divisions of the vestibulocochlear nerve. Dizziness in sports is often caused simply by anxious overbreathing, which causes reduced blood carbon dioxide that inhibits the nutritional balance of the balancing center. Dizziness may be caused by some vestibular system of dysfunction. One or both parts of the system may be involved. The causes of vertigo are, generally, 1 or more of the following: head injury; viral labyrinthitis (aural vertigo); lesions of the 8th cranial nerve; lesions of the brain stem, temporal lobe, or cerebellum; disorders of the forebrain (e.g., migraine and epilepsy); cerebrovascular disease; psychogenic dizziness (anxiety and hyperventilation syndromes); ocular vertigo; and motion sickness. Many drugs, such as alcohol and barbiturates, often give rise to dysequilibrium sensations. Infrequently, a metabolic process such as hypothyroidism may be involved.

vertigo, alternobaric. May occur during a diving ascent, as Eustachian tube blockage may cause a buildup of pressure in the middle ear, the "reverse squeeze" in which the eardrum sometimes ruptures. As the pressure builds up in the middle ear before the onset of vertigo, the diver may be aware of it and may slow down or stop the ascent until the air comes through the Eustachian tube, reducing the middle ear pressure. If not, then there may be a severe loss of orientation with a rotary vertigo. The feeling of disorientation may produce feelings of panic in the diver, but he or she usually reaches the surface. In some cases, if the diver can see his or her colleague, he or she may notice a shimmer effect, with the colleague seeming to be moving up an down owing to a vertical nystagmus. As the vertigo is usually overcome, the diver often learns to survive, with more care that future ascents are not as rapid and that care is taken not to dive when the Eustachian tubes are difficult to clear.

vertigo, diving. There are various forms of dizziness that may occur underwater. Overbreathing, leading to lowered blood carbon dioxide, may cause dizziness by reducing the blood supply to the balancing center by way of the intracranial vasoconstriction caused. Any anxiety state or mental tension may develop into a feeling of insecurity in a hostile underwater environment, giving a vague sense of imbalance or lightheadedness. True vertigo and loss of orientation may occur with some divers when they cannot see the bottom or when they are in a "whiteout" state. It is a visual disorder caused by there being nothing to fix the eye on. Under such circumstances, the diver should generally look for his bubbles and follow them up or close his or her eyes. In searching for nonexistent visual information, there may be a tendency to disregard other postural cues. Vertigo, mild to severe, can occur along with any of the disorders of the hearing mechanism possibly leading to deafness.

vision, photopic. Vision in bright light, which is a function of the cones, is generally thought to be of 3 kinds giving trichromatic vision. Each type is thought to have a different photosensitive pigment, with its own wavelength, to which it may be sensitive and by which it is broken down to form the chemical stimulus for the nerve impulse. Those photosensitive pigments in cones have not yet been isolated, but it is thought that "red" cones are probably stimulated by yellow-orange light; "green" cones may absorb green light; and "blue" cones may be sensitive to blue light. All 3 are probably stimulated in roughly equal proportions. There photopsins are split by the appropriate wavelengths of light, when white light falls on the retina; 2 or more in varying degrees when other colors fall on the retina. The various kinds of color blindness (e.g., red and green) could be explained by postulating the absence or deficiency of 1 or more of those photopsins in the cones. As the intensity of light is reduced, the cones generally cease to respond and the rods take over. When a person passes from darkness into bright light, he or she may be first dazzled by it. Gradually one adapts, and the initial discomfort passes off. Visual purple may break down rapidly with "bleaching." The adjustment or decrease in sensitivity of the rods on exposure to bright lights is called light adaptation.

vision, scotopic. Vision in dim light is a function of the rods. Rods are all of 1 type and give monochromatic vision, i.e., vision in black and white or in shades of gray. They contain rhodopsin (sometimes called scotopsin or "visual purple"). In dim light the pigment gradually splits to opsin (a protein) and retinene, the chemical stimulus to set off the nerve impulse. (In bright light, rhodopsin very rapidly breaks down with resultant "bleaching.") In darkness, retinene, regenerated from vitamin A, is then relinked with the opsin to reconstitute rhodopsin. When a person passes from a brightly lit scene to darkness, he or she is temporarily blinded. After about half an hour, visual purple is regenerated, and one may see well in the dark. That adjustment or increase in sensitivity is called dark adaptation. As light brightness or intensity increases, the rods gradually lose their sensitivity and cease to respond to stimulation by light and the cones take over.

vision, stereoscopic. When the eye looks at some object or landscape, the view seen by the right eye is slightly different from that seen by the left eye. The 2 dissimilar retinal images are fused in the visual centers of the brain to give a 3-dimensional picture, i.e., an appreciation of depth as well as of height and width. Other factors may also contribute to recognition of solidity, depth, and distance: (1) parallax. When the head is moved, objects near at hand appear to move in the opposite direction, while those farther off seem to move in the same direction as the eyes. (2) Colors appear to fade with distance, and details become indistinct. The far-off hills that we know to be green may appear blue or misty gray. This is due to the absorption by atmospheric haze of certain wavelengths of light. (3) The light and shade cast on the surfaces of solid objects and the shadows cast by them, occlusion or blocking out of parts of a distant object by things between it and the eye, perspective, the fact that straight lines known to be parallel appear to converge with distance, and the relative sizes of images cast on the retina (e.g., a box held in the hand, which is casting a large image on the retina, is known from experience to be a much smaller object than a hut in the background, which is casting a small image), we have learned to associate all of those factors in terms of distance, depth, and solidity. It is believed that subconscious interpretations of such phenomena may be contributing all the time to depth perception.

vitamins. Substances that are essential to the body for the maintenance of health and fitness. They are generally divided into two groups. Vitamins A, D, E, and K are the fat-soluble vitamins, and B and C the water soluble vitamins. Vitamin A, or carotene, is essential for the maintenance of normal epithelial tissue. It may also be necessary for the maintenance of normal night vision, since it is concerned in the regeneration of the pigment in the rods of the retina. Vitamin A is present in dairy products, eggs, fish oils, carrots, and tomatoes. Vitamin A is not a single vitamin, but a complex group of water-soluble vitamins. The exact function of some of these is still being researched and as yet is still not fully understood. The most important are thiamine (vitamin B_1), riboflavin, nicotinic acid, cyanocoblamin (vitamin B_{12}). Vitamin C (ascorbic acid) plays an important part in the immune system and is generally necessary for the maintenance of normal connective tissue. Vitamin C is present in fresh fruits and in green vegetables. Vitamin D is generally essential for the normal absorption of calcium from the alimentary canal. Vitamin E is a fat-soluble vitamin that is present in many dairy products and cereals and appears to play an important role in rebuilding and maintenance of healthy cells. The complete role in man is not fully understood. Vitamin K is generally necessary for the normal production of prothrombin as well as for the maintenance of the normal process of blood clotting. It is present in many green vegetables, tomatoes, and liver. The main mineral salts, which are essential to the body, are sodium, potassium, calcium, phosphorus, iron, and iodine. The mineral salts are generally recognized as ingested in the diet in soluble forms that are absorbed into the blood from the alimentary canal. Sodium is mainly present in the diet in the form of common salt, with sodium salts the main mineral salts found in the extracellular fluid. Potassium is present in most foods, with potassium salts, the main salts found in the intracellular fluid. Calcium is present in cheese, milk, eggs, and vegetables and is deposited in the organic matrix of bones and teeth. It is also necessary for maintaining their strength and necessary for the normal functioning of cardiac and voluntary muscle and nerves. Phosphorus is present in cheese, eggs, meat, and fish, and like calcium is generally necessary for maintaining the strength of bones. Iron is present in kidney, liver, beef, eggs, green vegetables, potatoes, and bread and is necessary for the formation of hemoglobin. Iodine is normally present in adequate amounts in drinking water, but in some areas where this source may be insufficient, sodium iodine may be added to table salt. Iodine is generally necessary for the formation of the hormone thyroxine.

W

warts. A common disease caused by the human papovarvirus (wart virus). Warts usually occur on areas that are unprotected by clothing. A long incubation period generally makes the transmission of the warts difficult to study. Epidemics have often been associated with communal bathrooms, gang showers, gyms, sharing of combs, and so forth. The appearance of the warts generally depends on the location. They vary primarily in degree of proliferation and keratinization. The common wart may be single or multiple and usually occurs on the hands and is 1 to 5 mm in diameter. The flat wart is a discrete, slightly elevated, felt papule occurring on the face, back of the hands, and anterior tibial surfaces. Hundreds may be present. They may have a potential for malignant transformation. Digitate warts often project as fingerlike structures. Plantar warts may occur on the undersurface of the foot. They may be painful on pressure and cause difficulty in walking. A polypoid growth occurring in genital and perianal regions is known as condyloma acuminatum. Athletic performance may be markedly effected when warts interfere with footwear comfort or appear on the hands or fingers.

water. The human body resides in a "sea of water." In a 70 kg person, two-thirds of body weight, or approximately 45 kg, is water. Body water exists in separate but continually interacting compartments. Two-thirds of total body water (about 30 kg) is intracellular. The remaining one-third is extracellular. The extracellular fluid (ECF) is divided into interstitial plasma spaces, which comprise three-fourths and one-fourth of the ECF, respectively. In a 70 kg person, interstitial volume is approximately 11 liters, and the plasma volume about 4 liters. The electrical charge of plasma proteins provides the attractive force of oncotic pressure for water, which maintains plasma volume. Body water, in a sense, is generally the most critical "nutrient." Some essential nutrients may be absent from the diet for days or months, without immediate serious effects. Not so with water. Without it, one cannot survive for more than a few days, and without adequate hydration, an athlete cannot compete in endurance events, such as marathon runs. Most problems encountered by marathon runners are generally the result of inadequate water replacement. Hormones, nutrients (amino acids, glucose, free fatty acids), antibodies, and waste products (urea, creatinine, CO_2) may all be transported in plasma to water that surrounds individual cells, and the body's more important chemical reactions are carried out in water and are generally less efficient when body water is depleted. Water is almost always of critical importance in regulating body temperature. Excessive heat produced with exercise is generally dissipated by sweating, which may function only if ample water is supplied to sweat glands. Daily water losses may be great with strenuous physical activity. Body water is generally replaced every 11 to 13 days. Most adults require 2.5 liters (about 10 8 oz glasses) of water per day, much of which is supplied in food and drinks. In addition, carbohydrates, protein, and fats are metabolized in CO_2 and water, contributing about one-fifth of the daily requirements. The greatest water loss is generally in urine and sweating. Water lost from the lungs in expired air and from the skin without obvious perspiration is called "insensible" water loss. The lower the humidity, the greater the insensible water loss.

water balance. In optimal health, the total quantity of body water (and salt) is kept reasonably constant, in spite of wide fluctuations in daily intake. A balance is usually struck between the fluid intake and the fluid output. Large quantities of fluid are constantly being filtered or secreted and consequently reabsorbed in various parts of the body; e.g., there is a large turnover of fluid in the secretion of the digestive tract. About 1,500 ml each of saliva, gastric, pancreatic, and intestinal juices are secreted into the tract each day, besides 800 ml of bile. Most of those secretions are reabsorbed to the blood stream from the gut. Only small amounts of water, salt, and potassium are lost in the feces. Similarly, vast quantities of fluid and electrolytes are filtered off in the glomerular tufts of the kidney.

water evaporation. To vaporize 1 cubic centimeter of water, 0.6 calories of heat is generally needed. That is true whether the evaporation takes place in a crucible over a bunsen flame or from the surface of the skin. In the latter case, 0.6 calories of body heat would be utilized. About 240 kc a day generally are used up vaporizing the water that may be lost from the lungs in expired air. And there is generally continual water loss of "seepage" or diffusion from the skin. This is called "insensible perspiration." About 500 kc a day are generally used up vaporizing this from the skin surface. In addition, the body may lose varying quantities of heat as required by the active secretion of sweat glands. For every gram of sweat allowed to lie on the skin surface, 0.58 kc of body heat may be used up in its evaporation. On a daily heat intake of about 3300 kc, with output as worked at about 300 kc, the heat balance chart may be completed thus: Heat Loss: (1) from the skin; by radiation, convection, conduction (2,100 kc); by evaporation of water (insensible perspiration) (500 calories). (2) From the lungs; by evaporation of water, and by warming inspired air (240 kc). (3) From the gut; by warming ingested food and fluid in feces (110 kc). (4) From the urinary tract; in urine (50 kc). Total 3,000 kc.

water on the knee. Completely encapsulating the knee joint and its articulating surfaces is a thin pouchlike membrane that secretes fluid into the joint, nourishes the articular cartilage, and aids in its lubrication. That membrane is called the synovium. It is overlaid with, and protected by, a layer of dense, tough, fibrous tissue; the overlay is called the capsule of the knee. The capsule not only protects the synovial membrane but also acts as an additional brace and support for the knee. The synovium is fed by the body's blood supply system. As blood passes through the synovial membrane, it produces in the membrane's tissues a clear plasma dialysate that then seeps into the joint and is resorbed, constantly lubricating and nourishing the interior parts of the joint. As with the bursa of the kneecap, when the synovium becomes irritated, owing to some abnormality or prolonged stress, the cells become inflamed and the synovium swells, often causing an excess of synovial fluid to fill the joint. And if the synovium is severely traumatized, blood will seep through its pores and join the fluid filling the joint. That, in essence, is the condition known as water on the knee, which tends to be an inaccurate explanation of the condition. What really occurs is not water on the knee, but excessive synovial fluid in the knee cap. The condition, water on the knee (in its chronic form), usually comes about when a chronic abnormality in the knee causes the synovial membrane to swell and release excessive amounts of synovial fluid into the knee joint itself. The excess fluid creates a kind of hydraulic or outward-expanding pressure on the interior surfaces of the joint, which in itself may produce further pain and may limit motion. Water on the knee is really the symptom of an ailment rather than the ailment itself.

water resistance. The resistance of water to the swimmer is constant for the portions of the body that are submerged. Resistance may be decreased by greater buoyancy, which occurs in salt water. Swimmers with a higher percentage of body fat are generally more buoyant and may be able to set records for endurance swimming, rather than for speed. Waves often act to impede the progress of a swimmer, tiring and slowing the individual down. Tides and other currents in the open water may aid or hinder depending on their direction. In long-distance swimming in open water, the best chances for record performance would be in still air with absence of waves.

weakness. Usually attributed to psychological disorders, physical disorders, or it may appear as a complication in an organic disease. Weakness, in the absence of further symptoms or signs, is generally indicative of an emotional problem, such as depression. However, weakness may be the only symptoms of an early systemic disease, such as Guillain-Barré syndrome. Weakness is often characterized by feelings of lassitude, tiredness, weariness, depletion, exhaustion, malaise, loss of energy or motivation. It may be general or local. If local, the weakness may be described in the lower or upper extremities, either distal or proximal. It may be localized in the trunk, head, or in respiration. It is important to analyze weakness in terms of body segments, because weakness generally follows a neuroanatomic distribution in organic disease. Neuromuscular defects are usually marked by weakness, and fatigue may be an early symptom in the myopathies. Weakness upon exertion that is progressive with muscular effort is called fatigability.

weight lifter's syncope. Weight lifter's occasionally complain of "blackout" during competition. Subjects studied during strenuous activity showed that they lowered their expired carbon dioxide levels through hyperventilation. During the lifts, tachycardia rather than bradycardia and extremely high intrathoracic pressures were recorded. Cardiac size was greatly reduced, and heart pulmonary artery and aortic actions were barely perceptible. Immediately after the weight was removed, pulmonary artery pulsations quickly normalized, but a delay was seen in the aortic pulsations (3 to 4 breaths). It is believed that the fainting may be the result of cerebral ischemia produced by a large transient fall in arterial pressure when the elevated thoracic pressure is suddenly released.

wrist injuries. The wrist covers the area from the distal end of the radius and ulna to the proximal end of the metacarpals. That includes the 8 carpal bones, the proximal articular surfaces of the metacarpals, the distal articular surface of the radius, and the fibrocartilage of the distal end of the ulna. There is no articulation between the ulna and the carpus, the 2 being separated by a fibrocartilaginous disk that also separates the wrist joint proper from the distal radio-ulnar joint. Injuries to the wrist that present pitfalls in diagnosis may produce pain and disability, but the seriousness of the injury can be easily overlooked. Fractures of the base of the 2nd and 3rd metacarpals are considered with the wrist, as symptoms are closely involved with wrist function. They are often associated with subluxation of the carpal-metacarpal joint and are tender in this area.

A fall on the outstretched hand may produce an avulsion fracture of the tip of the styloid process of the radius. Fracture of the navicular often occurs following a fall onto the outstretched hand, with pain and local tenderness at the base of the thumb and on the radial side of the wrist. Pain may be mild initially but usually increases with

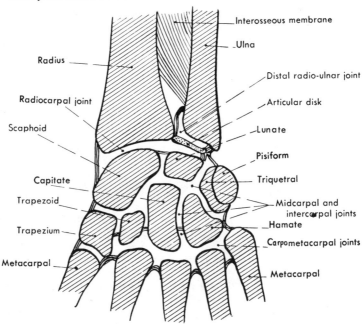

Radius

Radiocarpal joint

Scaphoid

Capitate

Trapezoid

Trapezium

Metacarpal

Interosseous membrane

Ulna

Distal radio-ulnar joint

Articular disk

Lunate

Pisiform

Triquetral

Midcarpal and intercarpal joints

Hamate

Carpometacarpal joints

Metacarpal

The bones and joint cavities of the wrist.

the use of the hand, especially in radial deviation and palmar flexion. Fracture of the triquetrum generally causes pain and sometimes clicking in the central area of the wrist on its dorsal surface. Pain in the central area of the wrist may also be produced by damage to the triangular wrist cartilage. Damage to that cartilage is usually characterized by a weak feeling in the wrist, and sometimes a click may be heard with motion. Fracture of the greater multiangular is generally produced by a force driving the thumb straight back against the wrist. It usually produces more early pain and disability than the navicular fracture. In dislocation of the lunate bone, the injury is often caused by acute dorsiflexion of the wrist while a force is being exerted against the extensor side of the forearm. A firm tender swelling may be palpable under the flexor tendons on the wrist and pain in the distribution of the median nerve may be severe. The wrist may not always be locked.

wrist joint movements. Movements that may occur at the wrist joint are flexion, extension, abduction, adduction, and circumduction. Flexion of the wrist joint is produced by the flexors carpi ulnaris and radialis, assisted by the long flexors of the fingers. The range of flexion at the wrist joint is usually not so great as it might appear, as a large amount of the apparent flexion occurs at the midcarpel joint. Extension is produced by the extensor carpi radialis longus and brevis and the extensor carpi ulnaris assisted by the extensors of the fingers. Abduction is produced by the flexor carpi radialis and the extensors carpi radialis longus and brevis. Abduction at the wrist joint is limited, and most of the apparent movement occurs at the midcarpal joint.

Z

zygoma fracture (mala fracture). The cause is a direct blow as from a punch, baseball, or hockey puck. Symptoms may include pain, numbness of the lip, difficulty in opening or closing the mouth, diplopia, and other disturbances varying with associated injuries. Signs may include external evidence of trauma to the cheek; edema, possibly involving the eyelids; cheek asymmetry; emphysema of the cheek; nasal bleeding; and other irregularities varying with associated injuries. Complications could lead to permanent deformity, permanent anesthesia of upper lip and possible visual impairment from associated orbital fracture.

Glossary

abdomen. That portion of the trunk located between the chest and the pelvis; the upper portion of the abdominopelvic cavity.

abduct. To draw away from the median plane of the body or one of its parts.

acetabulum. The rounded (cotyloid) cavity on the external surface of the innominate bone that receives the head of the femur.

Achilles tendon. The tendon of the gastrocnemius and soleus muscles of the leg. A flat, broad muscle of the calf of the leg.

acromioclavicular joint. An arthrodial joint between the acromion and the acromial end of the clavicle.

acromion. The lateral triangular projection of the spine of the scapula that forms the point of the shoulder and articulates with the clavicle.

adduction. Movement of a limb or eye toward the median plane of the body, or in case of digits, toward the axial line of a limb.

adductor. A muscle that draws toward the medial line of the body or to a common center.

adenitis. Inflammation of a gland or lymphnodes.

adenosine triphosphate (ATP). High energy molecule that provides the energy for muscle contraction.

adipose. fat; containing fat, as adipose tissue.

adipose tissue. Consists of fat-filled cells supported by strands of collagen fibers. Tissue forms a protective padding around organs. It forms the insulating layer in the hypodermis and serves as a fat depot for the body's reserves of "fuel."

adrenal. Located near the kidney; specifically the endocrine gland near the kidney.

aerobic. Requiring free oxygen for growth, as in the case of certain bacteria (aerobes).

aerobic activity or exercise. Exercise performed, using large muscle groups, at an intensity low enough so that all the energy (ATP) required for muscular work is produced from the complete metabolism of glucose and fatty acids with oxygen.

aerobic capacity. The amount of oxygen required or used by the body during peak or maximal muscular work; a measure of cardiovascular fitness.

aerobic power. The degree of physiological capacity to obtain and transport oxygen necessary for biological oxidation and provide the energy requirements of physical activity.

afferent. Carrying toward a center or main part; nerves that carry impulses toward the central nervous system or toward the ganglia.

albumen. One of the important proteins of the body, most of which circulates in the blood stream.

alkalosis. Condition characterized by an increase in blood pH above 7.4.

alkalosis, metabolic. Alkalosis resulting from the ingestion of alkaline drugs, for example, sodium bicarbonate; potassium depletion, some diuretics, or vomiting may be other causes.

alkalosis, respiratory. Alkalosis resulting from hyperventilation that results in depletion of carbon dioxide dissolved in the blood.

alveoli. Air sacs, clusters along the aveolar ducts. Lined with epithelium and covered with surfactant, forming parts of the respiratory membrane through which gas exchange occurs.

amino acid. A class of chemicals containing a carboxyl group (COOH) of an amino group (NH_2) plus a side chain. Basic constituents of proteins.

anaerobic exercise. Muscular activity of an intensity that exercising muscle's energy requirement (ATP) cannot be met aerobically. The extra energy is obtained by the metabolism of glucose without oxygen to lactic acid (lactate), which is toxic to the muscles.

anatomical snuffbox. Triangular area of the dorsum of the hand at the base of the thumb. When the thumb is extended, the tendons of the long and short extensor muscles of the thumb bound this area, which appears as a depression.

anemia. Decreased number of red blood cells or decreased amount of hemoglobin in red blood cells.

anesthesia. Partial or complete loss of sensation with or without loss of consciousness as a result of disease, injury, or administration of an anesthetic agent, usually by injection or inhalation.

aneurysm. A saclike enlargement of a blood vessel caused by a weakening of the wall.

angina. Pressure, discomfort, or actual pain in the front of the chest or arms, usually provoked by effort or tension. Angina occurs because of an inadequate supply of blood to the heart muscle. Almost all cases of angina are caused by narrowing or blockage of the coronary arteries by atherosclerosis.

angina pectoris. Severe pain and constriction about the heart, usually radiating to the left shoulder and down to the left arm.

ankylosis. Permanent consolidation, restriction of joint motion from abnormal fibrous or bony overgrowth.

anoxia. Lack of oxygen available to a tissue, often used interchangeably with hypoxia.

antagonist. A substance that binds to a receptor but does not activate it, in the process of blocking the binding of the natural agonist and so preventing its action.

antecubital. In front of the elbow; at the bend of the elbow.

antidepressant. Drug that results in behavioral and emotional simulation; may belong to 1 or 2 classes, the nonamine oxidase inhibitors or the tricyclic antidepressants.

antidiuretic hormone (ADH). Also called vasopressin. Octapeptide that increases water retention through its action on kidney tubules. Has marked effect on learning and motivation.

antiflexion. An abnormal forward curvature; a bending forward of the upper part of an organ, usually abnormal, but regarded as normal for the uterus.

antigravity muscles. Those muscles that oppose the effects of gravity and are involved in maintaining man's upright position.

antipyretic. Substance that counteracts the effects of a pyrogen, lowering the body temperature; aspirin is an effective antipyretic in subjects with a fever but does not lower normal body temperature.

anuria. Lack of urine excretion.

aorta. The main and largest artery of the body, connected directly to the left ventricle of the heart, which then branches, carrying blood to all parts of the body.

aortic stenosis. Narrowing of the aorta or its orifice because of lesions of the wall with scar formation; infection, as in rheumatic fever; or embryonic anomalies.

aphasia. The loss of power of expression by speech, writing, etc., or of comprehending what is said or spoken as a result of brain disease or brain injury.

apophysis. A projection, especially from a bone, an outgrowth without an independent center of ossification.

apoenzyme. The protein portion of an enzyme.

aponeurosis. A flat fibrous sheet of connective tissue that serves to attach muscle to bone or other tissues.

apraxia. Inability to perform useful movement correctly.

areflexia. Absence of reflexes.

arrhythmia. Irregularity of the pulse; too slow or rapid beating of the heart; or abnormality in the conduction of the heart's impulse to the different parts of the heart.

arrhythmia, sinus. Variation in rhythm of heartbeat dependent on interference with the impulse originating in the sinoauricular node; not associated with disease but with inspiration and expiration.

arterial blood pressure. Pressure in the large arteries of the body; usually measured in the brachial artery because it is about the level of the arch of the aorta and therefore indicative of aortic pressure.

arteriosclerosis. Hardening of the arteries caused by the deposition of calcium and lipids in the walls of the arteries, forming calcified plaques.

artery. A blood vessel that carries blood away from the heart to the rest of the body. All arteries, except those in the lungs, carry oxygen-rich red blood for use by the tissues.

arthritis. Inflammation of joints owing to infections, metabolic or other constitutional causes.

ascorbic acid (vitamin C). Strong reducing agent important for hemoglobin formation, the maturation of erythrocytes, and the development of interacellular substance, especially of bone and blood vessels.

aspirin. Acetylsalicyclic acid, which reduces inflammatory response by decreasing histamine and prostaglandin release; alleviates pain and fever also through its effect on prostaglandin production.

astigmatism. An irregularity of the cornea of the lens of the eye, causing the image to be out of focus and resulting in faulty vision.

ataxia. Failure or irregularity of muscular coordination, especially that manifested when voluntary muscular movements are attempted.

atelectasis. A collapsed or airless condition of the lungs.

atheroma. A fatlike cyst or tumor; a yellowish plaque that may be deposited in an artery wall, decreasing the size of the lumen (or channel).

atherosclerosis. Aging, damage, degeneration, and often thickening and infiltration by fatty substances of the inner layers of the arteries. If the process is severe enough, partial or complete blockage of blood flow through the arteries may occur. Although the term "hardening of the arteries" and "arteriosclerosis" do not have precisely the same meaning as atherosclerosis, most people use the terms interchangeably.

athlete's heart. A term describing the changes that regular high level of physical activity will produce in the normal heart. Once thought to be an abnormal condition, those changes are now known to be a normal response of the heart to exercise.

atrial fibrillation. An arrhythmia of the heart characterized by irregular, disordered beating of the atria (storage chambers) of the heart.

atrophy. A wasting away or decrease in size of a part; the result of a failure or abnormality or nutrition.

auditory ossicles. Three tiny bones, the malleus, incus, and stapes, that transmit vibrations from the tympanic membrane through the middle ear to the oval window of the inner ear.

autonomic nervous system. The part of the nervous system that is not under voluntary control. Its 2 major components, the sympathetic and parasympathetic nervous systems, control such functions as breathing, heart rate and function, blood pressure, and intestinal activity.

avascular. Lacking in blood vessels or having a poor blood supply, said of tissues such as cartilage.

avulsion. A tearing away forcibly of a part or structure.

ball of the foot. The prominent part of the bottom of the front of the foot, just behind the toes. It is composed of the ends or "heads" of the 5 metatarsal bones and forms the front part of the arch of the foot.

basal metabolic rate (BMR). Rate of activity of the tissues at rest, measured under controlled conditions of temperature, food intake, and activity and adjusted for body surface area, age, and sex.

basal metabolism. The minimum energy expenditure required to maintain life processes during a resting state.

biofeedback. Process by which information about subject's response (usually heart rate, blood pressure, or skin temperature) is relayed back to the subject as an auditory or visual signal. The subject can be taught to regulate these involuntary responses on the basis of the feedback.

biological clock. An intrinsic mechanism believed to reside in the pineal or hypothalamus or both that is responsible for the periodicity of certain biological rhythms.

bipartite patella. A congenital condition occasionally the cause of knee pain and secondary chondromalacia, particularly if a small piece is misaligned. Should be differentiated from a fracture.

Blocker's disease. The development of a bony growth at the middle third of the arm at or near the insertion of the deltoid from repeated contusions to that site; whether the complication is termed an exostosis or a traumatic myositis ossificans depends on the muscle tissue.

body "core." The central portion of the body that, for the purpose of assessing heat exchange, is assumed to be at a constant temperature. Rectal temperature is usually taken as a measure of "core" temperature.

brachial. Pertaining to the arm (the part between the shoulder and elbow).

bradycardia. Slow heart beat ranging from 50 to 60 beats per minute; nonpathologic if attributable to increased heart efficiency from endurance training.

bronchiectasis. A chronic disorder in which there is loss of the normal elastic tissues and dilation of lung air passages; characterized by difficulty in breathing, coughing, expectoration of puss, and unpleasant breath.

bursa. Fluid-filled sacs generally located where tendons (the ends of muscles) run over bony prominences near the joints. They are designed to cushion the tendons and prevent irritation and damage.

caffeine. Member of class of methylxanthines that increase calcium levels, inhibiting phosphodiesterase and prolonged cyclic AMP actions; also increases muscle contractibility.

calcaneal. Pertaining to the calcaneus, the heel bone.

calcaneus. The heel bone, or os calcis. It articulates with the cuboid bone and with the astragalus.

calculus. Commonly called stone, any abnormal concretion within the body. A calculus is usually composed of mineral salts, which can occur in the kidneys, ureter, bladder, or urethra.

callosity, callositas. Circumscribed thickening and hypertrophy of the horny layer of the skin.

callus. The thickening or overgrowth of the skin caused by chronic friction or irritation. The hard bonelike substance produced at the fracture line early in the healing phase of a fracture.

calorie. A unit of heat. When the term is used to describe the human body, it defines the heat produced by the metabolism or burning of energy sources, carbohydrates, fats, and proteins in food or body tissues.

capillaries. Tiny, thin-walled structures between arteries and veins, across which substances are transferred from the arterial blood to the cells or from the cells to be carried away in the venus blood.

capitellum. The round eminence at the lower end of the humerus, articulating with the radius; its radial head.

capsula. A sheath or continuous enclosure around an organ or structure.

carbohydrates. Substances containing only the elements carbon, hydrogen, and oxygen, arranged to form compounds called sugars, which in turn may be joined together in various combinations. Simple carbohydrates; substances containing only 1 or 2 sugar molecules (e.g., table sugar or honey). Complex hydrates; substances composed of many sugars linked together (e.g., starches and grains).

carbohydrate loading or packing. A method of increasing the muscle's glycogen (sugar) content by a major increase in the amount of carbohydrate eaten for several days before a track meet or long run.

carbon dioxide. Gas formed by tissue respiration; constitutes about 0.5 percent by volume of the atmosphere. Essential for stimulation of the respiratory centers.

carbon monoxide. Metabolic poison that combines firmly with hemoglobin, preventing hemoglobin from picking up oxygen and transporting it to the tissues.

carbuncle. An infection involving the skin and underlying connective tissues, tending to spread under the skin and to surface at various points.

carcinogenic. Stimulating or causing the growth of malignant cells or tumors (cancer).

carcinoma. A malignam spreading growth made of epithelial cells; a kind of cancer.

cardiac. Referring to the heart.

cardiac arrest. Absence of effective beating of the heart.

cardiac cycle. Period from the end of 1 heart contraction (systole) and relaxation (distole) to the end of the next systole and diastole.

cardiac output. A measure of heart efficiency. It is a direct measure of the total amount of blood pumped per unit of time (usually measured in liters per minute) and is a function of heart rate, degree of filling and heart volume.

cardiovascular. Referring to the heart and blood vessels that carry blood to the tissues (arteries) and from the tissues back to the heart (veins).

cardiovascular efficiency. The adaptive response of the heart to exercise. It is related to the efficiency of oxygen taken into the lungs and into the bloodstream and the ability of the heart to pump oxygenated blood to muscles for energy production and activity.

cardiovascular fitness. The capacity of the body to perform aerobic muscular exercise. Its level is defined by VO₂Max, the amount of oxygen consumed by the body at peak exercise. Cardiovascular fitness can be improved by the regular performance of aerobic exercise.

carotene. The orange or reddish pigment in foods such as carrots, sweet potatoes, leafy vegetables, and egg yolk; protovitamin A, which can be converted in the body to vitamin A.

carpal. Pertaining to the carpus or wrist. Carpal is any wrist bone.

caseous. Resembling cheese. Pertaining to transformation of tissues into a cheesy mass.

cauda equina. The terminal portion of the spinal cord and the roots of the spinal nerves below the first lumbar nerve.

cellulitis. Inflammation of cellular or connective tissue, spreading as in erysipelas. An infection in or close to the skin is usually localized by the body defense mechanism.

cerebration. Mental activity of the brain.

cervical. In the region of the neck or cervix.

cervix. Any neck or constricted portion of an organ, part, or region of the body.

cholesterol. One of the major fats or lipids contained in both food and the body's cells and fluids. Its level can be measured in the blood. High levels of cholesterol are associated with an increased risk of atherosclerosis. Precursor of the steroid hormones of the adrenal cortex, the sex hormones, and the bile acids.

chondral. Pertaining to cartilage.

chondromalacia. Literally "softening of the cartilage." The term here is used to describe the disease of the cartilaginous, inner surface of the patella commonly referred to as "runner's knee."

choroid. Pertaining to the thin, dark brown, vascular middle coat of the eyeball; also relating to the capillary fringelike parts of the pia mater that extend into the brain ventricles and produce cerebrospinal fluid.

circulorespiratory endurance. A degree of physiological eficiency involving the transporting functions of the circulatory system and the gaseous exchange function of the respiratory system.

cobalamin (vitamin B₁₂). Vitamin and coenzyme essential for normal maturation of erythrocytes; contains cobalt and is the intrinsic factor that can be absorbed only in the presence of the intrinsic factor, a glycoprotein in the parietal cells of the stomach. Absence of cobalamin generally results in pernicious anemia.

coccygodynia. Pain in the coccygeal region (small bone at the base of the spinal column in man, formed by 4 fused rudimentary vertebrae).

coccyx. Small bone at the base of the spinal column in man, formed by 4 fused rudimentary vertibrae.

condyle. A rounded protuberance at the end of a bone, forming an articulation.

convection. Exchange of heat between an object and the streaming currents of gas or liquid flowing past the object.

conjunctiva. The thin, delicate membrane that lines the eyelids and is reflected over the front of the eyeball.

conjunctivitis. Inflammation of the membrane that lines the eyelids and covers the front of the eyeball.

contrecoup. A French word that means "counterblow," especially referring to a skull fracture caused by a blow to the opposite side.

core temperature. The temperature inside the body itself, usually estimated accurately by obtaining the rectal temperature. Oral or mouth temperatures are often falsely low as a measure of core temperature.

cornea. Translucent front part of the outer coat (aclera) of the eye through which light rays enter; highly convex and a powerful refractive structure.

coronary. Applying to structures that encircle a part or organ, in a crownlike manner, as for example, the coronary arteries encircling the base of the heart.

coronary heart disease. An abnormal condition of the coronary arteries that impedes the adequate supply of blood to heart tissues.

cotton mouth. Sensation of discomfort associated with dry mouth from dehydration or emotional tension.

coxa. Hip or hip joint.

coxa vara. A deformity produced by a decrease in the angle made by the head of the femur with the shaft.

crepitus. The noise of gas discharged from the intestines.

cricothyroid. Pertaining to the thyroid and cricoid cartilage.

cruciate. Cross-shaped, as in the cruciate ligaments of the knee.

cyanosis. Slightly bluish, grayish, slatelike, or dark purple discoloration of the skin caused by the presence of abnormal amounts of reduced hemoglobin in the blood.

cyanotic. Pertaining to cyanosis.

dead space. The space in the air-conducting system of the respiratory tract; no gas exchange occurs in this area. It consists of the nose, pharynx, trachea, bronchi, and conducting bronchioles.

dehydration. Considered a potential source of debilitation in any events where considerable body sweat is elaborated. Football and basketball players may lose from 3 to 7 percent of their body weight during the course of a game. In this situation, a larger proportionate loss is sustained by the plasma volume than by other compartments of body fluid. Therefore, unequal loss of circulation to working muscles to the skin is curtained, which in turn leads to deterioration in performance. Salt is lost in relatively large amounts in sweat, so the individual daily requirements may be increased by 5 to 10 g under conditions where large amounts of sweat are lost per day.

deltoid. Shaped like the Greek letter delta; triangular.

dermis. Lower layer of the skin, containing specialized nerve endings for touch, temperature, and pain and rich plexuses of blood vessels. The hair follicles and skin glands also originate in the dermis.

diaphragm. The large muscle that separates the chest and abdominal cavities.

diaphragmatic breathing. Breathing caused by contraction and relaxation of the diaphragm. As the diaphragm contracts during inhalation, it moves toward the abdomen, enlarging the lung cavity and drawing air into the lungs. The abdominal contents are simultaneously pushed outward and down. As the diaphragm relaxes, it moves upward, reducing the volume of the lungs and expelled air from them (exhalation).

diaphysis. The shaft or middle part of a long cylindrical bone.

diastasis. In surgery, injury to a bone involving separation of an epiphysis. (A center for ossification of each extremity of long bones.)

diastole. The period in the cardiac pumping cycle during which the ventricles are relaxed and dilated and therefore receiving blood.

dietary fiber. Constituents of foods that cannot be digested (absorbed) by the body and are excreted largely unchanged in the stools. High fiber diets provide bulk for adequate stool production, often producing a satisfied or full feeling without excessive calorie intake, and are high in complex hydrates and low in fat.

diplopia. Double vision.

discoid. Like a disc.

distal. Farthest from the center from a medial line or from the trunk. Away from the point of origin.

diverticulitis. An inflammation of the abnormal sacs formed as a result of weakness in the muscle wall of a tubular organ, such as the colon.

dorsal. Pertaining to the back.

dorsiflexion. The act of drawing the toe or foot, finger or wrist, toward the dorsal aspect of the proximally cojoined body segment.

dorsum. The back or posterior surface of a part.

dural. Pertaining to the dura mater, the outer membrane covering the spinal cord (dura mater spinalis (NA) and brain (dura mater cerebri (NA) or dura mater encephali (NA).

dysesthesia. Sensations of the pricks of pins and needles or of crawling.

dysphagia. Inability to swallow or difficulty in swallowing.

dysphonia. Difficulty in speaking; hoarseness.

dysplasia. Abnormal development of tissue.

ecchymosis. A form of macula appearing in large irregularly formed hemorrhagic areas of the skin.

ecthyma. An infection of the skin. Usually a result of neglected treatment of impetigo.

ectopic. In an abnormal position.

edema. A local or generalized condition in which the body tissues contain an excessive amount of tissue fluid.

efferent. Conducting impulses from the central nervous system to the periphery; motor output.

effusion. Escape of fluid into a part, as the pleural cavity, such as pyothorac (pus), hydrothopax (serum), hemathorax (blood), chylothorax (lymph), pneumothorax (air), hydropneumothorax (serum and air) and pyopneumothorax (pus and air).

electromyogram. Record of the activity of the muscles.

elephantiasis. A disorder in which the lymph channels are obstructed, resulting in marked swelling and thickening of the skin.

embole. Reduction of a dislocation.

embolism. Blocking of an artery by a clot or air bubbles that have been transported through the blood.

emphysema. Chronic lung disease characterized by stretching, loss of elasticity, and overinflation of the lung tissue with breakdown and disruption of the alveoli or tiny air sacs where gas exchange in the lungs takes place (oxygen from the lungs into the bloodstream and carbon dioxide from the bloodstream to the lungs). Emphysema has many possible causes, but by far the most common is a combination of smoking and aging of the lung tissue.

empty calories. Food and drink generally containing simple sugars that offer no other nutritional benefits, such as minerals, vitamins, fiber, etc. Examples are hard candy, alcohol, and table sugar.

endocrine. Secreting to the inside, into either tissue fluid or blood. The opposite is exocrine.

endolyphatic. Related to the endolymph, pale transparent fluid within the labyrinth of the ear.

endothelium. A form of squamous epithelium consisting of flat cells that line the blood and lymphatic vessels, the heart, and various body cavities. It is derived from mesoderm.

enophthalmos. Recession of eyeball into orbit.

enzymes. Substances in the cells and body fluids that control the speed at which all biochemical reactions take place within the body.

epicardium. The membrane that forms the outer layer of the heart wall and is continuous with the lining of the sac that encloses the heart; the visceral pericardium.

epicondyle. The eminence at the articular end of a bone above a condyle.

epidermis. The outer layers of the skin.

epidermophytosis. A fungus infection of the skin, especially of the toes and soles of the feet, that is called tinea pedis (athlete's foot).

epinephrine. One of the important hormones, made chiefly in the adrenal gland, required for function of the sympathetic nervous system.

epiphyseal. Pertaining to or of the nature of an epiphysis, a center for ossification at each extremity of long bones.

epiphyses. The parts of bone in which growth occurs. In large bones they are usually located toward the ends of the bones near the joints.

epiphysis. A center for ossification at each extremity of longbone.

epigastric. Pertaining to the epigastrium, a region over the part of the stomach.

epistaxis. Hemorrhage from nose, nosebleed.

epithelia. Pertaining or composed of epithelium.

epithelium. The layer of cells forming the epidermis of the skin and the surface layer of mucus and serous membrane.

erythema. A form of macula showing diffused redness over the skin.

erythematous. Pertaining to or marked by erythema, a form of macula showing diffused redness over the skin.

estimated maximum heart rate. The calculated rate determined by subtracting one's age from 220.

Eustachian tube. The auditory tube extending from the middle ear to the pharynx, 3 cm to 4 cm long and lined with mucous membrane.

eversion. The act of rotating the pronated foot externally on the ankle. Turning outward.

exanthem. Any skin eruption or rash; visible skin lesions often accompanied by fever.

exercise test (exercise ECG, stress test). Measurement of the electrocardiogram and other cardiovascular functions during exercise. It is usually performed on a treadmill or bicycle with gradual increase in the level of exercise performed.

extension. A movement by which 2 parts are pulled apart toward a straightened position.

exogenous. Originating outside an organ or part.

exostosis. A bony growth that arises from the surface of a bone, often involving the ossification of muscular attachments.

exudate. Escaping fluid or semifluid material that oozes out of a blood vessel (usually as a result of inflammation), which may contain serum, pus, and cellular debris.

fascia. Specialized, fibrous tissues, usually extremely tough and strong, that support body structures and separate muscle groups.

fats. Chemical compounds that share a common property, the inability to dissolve in water or various body fluids. They are an important source of food and energy and are important parts of all body cells and tissues. Cholesterol and triglycerides are the most important fats.

fatty acids. Compounds composed of long chains of carbon atoms that serve as an important source of energy for the body. Fatty acids are part of the triglyceride molecule and are stored in fat tissue in this form. Fatty acids are "saturated" when all the bonds between the carbon atoms are filled and "unsaturated" when the bonds are incomplete.

febrile. Fever, feverish.

femoral. Pertaining to the thigh bone or femur.

femur. The thigh bone, extending from the hip to the knee. It is the longest and strongest bone in the skeleton.

fibrillation. Random, ineffective, disordered contractions of the heart muscle. Atrial fibrillation: fibrillation present in the upper heart chambers of the atria. Ventricular fibrillation: fibrilation present in the lower or pumping chambers. Unless immediately reversed, ventricular fibrillation is fatal.

fibrogen. Large asymmetrical plasma protein found in high concentrations in the blood; essential for blood coagulation (Factor I), it is split by thrombin into small fibrinopeptides that form a polymer, the large, insoluble fibrin molecule that cross links to form the fibrin clot.

fibrositis. A disorder in which there is inflammation of certain fibrous connective tissue layers around or near muscles, resulting in pain and stiffness.

fibula. The outer and smaller bone of the leg from the ankle to the knee, articulating above with the fibia and below with the fibia and talus. One of the longest and thinnest bones of the body.

fistula. An abnormal passage between 2 organs, or between the organ cavity and the outside, which may be formed by tissue injury and disintegration.

flatus. Gas, usually air, in the stomach or bowel (it means a "blowing" and so can refer to expelling air from the lungs).

flexion. The act of drawing a body segment away from a straight line with its proximally conjoined body segment or toward that joint's smallest acute angle.

flexion and extension. Flexion is the bending of a limb or body part at a joint. Extension is the straightening of that limb or body part.

fossa. A furrow or shallow depression.

folic acid. Vitamin essential for the normal growth and maturation of erythrocyte and a growth-promoting agent. Also called pteroylglutamic acid.

fossa. A hollow or depressed area; a valleylike region on a bone or other structure.

fovea. A small pit- or cup-shaped depression in the surface of a part or organ, as in the head of the femur and near the center of the retina of the eye; the point of clearest vision.

fremitus. Vibration tremors, especially those felt through the chest wall by palpation.

fulminate. Occurring suddenly and with severity. (A fulminating anoxia is a sudden reduction in the oxygen content of the blood causing collapse.)

fundus. The part of a hollow organ, farthest from the entrance.

funny bone (crazy bone). Contusion of ulnar nerve at the ulnar groove of the humeral medial epicondyle, producing a transiently disabling burning sensation and numbness along ulnar side of forearm and a hand.

furuncle. A boil; a painful nodule caused by infection and inflammation of a hair follicle or an oil gland.

galea. A helmetlike structure.

gastrocnemius. The large muscle of the posterior portion of the lower leg. It is the most superficial of the calf muscles. Extends foot and helps to flex knee upon thigh.

genu recurvatum. Hyperextensibility of knee; usually congenital in origin, may be predisposing factor in internal derangement of knee.

genu valgum (knock-knee). Deformity, usually congenital, but may be secondary to trauma; knees abnormally close together while the space between ankle is increased, curvature of leg with apex of convexity displaced medially at level of the knee; may be predisposing factor in development of recurrent subluxation of dislocation of patella or of medial collateral ligament sprain.

glaucoma. A disorder of the eye in which there is increased pressure because of an excess of fluid within the eye; results in atrophy of optic nerve and blindness.

gluconeogenesis. The formation of glycogen from noncarbohydrate sources, such as amino or fatty acids.

glucose. Six-carbon monosaccharide found in fruit and other foods and in the blood of all animals; chief source of energy for most living organisms.

glycogen. The storage form of sugar, primarily in the muscles and the liver. It is broken down to glucose to meet the body's energy needs.

glycemia. Presence of sugar (in the form of glucose) in the blood.

hallux valgus. The great toe. Displacement of great toe toward other toes.

hamstring. The group of muscles in the back of the thigh involved in movement of both the hip and knee joints.

heart burn. Burning sensation over heart area but coming from esophagus or stomach; related to reflux of gastric contents; frequently functional origin but organic cause may be present; nervousness, faulty digestion contributory.

heart monitoring. Procedure of palpating the radial artery at the wrist or the carotid artery at the end for a pulse rate count for 10 seconds immediately after a bout of exercise. This rate is multiplied by 6 to determine the approximate heart rate per minute for that intensity of work.

heart murmurs. Sounds heard through the stethoscope when one is listening to the heart. In most cases produced by increasing turbulence of the blood as it passes through the heart chambers. Some murmurs are benign or functional. (There is no underlying structural abnormality of the heart to account for them.) Other murmurs are organic and are caused by structural abnormalities with the heart.

heat, delayed. Biphasic burst of heat liberated from isometrically contracting muscle during the recovery period, after the muscle has relaxed; 1st phase is oxygen independent, the 2nd phase requires oxygen, is longer lasting, and liberates the most heat.

heat fatigue. Transient deterioration in performance from exposure to heat, humidity, and resulting in relative state of dehydration and salt depletion.

heat, initial. Two bursts of heat from an isometrically contracting muscle during the periods of contraction and relaxation, derived from the hydrolysis of ATP and CP. Independent of oxygen.

heat stroke. An acute, potentially lethal condition that results from excessive fluid loss and marked increase in body temperature usually caused by intense exercise performed in hot weather without adequate fluid replacement.

hemarthrosis. Bloody effusion into the cavity of a joint.

hematemesis. The vomiting of blood.

hematoma. A swelling or mass of blood (usually clotted) confined to an organ, tissue, or space and caused by a break in a blood vessel.

hematuria. Blood in the urine.

hemolysis. The disintegration of red blood cells that results in the appearance of hemoglobin in the surrounding fluid.

hemoptysis. Act of coughing up blood; caused by lesion of the lungs, trachea, or larynx.

hemothorax. Bloody fluid in the pleural cavity causing the rupture of small blood vessels, owing to inflammation of the lungs in pneumonia and pulmonary tuberculosis or to a malignant growth.

heparin. Powerful anticoagulant produced by many cell types, especially by mast cells in the liver.

hepatic. Pertaining to the liver.

herpes. A skin disease in which small blisters appear, often in clusters. (Herpes simplex may be referred to as cold sores or fever blisters and is caused by a virus infection involving mostly the lip borders and the nose. Herpes zoster, shingles, is also a virus infection but involves nerve trunk areas.)

hilum (hilus). An area, depression, or pit where blood vessels and nerves enter or leave the organ.

histamine. Amine produced by damaged cells, and by eosinophils and mast cells; potent vasodilator, increases gastric secretion, smooth muscle contraction, and capillary permeability. Antihistamine drugs reduce or prevent those reactions.

homeostasis. State of equilibrium of the internal environment of the body that is maintained by dynamic processes of feedback and regulation.

hormones. Substances produced by some of the glands in the body that then are carried by the blood to influence the activity of cells and tissues elsewhere. For example, the pancreas produces insulin, a hormone that regulates sugar metabolism in cells throughout the body.

hot spot. Early redness of the skin from friction that leads to blister formation if preventive measures are not taken.

humerus. Upper bone of the arm from the elbow (articulating with the ulna and radius) to the shoulder joint, where it articulates with the scapula.

hydrops. Dropsy or edema.

hypercapnia. Increased amount of carbon dioxide in the blood.

hyperemia. Congestion. An unusual amount of blood in a part. A form of macula; red areas on the skin that disappear on pressure.

hyperesthesia. Increased sensitivity to sensory stimuli, such as pain or touch.

hyperextension. Extreme or abnormal extension.

hyperkalemia. Excessive amounts of potassium in the blood.

hyperpyrexia. Elevation of body temperature above 106°F (41.1°C).

hyperreflexia. Increased action of the reflexes.

hypertension. Persistently high arterial blood pressure. A condition in which the individual has a higher blood pressure than that judged to be normal.

hyperthermia. Sharp rise in body temperature. Unusually high fever.

hypertomia. Abnormal tension of arteries or muscles.

hypertrophy. Increase in size of an organ or structure that does not involve tumor formation. Term is generally restricted to an increase in size or bulk not resulting from an increase in number of cells or tissue elements, as in the hypertrophy of a muscle.

hypesthesia. Lessened sensitivity to touch.

hyphemia. Blood in the anterior chamber of the eyes in front of the iris.

hypoglycemia. Deficiency of sugar in the blood. A condition in which the glucose in the blood is abnormally low.

hypokinesia. Decreased motor reaction to stimulus.

hypokinetic disease. The debilitating effects of insufficient physical activity. The whole spectrum of inactivity-induced somatic and mental derangements.

hypotonic. Pertaining to defective muscular tone or tension. A solution of lower osmotic pressure than another.

hypoxia. Deficiency of oxygen. Decreased concentration of oxygen in the inspired air.

ichthyosis. Condition in which the skin is dry and scaly, resembling fish skin. Because ichthyosis is so easily recognized, a variety of diseases have been called by this name.

idiopathic. Relating to any disorder than is of unknown origin or apparently of spontaneous origin; self-originating.

ileum. The last or distal part of the small intestine, ending at the cecum of the large intestine.

ileus. A twisting. Intestinal obstruction.

iliac. Pertaining to the ilium; 1 of the bones of each half of the pelvis.

iliopsoas. The compound iliacus and psoas magnus muscles.

infarct. An area of tissue in an organ or part that undergoes necrosis following cessation of blood supply. May result from occlusion or stenosis of the supplying artery.

inferior. Used medically in reference to the undersurface of an organ or indicating a structure below another structure.

inguinal. Relating to the groin region.

insulin. The hormone made by the pancreas that controls a variety of important body processes, including the uptake of glucose into the body's cells. Pancreatic hormone produced by the beta cells of the islets of Langerhans; lowers blood glucose by accelerating the passage of glucose into cells for storage as glycogen or oxidation to yield energy.

intercostal muscles. Respiratory muscles between the ribs. The internal intercostals elevate the ribs during inspiration; when they relax, passive expiration occurs. The internal intercostals lower the ribs in active expiration.

intrathecal. Within the spinal canal. Within a sheath.

intrinsic factor. A substance normally present in the gastric juice of humans. Its presence makes absorption of vitamin B_{12} possible. Absence of this factor leads to vitamin B_{12} deficiency and pernicious anemia.

inversion. Turning inside out of an organ. Reversal of normal relationship. The act of rotating the supinated foot medially on the ankle.

ischemia. Local and temporary deficiency of blood supply owing to obstruction of the circulation to a part.

ischial. Pertaining to the ischium, the lower portion of the innominate or hip bone.

islets of Langerhans. Islands of endocrine tissue found in the tail of the pancreas; produces insulin, glucagen, and somatostatin.

isometric contraction. Contraction of a muscle in which shortening or lengthening is prevented. Tension is developed but no mechanical work is performed, all energy being liberated as heat.

isometric exercise. Contraction of a muscle which is not accompanied by movement of the joints that would normally be moved by that muscle's action. The muscle length is not effected by this type of exercise.

isometric muscle. Contraction in which a muscle increases its tension without shortening.

isotonic. Having the same tension or tone. Shortening of a muscle while the tension generated remains relatively constant; as the muscle shortens, it moves a load a certain distance and work is done.

isotonic exercise. Contraction of a muscle during which the force of resistance to the movement remains constant throughout the range of motion.

jogging. A continuous noncompetitive program of exercise at any speed of running (from slow to fast) designed to improve or maintain physical fitness. Generally, a mile completed in more than 8 minutes is a mile jogged. Less than 8-minute mile is running. In jogging, the body is held in an upright position and the foot strike is flat, or heel-to-toe.

joint. The place of union or articulation between 2 or more bones. There are three types of joints; immovable, slightly movable and freely movable.

kidney. Paired organ in the lumbar region that filters the blood and through reabsorption and secretion, modifies the filtrate to produce the excreted urine.

kidney stones. Calculus or a crystalline mass present in the pelvis of the kidney. They are composed principally of oxalates, phosphates, and carbonates and vary in size from small granular masses to an inch in diameter.

kinetic. Pertaining to or consisting of motion.

knee. The anterior aspect of the leg at the articulation of the femur and tibia and the articulation itself, covered anteriorly with the patella or kneecap. Formed by the femur, tibia, and patella.

kneecap. The patella.

knee-jerk reflex. The reflex contraction or clonic spasm of the quadriceps muscle, produced by sharply striking the ligamentum patellae when the leg hangs loosely flexed at right angles.

lace bite. Painful inflammation of first metatarsal; develops usually from abrasive irritation of tightly locked footwear.

lactase. A sugar-splitting enzyme in the small intestine that splits lactose (milk sugar) into a glucose.

lactic acid. A colorless syrupy liquid formed in milk, sauerkraut, and in certain types of pickles by the fermentation of the sugars by microorganisms. It is also formed in muscles during activity by breakdown of glycogen.

lactose. A disaccharide which on hydrolysis yields glucose and galactose. Bacteria can convert it into lactic and butyric acids, as in the souring of milk.

ligament. A band or sheet of fibrous tissues which connects 2 or more bones, usually within a joint.

low back pain. Pain or soreness in the lumbosacral and spinal region.

lumbago. A general nonspecific term for dull, aching pain in the lumbar region of the back.

lumbar. Pertaining to the loins. The loin is the lower part of the back and sides between the ribs and pelvis.

lumbar plexus. Posterior swelling of the spinal cord representing the origin of the nerves innervating the legs.

lunate. A bone in the proximal row of the carpus.

lung cancer. Cancer that may appear in trachea, air sacs, and other lung tubes. It may appear as an ulcer in the windpipe, as a nodule or small flattened lump, or on the surface blocking air tubes. It may invade surface of tubes extending to lymphatics into blood vessels.

lung capacity. The maximum amount of air the lungs can inhale. Jogging and running can increase the capacity but not likely more than 10 percent. Smoking will decrease lung capacity.

lymph. A yellowish relatively clear watery fluid found in the lymphatic vessels; a liquid containing cells, most lymphocytes, and after a meal, fat globules; any clear watery fluid resembling true lymph.

lymph node. A rounded body consisting of accumulation of lymphatic tissue found at intervals in the course of lymphatic vessels. Lymph nodes vary in size from a pinhead to an olive and may occur singly or in groups. Produces lymphocytes and acts as a filter to localize bacterial and viral infections and entrap wandering malignant cells.

lymphocyte. Lymph cell or white blood corpusle without cytoplasmic granules. They normally number from 20 to 50 percent of total white cells.

lysis. The gradual decline of a fever or disease. Destruction of blood cells by a lysin, as when rabbit's red corpuscles are dissolved by dog's serum.

malleolus. The protuberance on both sides of the ankle joint, the lower extremity of the fibula being known as the lateral malleolus and the lower end of the tibia as the medial malleolus.

malunion. An abnormal healing of a fracture caused by faulty position, angulation, or other abnormality of alignment of the bone fragments.

maximum expected heart rate. The fastest heart rate for any age group. It tends to fall with age and is independent of fitness. It can be calculated approximately by subtracting the age from 220.

medial. middle.

mediastinum. A septum or cavity between 2 principal portions of an organ.

medulla. (1) The marrow. (2) Inner or central portion of an organ in contrast to the outer portion or cortex.

megoblast. A large primitive red blood cell that is usually found only in the bone marrow in pernicious anemia, but may also enter the circulation.

meatus. Opening or passage.

meningeal. Relating to the meninges. Membranes. The 3 membranes investing the spinal cord and brain; the dura mater (external), the arachnoid (middle), and pia mater (internal).

meniscus. Interarticular fibrocartilage of crescent shape, found in certain joints, especially the lateral and medial menisci (semilunar cartlageal of the knee joint.

metabolic equivalent (MET). A term describing in terms of oxygen consumption and corrected for differences in body weight, the oxygen requirement of physical activity. One MET, the oxygen requirement at rest, equals approximately the consumption of 3.5 milliliters of oxygen per kilogram of body weight per minute.

metabolic rate.   Heat produced within the body associated with chemical reactions. It is usually calculated indirectly from the consumption of oxygen (indirect calorimetry).

metabolism.   The sum of all physical and chemical changes that take place within an organism; all energy and material transformation that occur within living cells. It includes material changes, i.e., changes undergone by substances during all periods of life and energy changes, i.e., all transformation of chemical energy of foodstuffs to mechanical energy or heat.

metacarpal.   Pertaining to the bones of the metacarpus or bones of the hand.

metacarpus.   The part of the hand near the wrist, between the wrist and fingers; the 5 elongated bones in the hand.

metaphysis.   Portion of a developing long bone between the diaphysis or shaft and epiphysis; the growing portion of a bone.

metaplastic.   Pertaining to or formed by metaplasia (conversion of 1 kind of tissue into a form which is not normal for that tissue.)

metasasis.   The transfer of disease from 1 organ or part of the body to another part that is not connected with it.

metatarsalgia.   Severe pain or cramp in anterior portion of metatarsus.

metatarsus.   The region of the foot between the tarsus and phalanges. Includes the 5 metatarsal bones.

molluscum.   A mildly infective skin disease characterized by tumor formation on the skin.

mortise.   Ankle joint.

Morton's syndrome (Morton's toes).   A combination of abnormalities of the forefoot, the most obvious of which is a 1st toe which is shorter than the 2nd, which often causes excessive pronation of the foot during running. A variety of related injuries may be produced by this excessive foot pronation.

mucosa.   Mucous membrane lining the digestive and respiratory tracts; consists of a superficial layer of epithelium, a supporting layer of loose connective tissue, the lamina propria, and a thin layer of muscle, the muscularis mucosa. The epithelial cells secrete a protective lubricating solution, mucus.

mucus.   Protective lubricating solution produced by epithelial cells of the digestive and respiratory tracts; contains a protein, polysaccharide, mucin.

muscle atrophy.   Wasting away of muscle tissue, as the result of immobilization (casts), inactivity, loss of innervation, or nutritional disorder.

muscle cramp.   Painful involuntary contraction of skeletal muscle group; causes include salt depletion (heat cramp), fatigue, and reflex reaction to trauma.

muscle spasm.   A sudden violent, involuntary contraction of a muscle that at times is accompanied by pain and functional interference. It may occur during rest as muscles relax.

muscle tone.   A firmness of muscles caused by low intensities of contraction even in the relaxed state.

muscular endurance.   The ability of a muscle to contract repetitively without fatigue for a relatively long period of time. Endurance is developed by resistance exercises performed repeatedly for the increase of capillaries to supply additional blood to the muscles.

musculotendinous.   Composed of both muscle and tendon.

mycosis.   Any disorder caused by a fungus, such as dermatomycosis, a fungus infection of the skin.

myocardial.   Concerning the myocardian, the middle layer of the walls of the heart composed of cardiac muscle.

myocardial infarction. Necrosis in the myocardium caused by interruption of the blood supply to the area, as in coronary thrombosis.

myocardium. The middle layer of the walls of the heart, composed of cardiac muscle.

myofibril. Contractile element of a muscle fiber; composed of thick and thin filaments.

myosin. Elongated, 2-headed protein of muscle thick filaments; binds actin to form actomyosin and enzymatically binds and hydrolyzes ATP; contractile protein essential for muscle contraction.

myositis. Inflammation of muscle tissue, especially voluntary muscles.

myxedema. Condition resulting from hypofunction of the thyroid gland.

navicular. Shaped like a bone. Scaphoid bones in the carpus (wrist) and in the tarsus (ankle).

necrosis. Death of areas of tissue or bone surrounded by healthy parts; death in mass as distinguished from necrobiosis.

nephritis. Inflammation of the kidney, or any disorder resulting in degeneration of the kidney tissue.

nephrosis. Any disorder of the kidney, especially one that is not due to infection and inflammation (as in the case of nephritis); a degenerative lesion of the kidney with loss of function of the secreting epithelium of the cortex.

neuritis. Inflammation of a nerve, usually accompanied by pain, tenderness, and other symptoms, such as loss of sensation.

neurogenic. Originating from nervous tissue. Resulting from nervous impulses.

neuroma. Former term for any type of tumor composed of nerve cells.

neuron. Nerve cell; functional unit of the nervous system, specialized to respond to stimuli by electrical impulses that are rapidly conducted along the axon of the neuron to reach other cells with which the axon synapses.

norepinephrine (noradrenaline). A hormone-transmitter substance produced in the nerve endings of the sympathetic nervous system required for the production of most of the important effects of the sympathetic nervous system.

nystagmus. Involuntary, rapid movement of the eyes, consisting of a fast forward and a slow backward movement; enables the eyes to fix on an object while the head is moving.

obturator. Anything that obstructs or closes a cavity or opening.

occipital. Concerning the back part of the head.

olecranal. Concerning the elbow.

olecranon. A large process of the ulna projecting behind the elbow joint and forming the bony prominence of the elbow.

ophthalmia. A severe inflammation of the eye, or of the conjunctiva.

ophthalmic. Relating to the eye, as the ophthalmic arteries, veins, and nerves.

ophthalmitis. Inflamed condition of the eye.

opisthotonos. A form of severe muscle spasm in which the head and heels are bent backward and the body is arched forward.

orthotics. Devices or supports inserted into shoes to correct a variety of musculo-skeletal deformities.

Osgood-Schlatter's disease. The epiphysis of the anterior tibial tubercle become infarcted because of excessive pull from the patellar tendon. It is common in boys of 10 to 16 years and usually only persists for a few months, for once the epiphysis fuses the condition abates.

osseous. Bonelike, concerning bones.

ossicula. Little bones.

ossification. Formation of bone substances. Conversion of other tissue into bone.

osteoarthritis. Degeneration of articular cartilage from congenital traumatic, inflammatory, and aging factors.

osteochondritis. Inflammation of bone and cartilage.

osteochondritis dissecans. Condition affecting a joint in which a fragment of cartilage and its underlying bone become detached from articular surface.

osteogenesis. Formation and development of bone taking place in connective tissue or in cartilage.

osteomyelitis. Inflammation of bone, especially the marrow, caused by a pathogenic organism.

osteoporosis. Disease of the bone, occurring chiefly in older people, characterized by loss of calcium and supporting tissues and resulting in loss of bone strength, density and mass.

ostitis. Inflammation of a bone.

otitis. Inflamed condition of the ear.

oxygen consumption. The quantity of oxygen consumed or required by the body to function at any given time. The amount of oxygen required by a given activity is a method of estimating the intensity of the activity.

oxygen debt. The extra oxygen that must be consumed after strenuous exercise to oxidize accumulated lactic acid and to resynthesize ATP and CP.

oxygen saturation. The relationship between the oxygen content and the oxygen capacity of the blood. If the blood has an oxygen capacity of 20 volumes percent and an oxygen content of 10 volumes percent, the blood is 50 percent saturated.

palpable. Perceptible, especially by touch.

palpate. To examine by touch or feel.

palpation. Rapid, violent, or throbbing pulsation, as an abnormally rapid throbbing or fluttering of the heart.

palsy. A paralysis; a loss of impairment of nerve or muscle function; motor paralysis with muscle weakness and loss of function.

pancreas. Mixed endocrine and exocrine gland in abdominal area behind and below the stomach. Exocrine secretions are the digestive juices, endocrine secretions are insulin, glucagon and somatostatin.

papilloma. A projecting or branching type of benign tumor made of epithelial cells, such as warts.

papule. A small solid elevation on the skin; a pimple.

paraplegia. Extensive loss of neural function, both sensory and motor, below level of lesion of spinal cord at or below level of first thoracic vertebra.

paresis. Partial or incomplete paralysis.

paresthesia. Affected with or concerning paresis (partial or incomplete paralysis).

parietal. Pertaining to, or forming the wall of a cavity. Pertaining to the parietal bone.

Parkinson's disease. A motor disorder resulting from lack of the neurotransmitter dopamine. Treated therapeutically with L-DOPA, the dopamine precursor that can pass the blood-brain barrier. Characterized by a slow, weak voluntary movement or movements, muscular rigidity and tremor.

patella. A lens-shaped sesamoid bone situated in front of the knee in the tendon of the quadriceps femoris muscle.

patella bipartite. Failure of patellar ossification center to fuse in superolateral corner, thus producing 2 parts; usually bilateral symmetrical; usually asymptomatic.

Pellegrini-Stieda's disease. Consists of heterotopic calcification in the upper fiber of the medial collateral ligament; local tenderness and pain on springing the knee may be found. This condition may be due to faulty healing following partial avulsion of the super attachment of the medial collateral ligament.

pericarditis. Inflammation of the pericardium, the double membranous fibroserous sac enclosing the heart and the origins of the great blood vessels.

periarticular. Inflammation of area around a joint.

pericardium. Double membrane that surrounds the heart and fastens it to the mediastinum, a thick mass of tissue between the lungs.

perineal. Concerning or situated on the perineum, the structure occupying the pelvic outlet and comprising the pelvic floor.

periosteum. The fibrous membrane that forms the investing covering of the bones except at their articular surfaces.

peristalsis. A progressive wavelike movement that occurs involuntarily in hollow tubes of the body, especially the alimentary canal. It is characteristic of tubes possessing longitudinal and circular layers of smooth muscle fibers.

peritoneum. The serous membrane reflected over the viscera and lining the abdominal cavity.

peritonitis. Inflammation of the peritoneum, the membranous coat lining the abdominal cavity and investing the viscera.

peroneal. Concerning the fibula.

pes. The foot or a footlike structure.

pes anserinus. Three primary branches of the facial nerve after leaving the stylomastoid foramen.

pes cavus (hollow foot). Accentuated high longitudinal arch; may be congenital or result from neurological disorder, causing muscular imbalance; clawing of toes always associated and shortening of Achilles tendon frequently present; as a result, excessive weight is placed on metatarsal heads and calluses develop in the underlying skin.

phagocyte. A cell with the ability to ingest and destroy particulate substances, such as bacteria, protozoa, cells and cell debris, dust particles, and colloids.

phalangeal. Concerning a phalanx.

phalanges. Bones of a finger or toe.

phalanx. Any one of the bones of the fingers or toes.

pharynx. Chamber into which the mouth, the back of the nose, and the Eustachian tubes open; both the esophagus and the trachea lead from the pharynx.

phosphagenic exercise (activity). High-intensity exercise performed for a brief period that uses ATP already stored in the exercising muscles.

phrenic nerves. Motor nerves originating in the cervical spinal cord, from the 3rd, 4th and 5th cervical nerves, to innervate the diaphragm.

plantar. Concerning the sole of the foot.

plantar fascia. The fascia that supports the arch and bottom of the foot.

plantarflexion. Extension of the foot so that the forepart is depressed with respect to the position of the ankle.

pleura. Delicate membrane investing each lung; consists of 2 layers, the visceral pleura that is attached to the lung surface and the parietal pleura that lines the chest wall.

pleurisy. Inflammation of the serous membrane covering the lungs and lining the chest cavity (the pleura).

pleurodynia. Pain of sharp intensity in the intercostal muscles caused by chronic inflammatory changes in the chest fasciae; pain of the pleural nerve.

pneumonitis. An acute localized inflammation of the lung without the serious generalized symptoms seen in lobar pneumonia.

pneumothorax. A collection of air or gas in the pleural cavity.

polyp. A protruding, often grapelike growth from a mucous membrane, such as the lining of the nose or the uterus.

popliteal. Concerning the posterior surface of the knee.

postconscious syndrome. Persistent variable symptoms of headache, tinnitus, dizziness, and confusion subsequent to a cerebral concussive incident.

posterior. Toward the rear or back.

precursor. A forerunner; something that goes before.

premature beats (extra systoles). Heartbeats that come earlier than expected, causing an irregularity of the heartbeat or pulse, which may be felt as palpitations. Premature beats may be single or repetitive, occasional or very frequent. They may arise from many parts of the heart and often may be accurately diagnosed by electrocardiography.

presbyopia. A visual change owing to advancing age; loss of elasticity of the lens in the eye.

pronate. To rotate inward.

pronation. The act of lying in a face-down or prone position. (In the case of the hand, it is the act of turning the hand so that the palm faces backward.)

proprioceptive. Receiving stimulations within the body tissues, especially in muscles, tendons, and in the inner ear.

protein. Large chemical molecules made up of various amino acids. Adequate protein intake in the diet is necessary to allow the body to produce the cell and tissue proteins necessary for normal body function.

proximal Nearest the point of attachment, center of the body, or point of reference.

pruritis ani. Intractable itching in anal area often resulting from unknown causes; may be associated with local infection; hemorrhoids, or other local conditions; poor anal hygiene, contributory; possible allergy, emotional and tension states.

psoriasis. A chronic recurring skin disorder characterized by the appearance of scaly red or silvery patches, sometimes elevated and other times like plaques.

ptosis. A drooping or falling down or a part or organ, such as the eyelid, the kidney, stomach, and intestine.

pulmonary. Relating to the lungs.

pulmonary gas exchange. The transfer of oxygen from atmosphere to blood and of carbon dioxide from blood to atmosphere.

pulmonary stenosis. Narrowing of the opening into the pulmonary artery from the right cardiac ventricle.

pulse. The expansion of blood vessels, felt as an impulse or beat, caused by each contraction of the heart. Arterial pulse, commonly called "the pulse." The pulse felt when an artery is lightly palpated or touched.

pulse rate. Number of pulsations per minute measured in an artery in response to the contraction of the heart; usually measured in the wrist, where the radial artery pulsates against the radius. Equivalent to the heart rate.

punched nerve syndrome (nerve contusion). Term used to describe transient rootlike pain and other manifestations resulting from injury to the neck as in blocking and tackling.

purpura. A disorder in which hemorrhages occur in the skin and mucous membranes, often accompanied by a low platelet count.

pustule. A small pus-containing elevation on the skin; a pimple that is filled with pus.

pyrogen. A chemical agent that raises the body temperature.

quadriceps muscle. The 4 muscles in the front of the thigh. They attach to the lower leg below the knee and extend (straighten) the lower leg.

rales. Abnormal breathing sounds heard (usually with a stethoscope) in certain disorders of the lung; rattling, bubbling, whistling, or crackling sounds heard in the chest.

rectus. Straight, not crooked.

reduction. Restoration to normal position, as a fractured bone or a hernia.

reflex, accommodation. Integrated adaptation of the eye for near vision; it includes increased convexity of the lens, constriction of the pupils, and convergence of the eyes.

renal. Pertaining to the kidney.

reflex, axon. A triple response of the skin to a simple stimulus, such as a scratch, caused by antidromic conduction along a branch of the stimulated sensory nerve axon, resulting in vasodilation of the blood vessels in the skin.

reflex, conditioned. Reflex response to a stimulus that has replaced the physiological stimulus.

reflex, flexor. Contraction of the flexor muscles in response to a harmful or unpleasant stimulus, resulting in a rapid withdrawal of the stimulated limb or flexions of the torso.

rhinitis. Inflammation of the lining of the nasal cavities.

rhinorrhea. Thin, watery discharge from the nose.

root. Proximal end of a nerve. Portion of an organ implanted in tissue.

rosacea. A skin disorder in which the capillaries of the nose, forehead and cheeks are dilated, causing flushing and redness, and accompanied by a breaking out of pustules and papules.

sacroiliac. The triangular bone situated dorsal and caudal from the 2 ilia between the 5th lumbar vertebra and the coccyx. It is formed of 5 united vertebrae and is wedged between the 2 innominate bones, its articulations forming the sacroiliac joint.

sagittal. Arrowlike; in an anteroposterior direction.

sartorius. A long, ribbon-shaped muscle of the thigh. The longest muscle in the body, it aids in flexing the knee.

scapula. The large flat, triangular bone that forms the posterior part of the shoulder. It articulates with the clavicle and the humerus.

scapulodynia. Inflammation and pain in the shoulder muscles.

sciatica. A term referring to symptoms, usually pain, caused by irritation or damage to the sciatic nerve, which runs from the lower back and pelvic area down the back of the leg.

sclera. The tough opaque white coat that forms the outer protective layer of the eyeball. (It is continuous with the transparent colorless cornea at the front.)

scleroderma. A chronic disease of unknown etiology that causes sclerosis of the skin and certain organs including the gastrointestinal tract, lungs, heart, and kidneys.

sebaceous. Secreting or pertaining to oil or an oily substance called sebum.

septum. A wall dividing 2 cavities.

sequestrum. Fragment of a necrosed bone that has become separated from surrounding tissue.

septum, deviated. Posttraumatic or congenitally deformed nasal septum causing a degree of nasal passage obstruction.

serosangineous. Containing or of the nature of serum and blood.

serous. Thin, watery. A serous membrane is thin and produces a waterly fluid.

sesamoid bone. An oval nodule of bone or fibrocartilage in a tendon playing over a bony suture. The patella is the largest one.

shin splints. Generally, a pain in the shin near the bone, caused by injury to structures in that area. Specifically, tears in the shin muscle fibers where they attach to the prominent bone in the front, inner part of the shin.

shock. A critical clinical condition characterized by variable signs and symptoms that arise when the cardiac output is insufficient to fill the arterial tree with blood under sufficient pressure to provide organs and tissues with adequate blood flow; often present with severe trauma and hemorrhage.

sinus. A canal or passage leading to an abscess. A cavity within a bone. Dilated channel for venous blood. Any cavity having a relatively narrow opening.

sinus arrhythmia. Irregular heartbeat occurring commonly in children or in the aged in which the rate alternately increases and decreases.

sinusitis. Inflammation of a sinus, especially a paranasal sinus.

soleus. A flat broad muscle of the calf of the leg.

spearing. Act of butting head into midsection or chest of an opponent; hazardous to spearer (cervical spin injury) as well as to opponent (direct trauma).

sphincter. Circular muscle constricting an orifice.

sphygmomanometer. Instrument for determining arterial blood pressure indirectly.

spleen. Large lyphoid organ used as blood reservoir and filter.

sprain. Injury to a joint usually involving the ligaments or tendons without fracture or dislocation of the bones that form the joints.

spur. A sharp horny outgrowth of the skin. A sharp or pointed projection.

snuffbox, anatomical. Triangular area of the dorsum of the hand at the base of the thumb. When the thumb is extended, the tendons of the long and short extensor muscles of the thumb bound this area, which appears as a depression.

squamous. Scalelike.

stenosis. Constriction or narrowing of a passage or orifice.

stress test. Measurement of cardiac reserve, heart rate, blood pressure, ECG, and oxygen consumption during strenuous exercise, usually measured with subject on a treadmill or exercise bicycle.

stroke. Abnormal function in 1 or more parts of the brain owing to interference with its blood supply. Symptoms may include paralysis, altered sensation, inability to speak, or many others. The blood supply may be reduced by narrowing or blockage of the arteries by atherosclerosis, rupture of the artery (ruptured aneurysm), or a blood clot formed in the heart or large arteries and carried to the brain in the bloodstream (embolus).

styloid process. (1) A pointed process of the temporal bone, projecting downward, and to which some of the muscles of the tongue are attached. (2) A pointed projection behind the head of the fibula. (3) A protuberance on the outer portion of the distal end of the radias.

subcutaneous emphysema. Follows an escape of air from a damaged lung or air passage that then finds its way into the chest wall, mediastinum and subcutaneous tissues by the way of a tear in the parietal pleura. It is occasionally associated with an open chest wound.

subluxation. A partial or incomplete dislocation.

sulcus. A furrow, groove, slight depression, or fissure, especially of the brain.

supinate. To turn the forearm or hand so that the palm faces upward. To rotate the foot and leg outward.

suppuration. The process of pus formation.

supramalleolar. Located above either malleolus.

sympathetic nervous system. That part of the autonomic nervous system that originates in the thoracolumbar region of the spinal cord, synapses in the chain of sympathetic ganglia with neurons that release norepinephrine in the organs they innervate; in general the sympathetic nervous system prepares the body for activity in emergency.

synapse. The point of junction between 2 neurons in a neutral pathway, where the termination of the axon of 1 neuron comes into close proximity with the cell body or dendrites of another.

syncope (fainting). A mild and transient form of shock with a short period of unconsciousness from which rapid recovery is made upon assuming a horizontal position; in the emotional or psychogenic type, vasovagal reflexes slow the heart and bring on peripheral vasodilation, thereby diminishing cardiac output.

synosteosis. (1) Articulation of osseous tissue of adjacent bones. (2) Union of separate bones by osseous tissue.

synovial. Relating to a thick fluid found in joints, bursae, and tendon sheaths. The lubricating fluid of the joints.

synovitis. Inflammation of a synovial membrane.

systemic. Affecting the whole body; generalized.

systole. The period during the heart cycle when the heart contracts and expels blood into the arteries.

systolic blood pressure. The pressure measure in the arteries when the heart contracts during systole.

tachycardia. An excessive rapid heart rate. (It is usually applied to a pulse rate over 100 a minute).

talus. The ankle bone articulating with the tibia, tibula, calcaneus, and navicular bone.

target heart rate. (1) Generally, that heart rate which defines aerobic activity intense enough to produce a training effect. (2) Specifically, between 70 and 85 percent of the age corrected maximum expected heart rate.

tarsal. Pertaining to the tarsus or supporting plate of the eyelid. Pertaining to the ankle or tarsus.

tarsitis. Inflammation of a bone in the instep of the foot, or inflammation of the eyelid edge.

tendinitis. Inflammation of a tendon.

tendon. Tough, inelastic cords of dense fibrous tissue that attach muscle to bones. Their direction of pull tends to impose a parallel arrangement on the bundles of collagen fibers. The tendon cells are found lying between bundles of dense fibrous tissue.

tensor. Any muscle that makes a part tense.

tentoriam. A tentlike structure or part.

tetra. Combining form meaning 4.

tetraplegia. Paralysis of both arms and legs.

thermalgesia. A condition in which pain is experienced upon the application of heat.

thoracic. Relating to the chest portion of the body.

thorax. The chest; the part of the body between the neck and the abdominal cavity (from which it is separated by the diaphragm).

thrombophlebitis. A disorder in which inflammation of a vein wall is followed by the formation of a blood clot (thrombus).

thrombus. A blood clot that obstructs a blood vessel or a cavity of the heart.

tibia. The inner and larger bone of the leg between the knee and ankle articulating with the femur above and with the talus below.

tinnitus. The sensation of a ringing in the ears from traumatic or other causes.

tonus. Constant, low-grade contraction of muscle, essential background activity for voluntary contractions, maintenance of posture, and venous return to the heart (muscle pumps).

trapezius. A flat, triangular muscle covering posterior surface of neck and shoulder.

trigger point. A focal point of irritation that when stimulated sets off a painful reaction referred to a distant area or areas.

trachea. A membranous and cartilaginous tube, commonly called the windpipe, extending from the larynx (the voice box) to its 2 branching bronchi.

trachiostomy. Incision of the trachea through the skin and muscle of the neck overlying the trachea.

transpiration. The discharge of air, vapor, or sweat through the skin.

transverse. Lying at right angles to the long axis of the body; crosswise.

triglycerides. Important fats (lipids) that constitute a major source and storage form of energy. Each triglyceride molecule is made up of 3 fatty acid molecules attached to a compound called glycerol.

trochanter. Either of the 2 bony processes below the neck of the femur.

trochlea. A structure having the function of a pulley; a ring or hook through which a tendon or muscle projects.

tubercle. A small rounded elevation or eminence on a bone.

tuberosity. An elevated round process of bone. A tubercle or nodule.

valgus. A term denoting position, meaning "bent outward" or "twisted," applied especially to deformation in which a part is bent outward and away from the midline of the body.

varicose veins. Dilation of superficial veins, usually in the leg, from valvular incompetency producing pain and discomfort.

varus. (1) Turned inward. (2) A condition in which a club footed person walks on the outer border of the foot.

vascular. Referring to the blood vessels, arteries, capillaries and veins.

vasodilation. Dilation of blood vessels, especially small arteries and arterioles.

vasopressin. Produced in the supraoptic and paraventricular nuclei of the anterior hypothalamus and its granules are stored in the posterior pituitary gland (neurohypophysis). The primary function is to preserve body fluids, and its secretion is regulated primarily by changes in plasma osmolality.

venous. Pertaining to the veins or blood passing through them.

ventricles. The lower, muscular pumping chambers of the heart. There are two ventricles: (1) The left ventricle pumps blood rich in oxygen to the rest of the body tissue. (2) The right ventricle pumps blood poor in oxygen to the lungs.

ventricular fibrillation. A condition similar to atrial fibrillation resulting in rapid, tremulous and ineffectual contraction of the ventricles. May result from mechanical injury to the heart, occlusion of coronary vessels, effects of certain drugs such as excess of digatalis or chloroform, and electrical stimuli.

viscera. Internal organs enclosed within a cavity, especially the abdominal organs.

VO₂Max (maximal oxygen consumption). The maximum amount of oxygen the body can use; that is, the amount of oxygen consumed during maximal physical activity. Also called maximal aerobic power or capacity.

volar flexion. The act of drawing the fingers or hand toward the palmar aspect of the proximally conjoined body segment.

whiplash. Popular term for hyperextension-hyperflexion injury to the cervical spine; does not imply any specific resultant pathology.